W0050872

Diagnostic Neuropathology
Volume II

Diagnostic Neuropathology
Volume II

Editors

Julio H. Garcia, M.D.
The University of Alabama at Birmingham, U.S.A.

Julio Escalona-Zapata, M.D.
Universidad Complutense de Madrid, Spain

Uriel Sandbank, M.D.
University of Tel-Aviv, Israel

Jorge Cervós-Navarro, M.D.
Free University, Berlin, F.R.G.

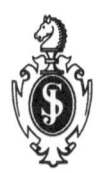 Springer-Verlag London Ltd.

Copyright © 1990, Springer-Verlag London
          Originally published by Field & Wood, Medical Publishers, Inc. in 1990
          Softcover reprint of the hardcover 1st edition 1990

All rights reserved. No part of this book may be reproduced or
transmitted in any form or by any means, electronic or mechanical,
including photocopying, recording, or any other information storage
and retrieval system, without permission in writing from the
Publisher.

ISBN 978-3-662-06587-7   ISBN 978-3-662-06585-3 (eBook)
DOI 10.1007/978-3-662-06585-3

Contents

7

Nerve Biopsy   123
Thomas W. Bouldin

8

Muscle Biopsy   203
Hans H. Goebel

Contributors

Thomas W. Bouldin, M.D.
Associate Professor of Pathology
University of North Carolina
Chapel Hill, North Carolina, USA

J. Cervós-Navarro, M.D.
Professor of Neuropathology and
  Director
Institute of Neuropathology
Klinikum Steglitz, Freie Universität
Berlin, Federal Republic of
  Germany

J. Escalona-Zapata, M.D.
Professor of Pathology and
  Director
Department of Anatomical
  Pathology
Hospital Provincial
Madrid, Spain

J. H. Garcia, M.D.
Professor of Pathology
University of Alabama at
  Birmingham
Birmingham, Alabama, USA

Hans H. Goebel, M.D.
Professor of Neuropathology
Johannes Gutenberg Universität
Mainz, Federal Republic of
  Germany

Preface

Every year dozens of physicians-in-training face, for the first time, the responsibility of examining and diagnosing central nervous system tumors or biopsies of the central nervous system, the peripheral nerves or muscles, whose surgical resection has been decided on both as a form of treatment (in the case of tumors) and as means to confirm a presumptive diagnosis. The selection of the most appropriate form of post surgical treatment for most tumors is predicated on the precise identification of the tumor cells.

The evaluation of the specimen, by a pathologist, will not only determine whether the lesion is truly neoplastic, but also whether there are histologic indicators of malignancy. Moreover, in some cases, the pathologist will be asked to determine whether the tumor cells contain certain hormone precursors or receptors, as an example.

Recognition of many of the features that one must search for requires the judicious application of methods that may not be readily known to the physicians involved in the various diagnostic procedures.

The handling and processing of the tissues as they arrive in the pathology laboratory for the above reasons vary as a function of the organ (or site) of origin of a given tumor as well as a function of the presumptive clinical diagnosis.

The material contained in this book series has been organized in an attempt to help the pathologists-in-training, the general pathologists, the neurosurgeons, and neurologists to understand the logic behind such special requirements.

The book attempts to answer questions of how to handle biopsy material derived from the CNS, peripheral nerve and skeletal muscle in order to arrive at a definite diagnosis.

Some of the specific questions this book attempts to answer are:

- What differences are there in the handling of brain biopsies, nerve biopsies, and muscle biopsies?
- What diseases can be diagnosed through the appropriate evaluation of these tissues?
- What are the consequences of not following the recommended procedures?
- What is the minimum number of histologic or electron microscopic features that are required to diagnose a specific tumor, eg: meningioma?
- What is the appropriate way of reporting, coding, and filing a diagnosis in neuropathology?

The book is directed to specific groups of physicians, namely those involved in the diagnosis of neuromuscular diseases.

1. The neurologists who define the list of most probable· diagnoses on the bases of the clinical history and the physical examination;
2. The neuroradiologist, who on the bases of contrast studies, either expands or narrows the list of diagnostic possibilities;
3. The neurosurgeon who obtains the brain, muscle, nerve biopsy; and
4. The pathologist who takes the ultimate responsibility for assigning a specific diagnosis to a given patient.

We assume that the average reader will want to know what fixatives should be used, when tissues should be frozen instead of fixed, what can be expected from the application of special methods such as immunocytochemistry and electron microscopy, what elements should be incorporated in a microscopic description, and how the final diagnosis should be composed.

Most textbooks on pathology provide descriptive information on specific disease processes. For example, these books may discuss the entity of cerebellar astrocytoma from the standpoint of incidence in certain age groups, common clinical symptoms, radiographic features, and gross microscopic characteristics of the neoplasm. This information is useful for someone who already knows that the patient has a cerebellar astrocytoma. But, to persons who aspire to become pathologists or to a practicing pathologist who is charged with the responsibility of providing diagnoses on the basis of microscopic evaluation of small samples, the average textbook presentation may not be so useful.

The contributors to *Diagnostic Neuropathology* have provided all the information necessary for arriving at a prompt diagnosis, on the basis of microscopic evaluation. They have striven to present visual evidence of the elements considered indispensable to arrive at a final diagnosis, e.g., pseudopalisading in glioblastoma multiforme or perivascular pseudorosettes in ependymomas. Thus, definitions of terms commonly used by pathologists are provided in abundant, well chosen illustrations.

I am pleased to acknowledge the intellectual contributions made to this book series by my former mentors, Professor S. M. Aronson (Brown University) and Professor H. Okazaki (Mayo Clinic School of Medicine); my former trainees; and the entire personnel of the Department of Pathology at UAB.

The continued support and trust of several of my colleagues, in the United States and abroad, has made my editorial task relatively manageable. I am much indebted to the contributors who have participated in this series' production.

The Alexander von Humboldt Stiftung of Bonn, Federal Republic of Germany, provided me with the support that made possible my initiation in a new job; for this, I am especially grateful to my colleagues in the Bundesrepublik Deutschland.

I am pleased to announce that plans are under way to publish additional volumes in this series. Some of the topics to be covered in future volumes include perinatal neuropathology, neuropathology of AIDS, application of immunocytochemistry to the diagnosis of tumors, neuropathology of dementia, and neuropathology of trauma.

Julio H. Garcia, M.D.
Birmingham, Alabama

Diagnostic Neuropathology
Volume II

5

Tissue Culture in the Diagnosis of Brain Tumors

J. Escalona-Zapata

Introduction

This chapter outlines the diagnostic usefulness of some tissue culture methods and their contribution to one of the most difficult challenges that pathologists face: i.e., to establish the origin of the cells of a given tumor. The methods are difficult to apply to specific individual cases; they are also time-consuming. These objections, however, can be also applied to other special methods used in diagnostic histopathology, such as electron microscopy. By comparison with the latter, the cost of installing a facility appropriate for tissue culture is relatively low. The practical applications of tissue culture to the study of brain tumors are emphasized in this chapter.

Historical Note

Tissue culture, as applied to brain tumors, began in the neurosurgical clinic of Cushing with Kredel,[56] Buckley and Eisenhardt,[9] and Russell and Bland.[84,85] Canti et al[11] and Bland and Russell[6] studied meningiomas and astrocytomas and introduced the technique of time-lapse cinematography. In the United States, Murray and Stout[68–71] (1940–1948) primarily studied peripheral nervous system tumors; while Pomerat,[76] Costero, and Lumsden applied the tissue culture methods to the study of meningiomas, oligodendroglioma, and normal nervous tissue.[14–16,62,76,78] In the late 1960s and early 1970s, Kersting, Scharenberg, Liss and Lumsden succeeded in applying the tissue culture techniques to the study of large numbers of tumors.[51–53,60,61,86] Rubinstein and his associates have continued the study of brain tumors by various culture techniques. They introduced the organ culture method to the study of brain tumors in the early 1970s.[82,83,87,90] In Europe, only a handful of investigators working at three or four different laboratories have applied tissue culture methods to the diagnosis of brain tumors.[31]

One of the main purposes in establishing a specific diagnosis for a tumor is to determine the degree of malignancy, thereby predicting the biologic behavior of the tumor. Some authors have described differences in the in vitro rhythm of growth as an indicator of malignancy, but most believe that in terms of prognosis, the study of growth patterns in tissue culture is not a reliable method to predict the biologic behavior of tumors. The analysis of conventional histologic preparations provides a more accurate approach to predict the growth pattern of a given tumor.

Identifying cells of origin in tissue culture is predicated on the ability to: (1) separate uncontaminated cell populations of a tumor. Non-neoplastic cells such as leukocytes disappear from the culture in a few days. A pure cell line may presumably be obtained only through cloning, but in practice, the separation of neoplastic cells from non-neoplastic ones is a relatively easy task; (2) maintain the primary neoplastic characteristics with elimination of secondary and tertiary structures; and (3) enhance in vitro simplification[14,16] and, in some cases, induce a variable degree of maturation, thus facilitating the identification of the cell of origin.

In this way, in vitro culture provides a tumor image that is relatively uncontaminated by stromal elements, which can be studied by various conventional methods (observation with phase contrast optics, staining with H&E, Giemsa, and other methods), and with special techniques such as cytohistochemistry and electron microscopy. The application of immunohistochemical methods to tissue culture at present remains incompletely defined.

Tissue culture is of major importance in defining the cell of origin in certain tumors that are otherwise difficult to classify. This method is also important for identifying individual cell populations in tumors, which in conventional histologic preparations appear to have single cell derivation.

Limiting Factors

The limitations of tissue culture methods include the inability to obtain growth in a significant percentage of cases, the necessity to select only one growth technique for the purpose of standardizing results, and the long period of time necessary to induce the required growth. The diversity of available techniques presents a serious obstacle to the standardization of methods. Another limiting factor is the need for specialized facilities and personnel.

Short-term tissue cultures, in our hands, are superior to the techniques based on monolayer and trypsinization;[60,86] the use of short-term cultures ensures that the cells under study are the original neoplastic cells. These tend to maintain their morphologic features, and therefore, the short-term culture provides images comparable to those visible in conventional histologic preparations. In his laboratory, the author applies the technique of Gey modified by Kersting.[51]

Tissue Culture Evolution

Tissue cultures evolve through two phases. In the initial phase, the cells migrate in divergent directions from the explant. At the beginning, the cells grow in a plasma coagulum and tend to be fusiform and arranged radially, with the exception of lymphocytes, macrophages, and epithelial cells, which maintain patterns of separation/cohesion, characteristic to each of these groups. In a second phase of stabilization, the cells arrange themselves in a layer over the glass surface and adopt a cellular pattern of association that is peculiar to each cell group. The images in the first phase are mostly nonspecific, and for this reason it is necessary to wait until the second phase develops, when the primary growth features characteristic of each group of tumors are more easily recognized.

Patterns of Growth

The morphologic analysis of tissues grown in vitro is based on the recognition of growth patterns (characteristic to each cell type) and the identification of association patterns determined by the cell of origin. Willmer[93] described six patterns: (1) *epitheliocytic,* resulting in the formation of a mosaic in which cells are apposed to one another; (2) *mechanocytic* (fibroblastic), in which cells grow as fusiform-shaped units unattached to one another, except in the case of the endothelial cells, which maintain some degree of cohesiveness; (3) *amoebocytic,* consisting of cells having active movements (the most typical representative is the macrophage); (4) the *neuronal* pattern, applying to cells having scant mobility, but endowed with very long axonal processes; (5) *neuroglial* cells, growing initially as unattached fusiform cells, and later adopting a typical plexiform arrangement; and (6) *lymphocytic,* round small cells, which abandon the explant early and disappear within a few days.

The majority of tumors of the central nervous system grow according to patterns that can be classified into four groups: (1) *neuronal pattern,* peripheral and central ganglioneuromas and neuroblastomas; (2) *reticular* or *plexiform pattern,* similar to the neuroglial pattern of Willmer (astrocytomas, oligodendrogliomas, and medulloblastomas); (3) *epithelial pattern* (tumors of the choroid plexus and ependymomas, craniopharyngiomas, and metastatic carcinomas); and (4) *mechanocytic patterns* (meningiomas, hemangioblastomas, schwannomas, and sarcomas).

Tumors of Neuronal Pattern

Tumors derived from nerve cells are rare; however, their growth patterns have been thoroughly documented.[10,36,37,43,44,60,70,71] Among these neoplasms one must be able to recognize neuroblastoma, ganglioneuroblastoma, and differentiated ganglioneuroma; each of these subtypes behave differently both in vitro and in vivo.

NEUROBLASTOMA

The initial observations on the neuroblastic tumors of Murray and Stout[70] were based on those of Harrison.[48] Two facts are characteristic: (1) the lack of migration of the nervous cells in the explant. Cellular plaques at the periphery of the explant have been intrepreted as Schwann cells or fibroblasts. Neurites grow from the explant and can be demonstrated as early as 24 hours after the start of the culture; (2) the formation of a dense tangle of axons arranged as a corona around the explant appears within 2–3 days. These neurites are easily observed in material fixed in aldehydes and stained with H&E and are readily apparent with phase contrast microscopy as slender, straight processes with occasional nodular surface varicosities. This behavior is constant, develops early, and allows prompt identification of the tumor (Fig. 5-1).

This type of culture is valuable in the diagnosis of small undifferentiated cells, especially when the growth is retroperitoneal and the differential diagnosis includes lymphoma, extraskeletal soft-tissue Ewing tumor, and neuroblastoma.

GANGLIONEUROMAS

Ganglioneuromas of the peripheral nervous system have been infrequently studied by culture methods,[60,71] possibly because they are rare tumors and their identification by conventional means is not difficult. The explanted nerve cells have a great capacity to migrate; moreover, multipolar cells, resembling adult neurons, are common at some distance from the explant. It is doubtful that these cells really divide; rather, the neurons are perhaps passively displaced on the glass surface. The development in ganglioneuromas of neurites similar to those of a neuroblastoma is the most important identifying feature in tissue culture. These neurites are equally distributed in a radial fashion, and through rapid growth, some reach great lengths (Fig. 5-2).

The migration and proliferation of fusiform cells, probably derived from Schwann cells, is common in ganglioneuromas. This feature permits distinguishing ganglioneuromas from neuroblastomas as this migration and proliferation rarely occur in the latter group of tumors.

The cerebral ganglioneuroma or ganglioglioma is even more rare than the two previous ones, therefore, this neoplasm has been studied by tissue culture only

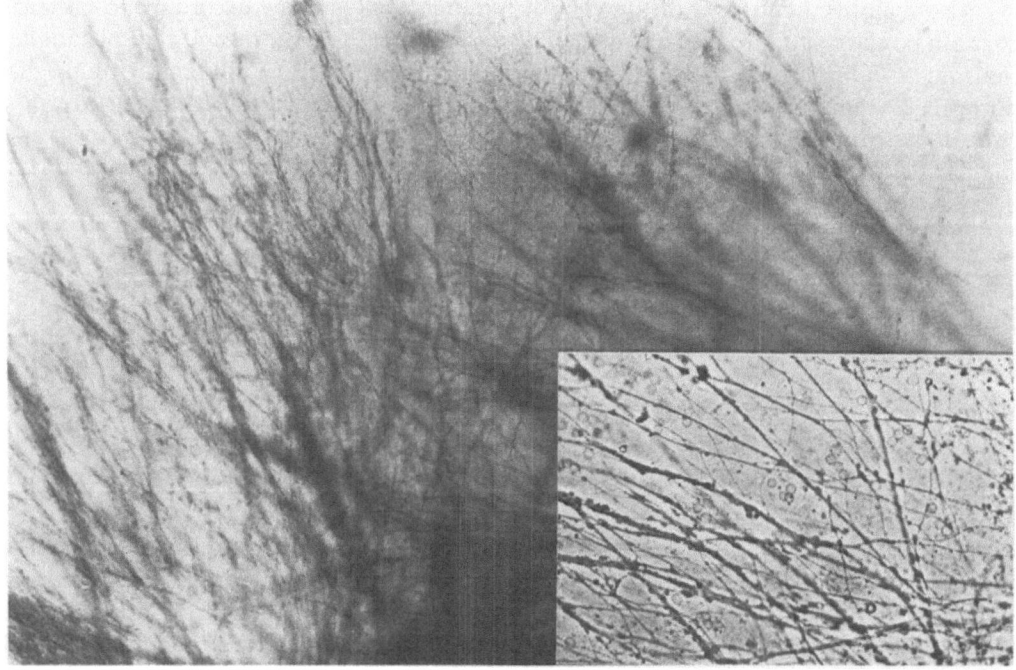

Fig. 5-1. Retroperitoneal neuroblastoma. The halo of growth is formed by neurites sometimes associated with one another in parallel arrays. After two days of culture, there is no cell migration (original magnification ×200). *Inset:* Cell processes as seen with phase contrast. The neurites are elongated and some show varicosities (×400).

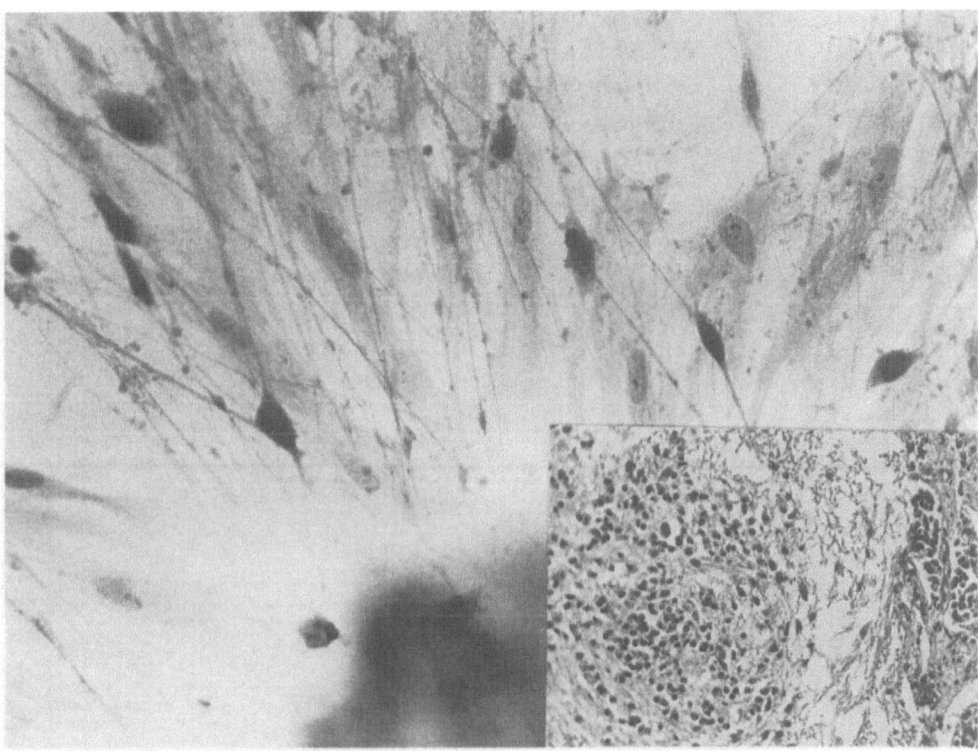

Fig. 5-3. Cerebral ganglioneuroma after 2 days of culture. Neurites emerging from the explant and with a radial disposition can be seen to the left. There is no cell migration. (H&E, ×400.) *Inset:* Histologic preparation of the original tumor (×200).

occasionally.[41] The in vitro cellular behavior of cerebral ganglioneuroma is similar to that of the peripheral neuronal tumors. The neoplastic cells remain within the explant and, as it happens in the peripheral ganglioneuromas, only occasionally can one find a few cellular elements having a ganglion-like appearance at the periphery. These cells do not proliferate; instead they appear to be passively displaced to the periphery (Fig. 5-3).

The halo of growth of the explant is formed by fine expansions of great length that sometimes display surface knobs or varicosities; these processes are neurites (Fig. 5-4). Occasionally, there is concomitant growth of glial cells; these probably accompany cells that quickly degenerate and disappear. In the authors' experience, explants of mixed tumors (gangliogliomas) do not grow simultaneously as a mixture of neuronal and astrocytic elements. Instead, one or the other cell type predominates and overcomes the companion one.

Tumors of Reticular or Plexiform Pattern

The reticular pattern in tissue culture is most typical of the gliomas and is characterized by the arrangement, in a plexiform fashion, of cells that are either bipolar or

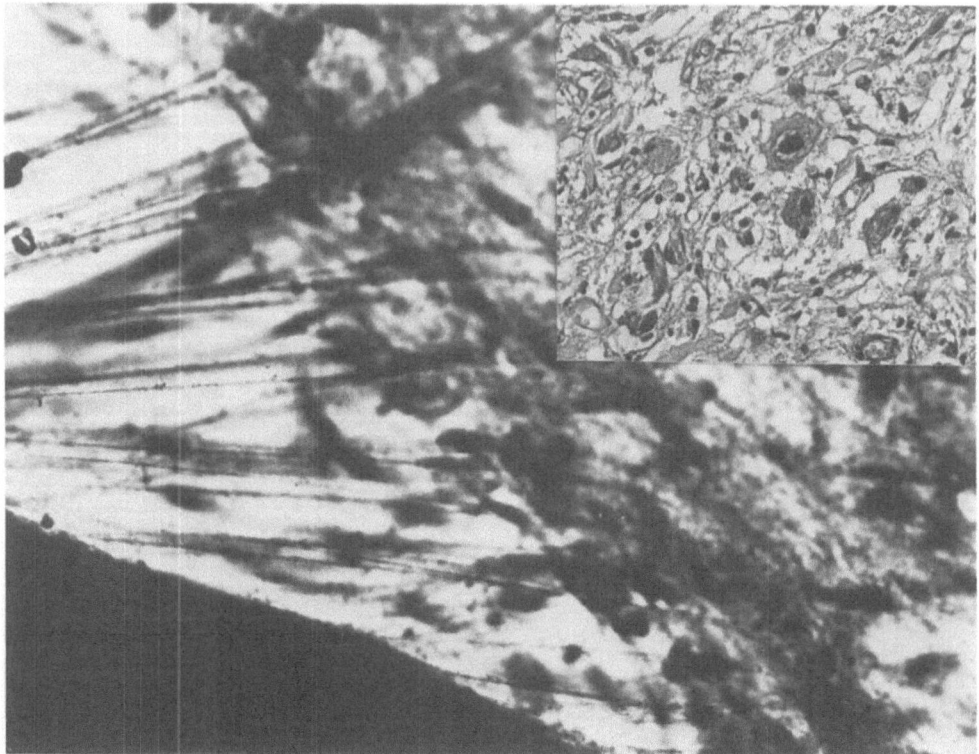

Fig. 5-3. Cerebral ganglioneuroma after 2 days of culture. Neurites emerging from the explant and with a radial disposition can be seen to the left. There is no cell migration. (H&E, ×400.) *Inset:* Histologic preparation of the original tumor (×200).

multipolar. This architecture reproduces the normal neuropil and is found in astrocytomas, oligodendrogliomas, and medulloblastomas. In ependymomas, a mixture of the reticular pattern and an epithelial pattern are readily visible within the network of the cellular processes. In every case, these cultures go through an initial bipolar phase in which the reticular pattern is only suggested.

ASTROCYTOMAS

A number of investigators have studied astrocytic tumors by tissue culture.[34,49,82,87,94] The following conclusions have been reached in the authors' laboratories:

1. Two tissue culture patterns are seen in astrocytomas. One pattern applies to the astrocytomas of the cerebral hemispheres; the second pattern is seen in astrocytomas of the midline including those originating in the cerebellum, diencephalon, optic nerve, brain stem, and spinal cord.[29]

2. The malignant astrocytomas represent different modulations of the same basic process, (i.e., the neoplastic growth of astrocytes). Regardless of their site of origin, cerebral hemispheres or midline astrocytomas reproduce a characteristic growth pattern in tissue culture.[29,30]

3. The glioblastoma multiforme is a tumor derived from astrocytes. The cerebral hemispheric glioblastomas and the cerebellar glioblastomas behave in vitro accord-

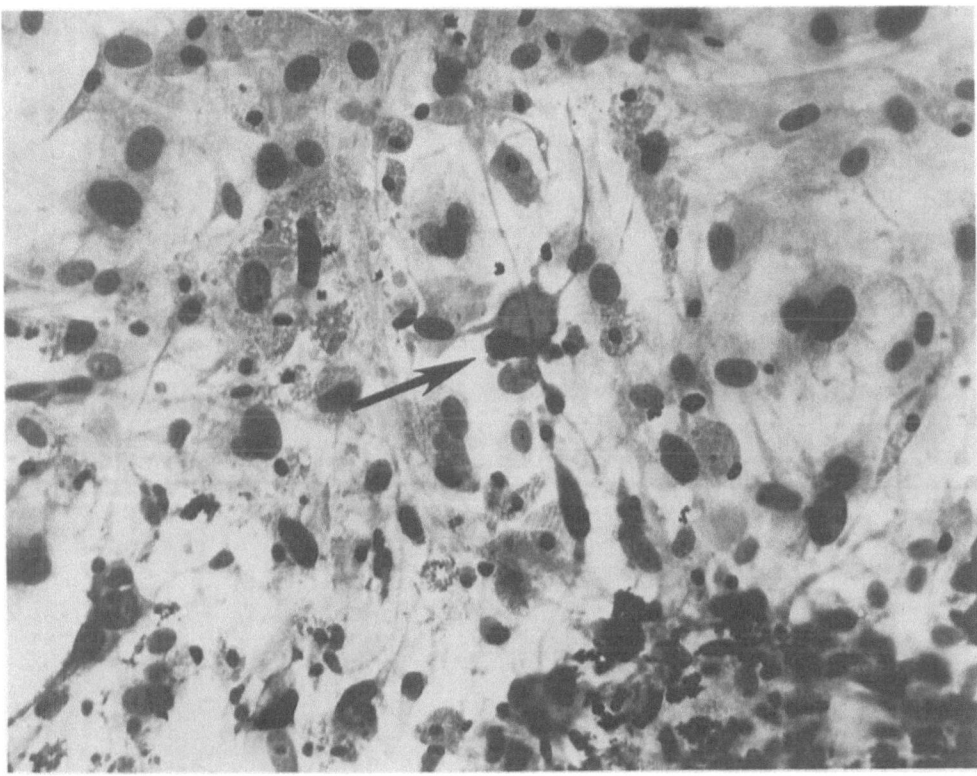

Fig. 5-4. Cerebral ganglioneuroma. Same case as in Fig. 5-3, after 6 days of culture. Fibroblasts are visible near the explant (right lower corner). Among these, there is a multipolar neuron (arrow) with eccentric nucleus and abundant Nissl substance (H&E, ×400).

ing to the respective patterns of each of the original forms. They are, therefore, two distinct groups of neoplasms.[25,28,29]

HEMISPHERIC ASTROCYTOMAS OF LOW MALIGNANCY

This group includes astrocytomas of the cerebral hemispheres having a minimal histologic degree of malignancy. There are three types: fibrillary, protoplasmic, and pilocytic.

The explants have a monotonous development, with migration of the dominant bipolar cells in the first days of culture. The cellular nuclei are oval and the elongated and narrow cytoplasm is endowed with bipolar processes of which a proximal one retains contact with the explant. The result of this migration is a radial disposition of the cells (Fig. 5-5).

Multipolar cells appear after the first weeks, which at first have scarce processes, but at the end, each cell has a distinct stellate morphology. At this stage, the nucleus is round and centrally situated in the perikaryon. The cytoplasm is eosinophilic and endowed with long, fine processes that occasionally have triangular endings. The more mature cells lose their initial radial association and adopt a reticular pattern. The radial disposition persists only in the proximity of the explant (Fig. 5-6).

This pattern of growth is common to all hemispheric astrocytomas and follows the behavior of the diffuse variant. The tumors with protoplasmic pattern have the

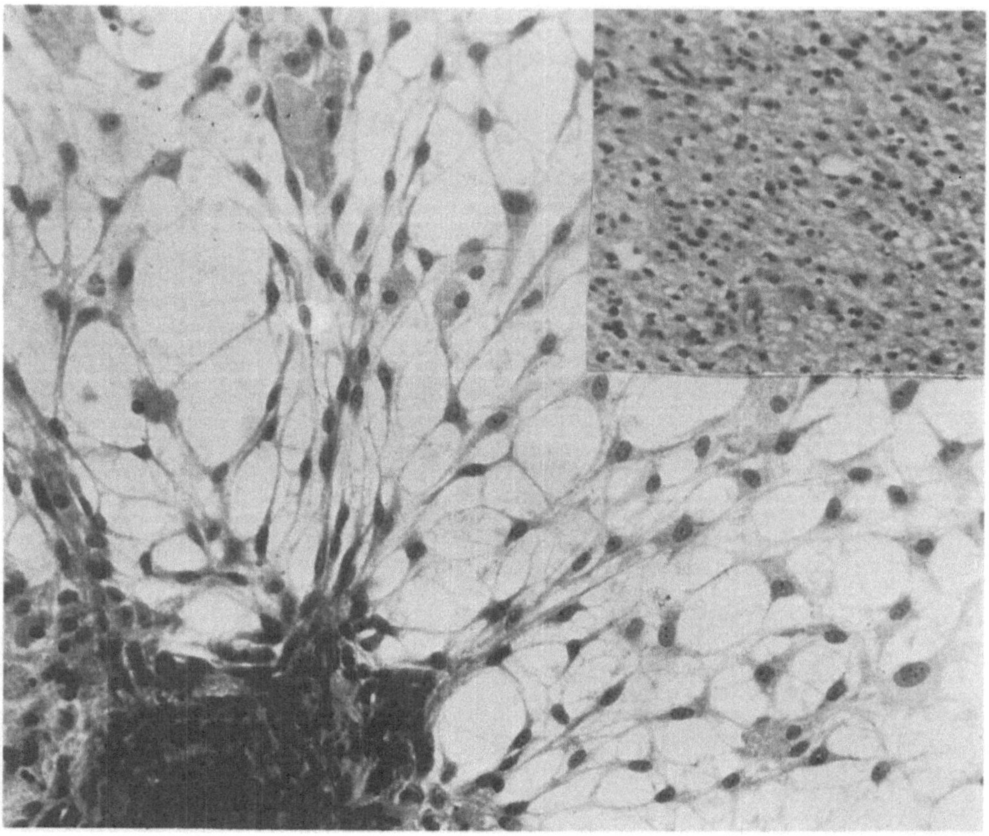

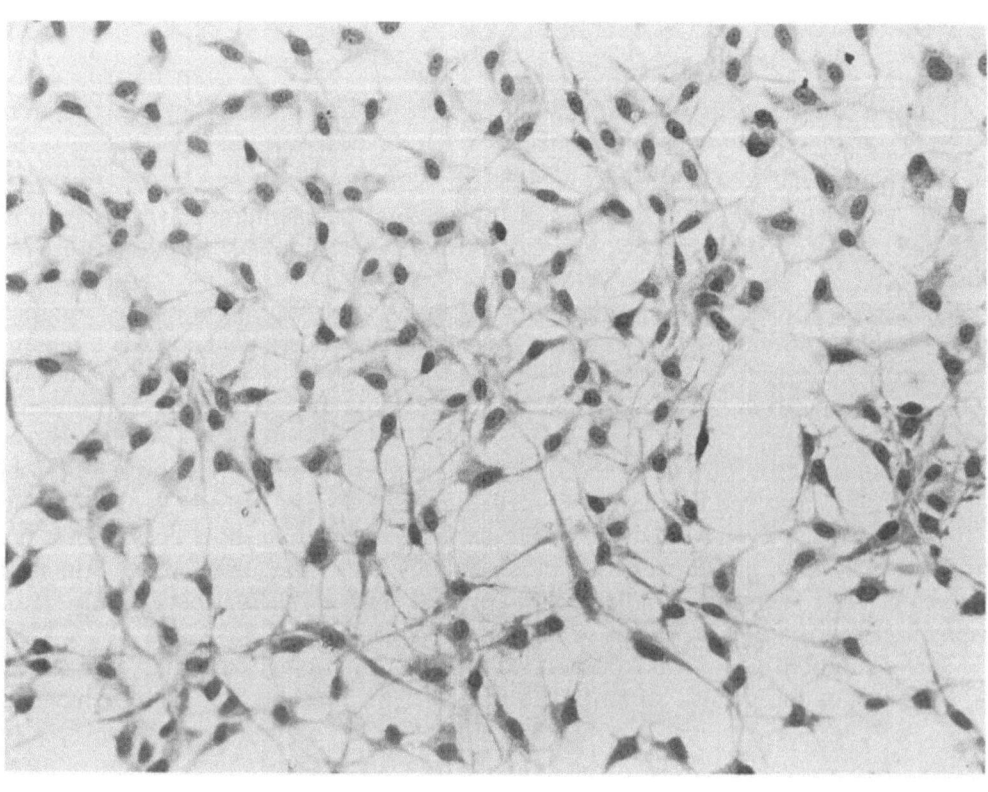

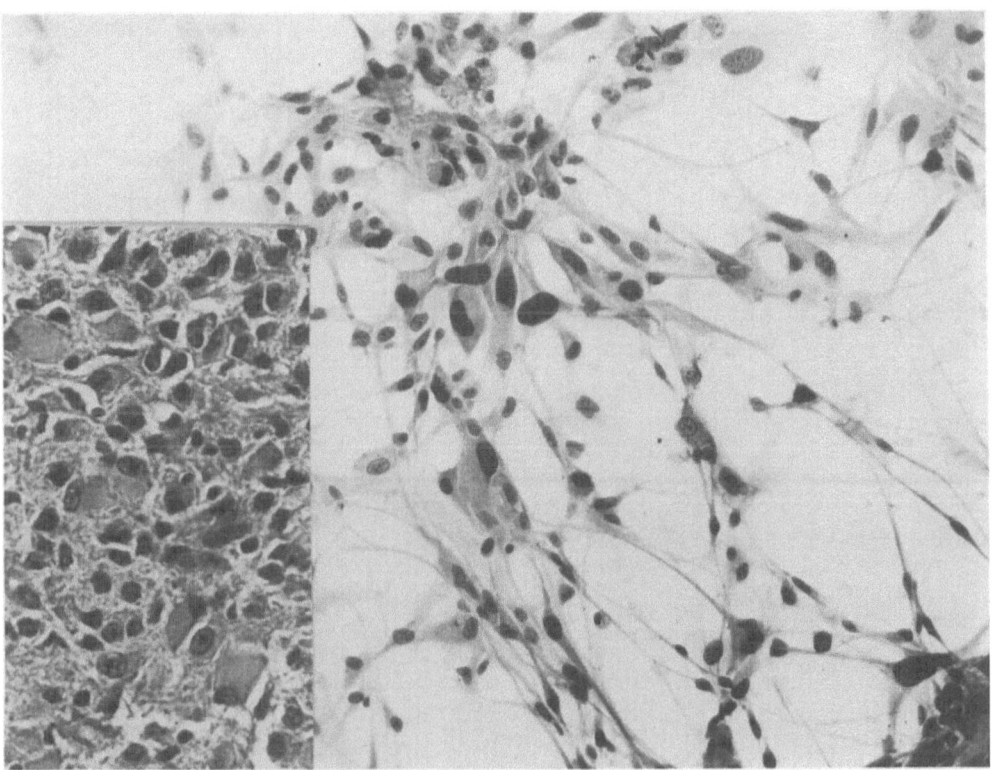

Fig. 5-7. Cerebral hemisphere astrocytoma after 21 days of culture. The most peripheral cells have a reticular arrangement. The plump nature of the tumor cells (*inset*) is faithfully reproduced in the tissue culture. (H&E, ×200.) (Reproduced with permission from *Patologia* [*Madrid*] 16:23–45, 1983).

same behavior, which is modified only by the much larger and intensively eosinophilic cytoplasm containing an eccentrically placed nucleus. The cytoplasmic processes are thicker than in the previous variety, but they are numerous and long. The fusiform variant has the same features except that the cytoplasm is less abundant, and the processes are longer and less numerous than in the protoplasmic type (Fig. 5-7, 5-8). Astrocytomas are characterized in the initial phase by bipolar cells migrating in a radial fashion. During the stabilization phase, these cells become multipolar and adopt a reticular pattern.

Fig. 5-5. Cerebral hemisphere astrocytoma after 9 days of culture. The migrating cells are bipolar and arranged in a radial fashion. They acquire a multipolar or stellate shape at the most peripheral fields. H&E, ×200.) *Inset:* Histologic preparation of the original tumor. (H&E, ×100.) (Reproduced by permission from *Acta Neuropathol* [*Berlin*] 53:155–160, 1981).

Fig. 5-6. Cerebral hemispheric astrocytoma. Same case as in Fig. 5-5, but shown after 20 days in culture. The cells have migrated a considerable distance from the explant and have acquired a clearly multipolar or stellate appearance, typical of adult astrocytes. (H&E, ×200.) (Reproduced by permission from *Histopathology* 5:639–650, 1981).

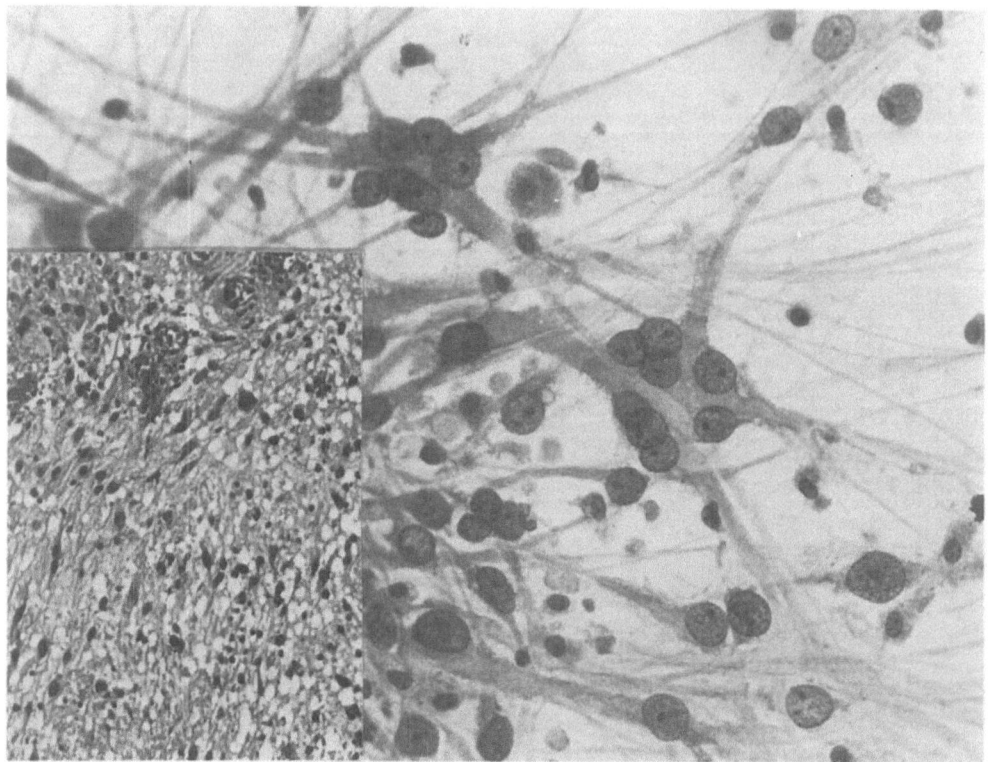

Fig. 5-8. Cerebral hemisphere astrocytoma after 18 days of culture. The cells are multipolar, but their processes are long and slender. The perikaryon is scanty. (H&E, ×400.) *Inset:* Histologic preparation of the original tumor (H&E, ×120) (Reproduced with permission from *Patologia* [*Madrid*] 16:23–45, 1983.)

ANAPLASTIC ASTROCYTOMA

In this group, the association pattern is also maintained in vitro; there is initial bipolar migration with subsequent predominance of multipolar cells. The anaplasia of these neoplasms is translated in the culture in the maintenance of cellular pleomorphism, which is consonant with that prevailing in the original tumor. In addition, the bipolar phase lasts longer than it does in the astrocytomas of low malignancy (Fig. 5-9).

The pattern of growth in tissue culture is repetitive and characteristic for cerebral hemispheric tumors of astrocytic origin. The differences among the subgroups are minimal and involve only slight variations in the duration of the bipolar phase with respect to the multipolar phase.

ASTROCYTOMAS OF THE MIDLINE

These astrocytic tumors grow at the expense of glial cells located in midline structures, (e.g., pontine astrocytoma). The author proposes to include cerebellar astrocytoma because the in vitro behavior of this tumor is well defined and is significantly different from that of the cerebral hemispheric astrocytomas. Most publications on this subject deal with cytologic aspects,[11,21,63,85] in which the authors describe astrocytes whose morphology varies depending upon the technique employed.

A great number of microvilli and undulating membranes have been described in the cells of cultured cerebellar astrocytomas studied ultrastructurally.[67] Kersting and

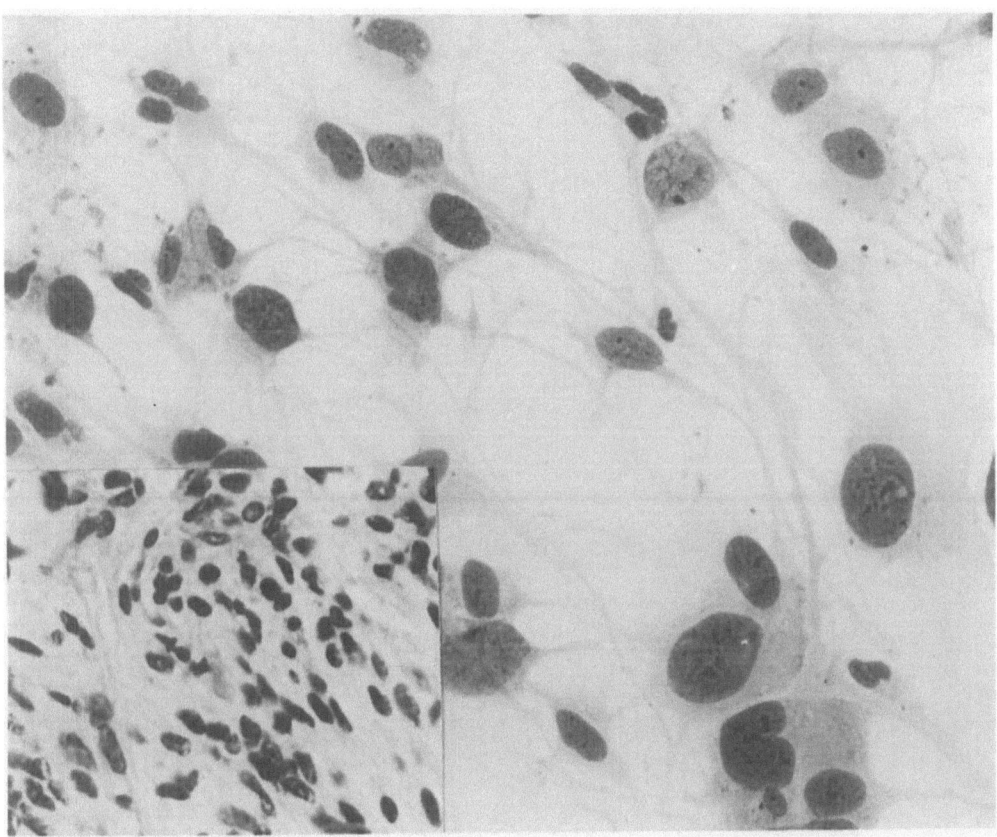

Fig. 5-9. Malignant cerebral hemisphere astrocytoma after 21 days of culture. The cells can be identified as astrocytic, but there is considerable nuclear pleomorphism; chromatin patterns are apparent. (H&E, ×400.) *Inset:* Histologic preparation of the original tumor (×125). (Reproduced with permission from *Patologia* [*Madrid*] 16:23–45, 1983).

others[17,19,29,38,42,47,51,53] have confirmed these observations. These publications have led to the establishment of criteria for the in vitro identification of cerebellar and brain stem astrocytomas, as well as astrocytomas of the diencephalon, optic nerve, and spinal cord. The formation of *Rosenthal fibers* in tissue cultures of these tumors has also been documented.[29,42]

As early as the third day after beginning the culture, there is profuse migration of narrow, elongated cells whose nuclei are oval and the cytoplasm is brightly eosinophilic. These cells are associated with the coagulum in a clear, radial disposition, remaining constantly independent of one another. These features persist during the first 2 weeks providing the culture with a clear countenance in which a growth halo is very wide and contains elongated cells devoid of multipolar components (Fig. 5-10). Subsequently, the radial disposition of the astrocytoma cells is less regular; the cells tend to be associated with one another in a reticular pattern, which acquires a maximal intricacy within the last week of the culture's life. Even within this busy reticular pattern, the majority of the cells are bipolar, elongated, and only in the very last days can multipolar astrocytes be found (Fig. 5-11).

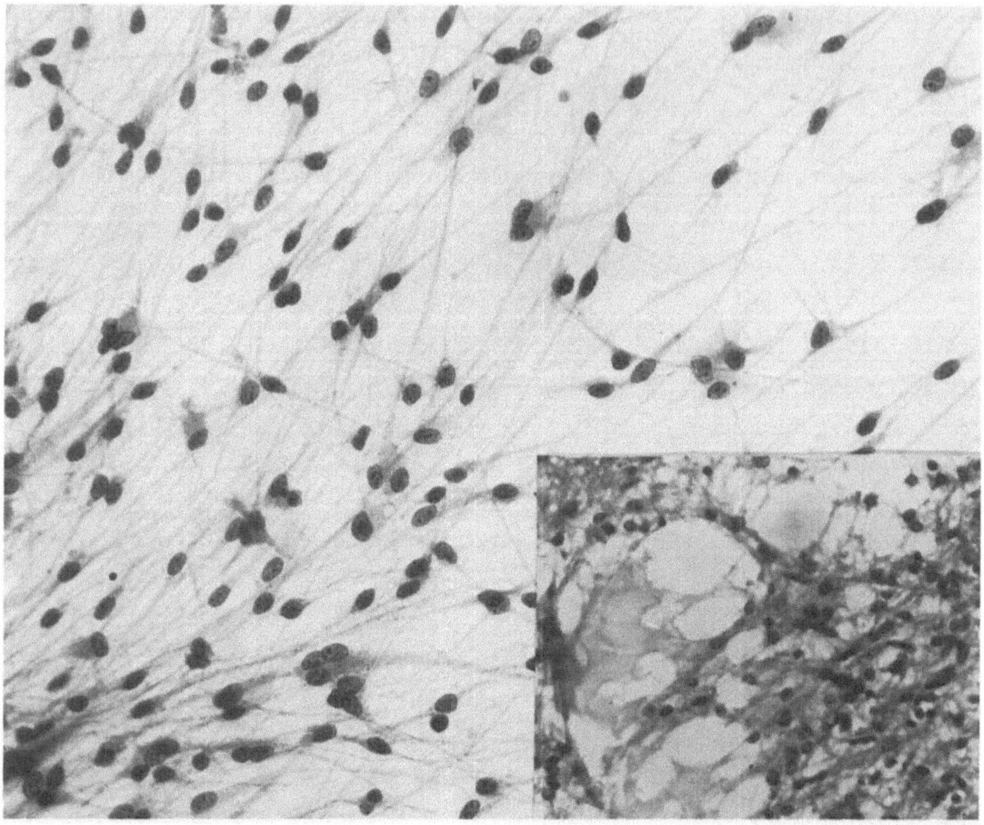

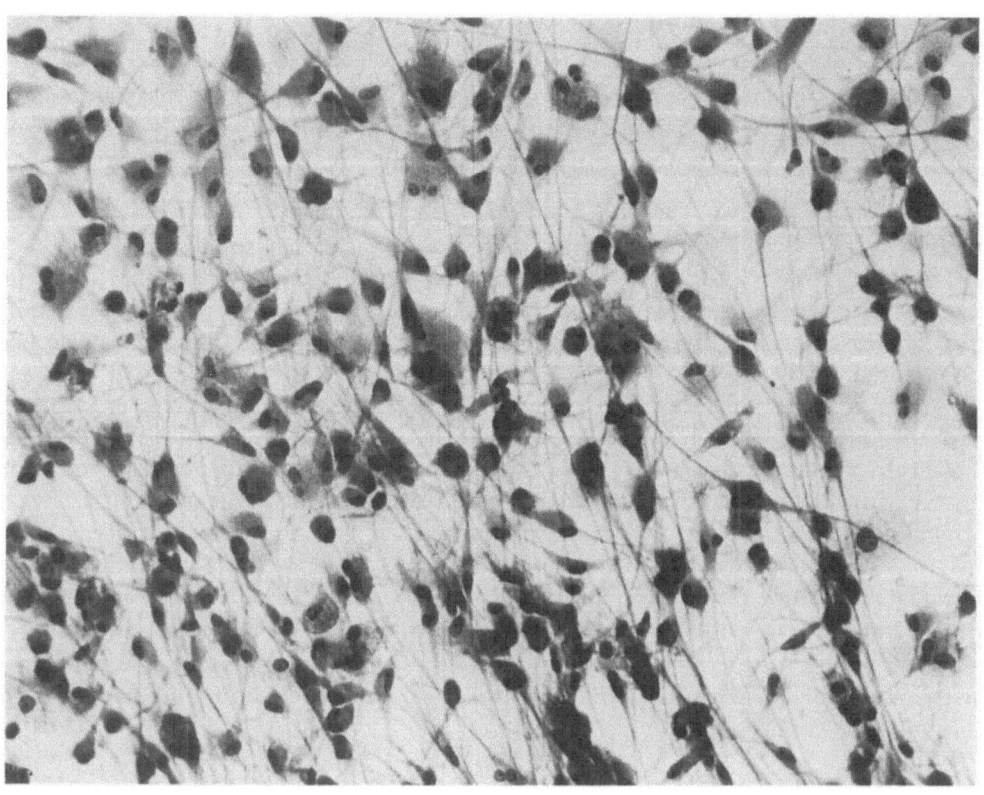

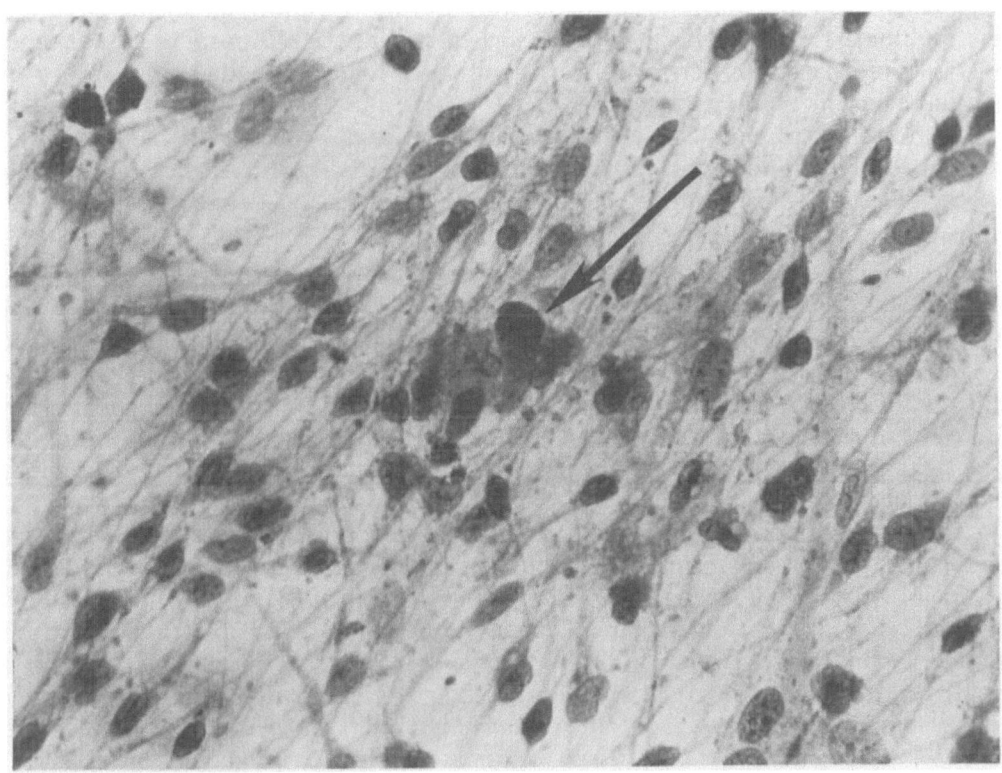

Fig. 5-12. Cerebellar astrocytoma after 48 days of culture. Multiple bipolar cells with an occasional stellate element. The club-shaped, dense, eosinophilic structure in the center (arrow) is a Rosenthal fiber. (H&E, ×400.) (Reproduced with permission from *Histopathol* 5:639–650, 1981).

When the culture is maintained beyond the usual 4 weeks, the cells begin to degenerate; masses of PAS-positive amorphous material can be seen both inside and outside the cells. These amorphous structures correspond to the *Rosenthal fibers* of conventional microscopy (Fig. 5-12).

With slight variations (of which the most outstanding is the tendency to develop multipolarity in the tumor cells derived from the cerebellum), this pattern is common for these astrocytomas as well as for those growing in the hypothalamus, optic nerve, brain stem, and spinal cord. This growth pattern defines a type of astrocytic neoplasm that is peculiar to the midline and is distinct from the tumors of the cerebral hemispheres. Cultures of midline astrocytoma are characterized by: (1) Migration of bipolar elongated

Fig. 5-10. Cerebellar astrocytoma after 8 days of culture. Isomorphic cells migrate actively and retain a bipolar appearance; the cells have long processes and scanty perikaryon. (H&E, ×200.) *Inset:* Histologic preparation of original tumor (×125). (Reproduced with permission from *Histopathol* 5:639–650, 1981).

Fig. 5-11. Cerebellar astrocytoma after 24 days of culture. The cells maintain their basic bipolar appearance, but there is a reticular pattern and occasional cells show a stellate or multipolar appearance. (H&E, ×200.) (Reproduced with permission from *Patologia* [*Madrid*] 16:23–45, 1983).

cells that remain independent of one another during the entire life of the culture. A few multipolar cells develop only after several weeks; (2) Disposition of the tumor cells in a radial pattern persisting for a long time, followed in the last week by the development of a reticular pattern.

Cultures of malignant cerebellar astrocytomas retain the growth pattern that is peculiar to all midline astrocytomas.[30] The tissue culture characteristic of optic nerve astrocytomas are similar to those of midline astrocytomas.[47,51]

GLIOBLASTOMA

Tissue cultures were applied to the study of glioblastoma several decades ago.[8,16,51,53,60,61,84,94] Later, Wilson et al.,[94] Kersting,[51–53] and Lumsden[60,61] expanded the previous observations. These works provide detailed descriptions of bipolar astrocytic cells and gigantic cells. However, slight attention has been paid to the reciprocal relationships among these cells, and the variations in behavior as a reflection of the time course have received slight attention. According to several authors, tissue cultures of glioblastomas contain many cell types; therefore, these tumors are considered by them as being of multiple cell origin.[21,59,63,64,86]

The astrocytic derivation of the glioblastoma is supported by several workers, especially Lumsden,[60] who groups all astrocytomas in what he calls "the astrocytoma–glioblastoma sequence." Only Kersting[51] suggests that some of the so-called glioblastomas of round cells may represent malignant oligodendrogliomas. This has not been confirmed in other laboratories.

The authors have observed significant cellular differentiation in tissue cultures of glioblastoma and on this basis, have concluded that the origin of the neoplastic cells is purely astrocytic.[28] The tissue cultures of hemispheric glioblastomas show a similar behavior to that of the hemispheric astrocytomas. In these cultures, one observes the same dual cell population in which the sequence from bipolar to multipolar is repeated. The reticular association pattern appears much later than in hemispheric astrocytomas. The difference between the glioblastomas and the astrocytomas is really a subtle one; it consists of a maximal lengthening in the duration of the bipolar phase of cellular evolution. The multipolar cells appear only in the late phases of the culture. Surprisingly, the existence of a final multipolar phase is especially prominent in the fusiform glioblastomas, a group which in histologic preparations represents one of the least differentiated ones. Two cultures showing a spatial coexistence of malignant astrocytoma and glioblastoma, displayed no variations with respect to the general growth pattern (Figs. 5-13 and 5-14).

Explants from a cerebellar glioblastoma showed, in contrast, cells that were oriented radially and exhibited long distal bipolar expansions. As early as the ninth day of culture, a 2–3-mm-wide halo developed with bipolar cells, not purely arranged in a radial fashion, but with a definite tendency to form a reticular pattern. After 15 days

Fig. 5-13. Cerebral glioblastoma multiforme after nine days of culture. The cells are large, the nuclear features are irregular and pleomorphic. The cytoplasm is bipolar, scanty, and the cells are arranged in a radial fashion during this early stage. (H&E, ×400.) *Inset:* Histologic preparation of original tumor (H&E, ×100).

Fig. 5-14. Cerebral glioblastoma multiforme after 21 days of culture. Eventually, the bipolar cells become multipolar elements with all the features of adult astrocytes arranged in a reticular fashion. (H&E, ×400.) (Reproduced with permission from *Acta Neuropathol* [Berlin] 53:155–160, 1981).

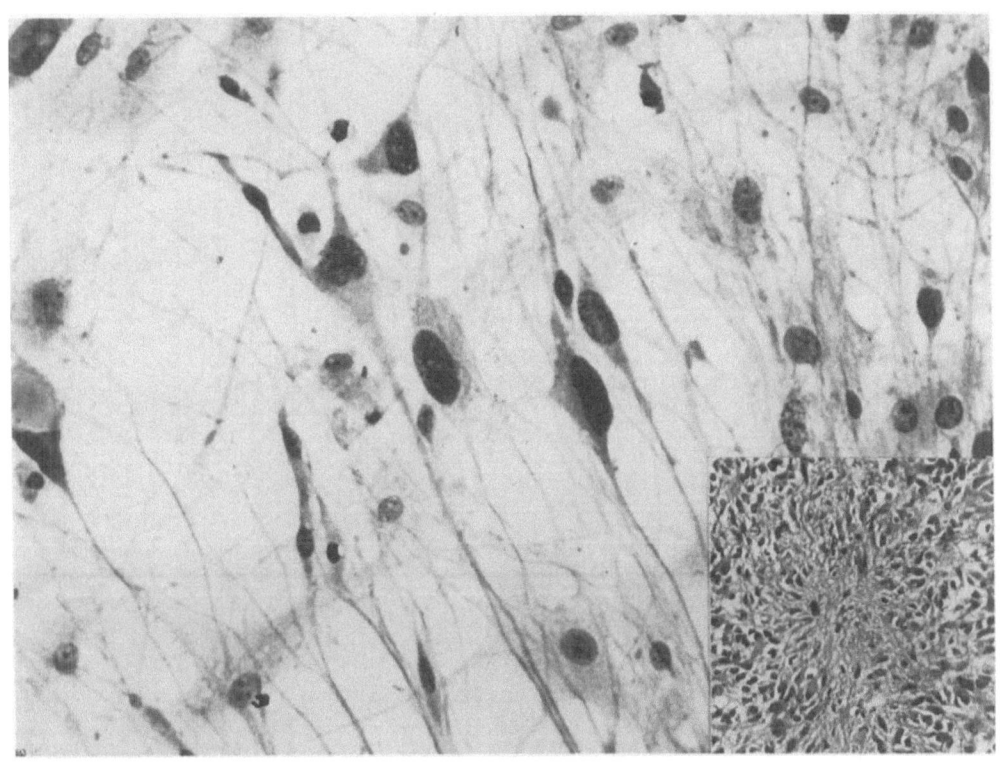

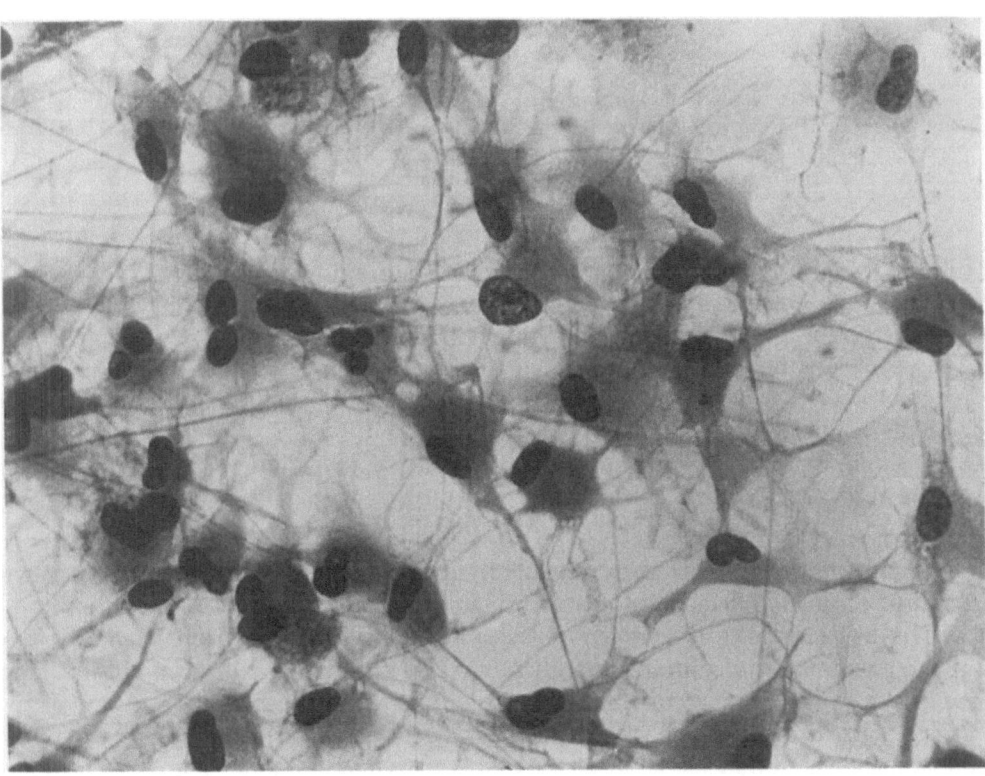

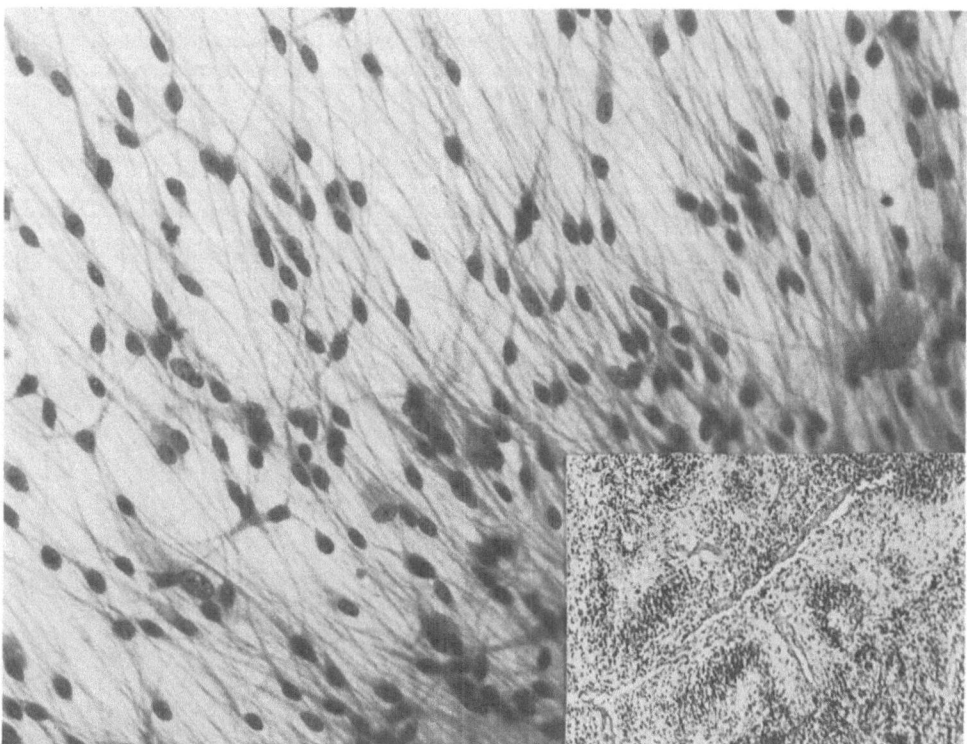

Fig. 5-15. Cerebellar glioblastoma multiforme after 12 days of culture. The in vitro growth patterns of this tumor are similar to those of the cerebellar astrocytomas. There are numerous elongated bipolar cells arranged in a radial fashion. (H&E, ×200.) *Inset:* Histologic preparation of the original tumor showing pseudopallisading in the molecular layer of the cerebellum (H&E, ×100).

of culture, there were several multipolar cells. Therefore, the in vitro behavior of cerebellar glioblastoma was identical to that of the cerebellar astrocytomas and different from that of the cerebral hemispheric astrocytomas (Fig. 5-15).

These observations also suggest that the glioblastoma multiforme is a malignant astrocytic tumor that follows two growth patterns, depending upon whether the tumor is located in the cerebral hemispheres or in the midline. In spite of its pronounced lack of differentiation, the neoplastic components of the glioblastoma can mature in vitro into recognizable adult cells.

SPECIAL FORMS OF ASTROCYTOMA

In *subependymal giant cell astrocytoma*,[44] the cells maintain their typical plump cytoplasm and eccentric nucleus, and the tendency to group themselves in clumps of 4–6 cells. The bipolar phase is very short (Fig. 5-16). Cells with neuronal features have not been encountered in cultures of subependymal giant-cell astrocytoma even though some cells of these tumors contain S-100 protein and neurosecretory granules.[72]

Observations made by electron microscopy and by the culture of tissues and organs support the concept that *subependymomas* (subependymal glomerate astrocytomas) have a mixed ependymal and astrocytic origin.[12,33] In observations of the author, limited

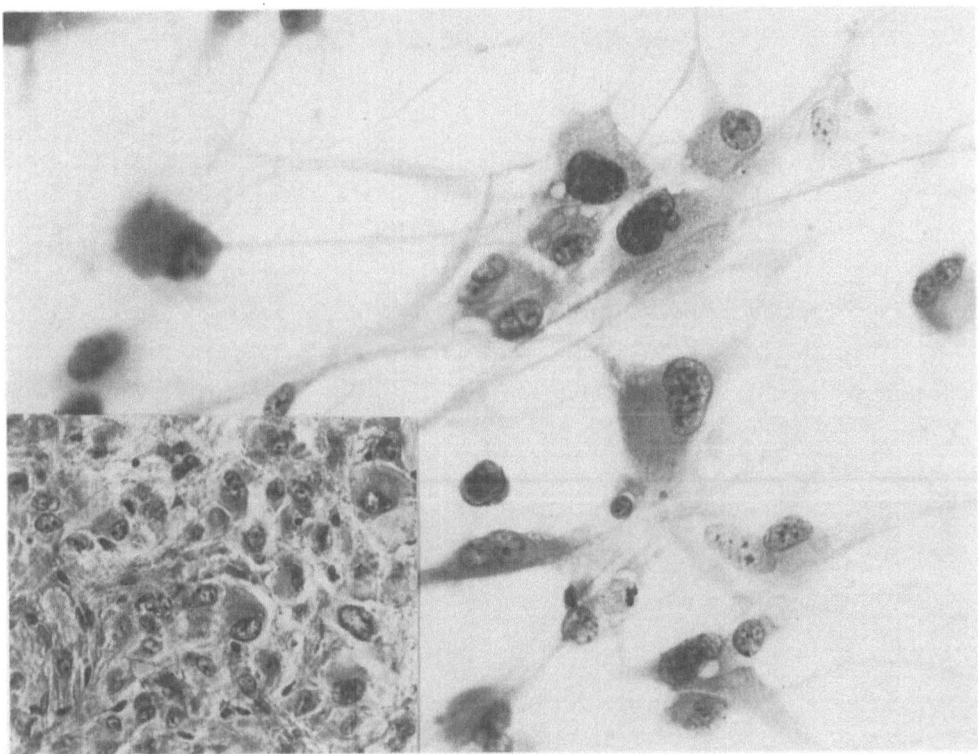

Fig. 5-16. Subependymal giant cell astrocytoma after 12 days of culture. The cells have a clear astrocytic appearance including the presence of multiple cell processes and abundant perikaryon with an eccentric nucleus. (H&E, ×400) *Inset:* Histologic preparation of the original tumor (H&E, ×200).

to one subependymoma studied by tissue culture, the only cell type was a narrow elongated cell that showed a latent tendency to adopt reticular disposition and an absence of a multipolar component. Epithelial or ependymal components were not observed in any of the explants (Fig. 5-17).

OLIGODENDROGLIOMA

The honeycomb pattern present in most oligodendrocytic tumors makes the diagnosis of oligodendroglioma usually simple. There are diagnostic difficulties in the atypical forms of the tumor,[24] which include pleomorphic oligodendroglioma, the eosinophilic, fusiform, and pseudoglioblastomatous variants of oligodendroglioma. Of special interest are the difficulties offered by the mixed tumors that have elements of both oligodendroglioma and astrocytoma. The precise identification of unusual variants of oligodendroglioma could be important in those instances in which the histologic features are strongly suggestive of malignancy.

The morphology of normal oligodendroglia in tissue cultures has been studied by Pomerat,[76] Lumsden and Pomerat,[62] and Pomerat et al.[77] The more important features, as seen with the phase contrast microscope, include: round cells having dense and glistening cytoplasm and short cytoplasmic processes reminiscent of the image originally described by del Rio-Hortega; these cells have pulsatile activity.

Several studies[5,11,17,19–22,40,51,53,60,61,73,86] have defined the in vitro behavior of oligo-

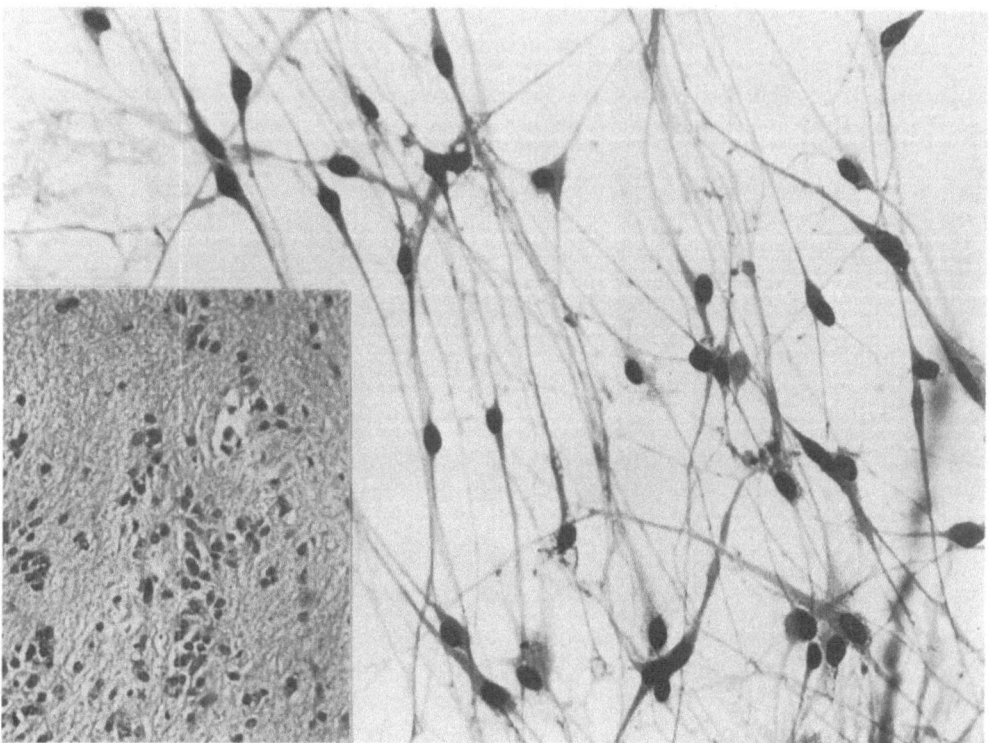

Fig. 5-17. Subependymoma (glomerate subependymal astrocytoma) after 12 days of culture. This image is unique for this tumor, which is made of elongated bipolar cells with scanty cytoplasm. From the beginning the cells tend to have a reticular association pattern. (H&E, ×200.) *Inset:* Histologic preparation of the original tumor (H&E, ×125).

dendrogliomas. The cellular migration is slow. Small cells having a round nucleus, sometimes eccentric in location and surrounded by scanty cytoplasm, are seen in the primary stage. At first, the cytoplasm retains a clear aspect, but gradually it turns dense, and with phase contrast microscopy, it is intensely brilliant. The cytoplasmic processes become more evident. They are scanty, short, and straight, and emerge abruptly from the perikaryon. This morphology barely varies throughout the life of the culture (Fig. 5-18).

The cellular association is initially markedly reticular. The cells begin to separate from the explant and are initially arranged in a densely packed pattern; slowly, they become disaggregated. This is due, in part, to the active digestion of the coagulum, and also to the spatial rearrangement of the migrating cells. Halos or vacuoles limited by packed fibers with some perikarya are seen within the reticular network. Other times small groups of oligodendrocytes remain isolated either at the periphery of the explant or within the large vacuoles. These oligodendrocytes have radial processes that contact through their ends with the fibers limiting the vacuoles. Through time-lapse cinematography, these cells are seen moving from one edge of the vacuole to the other to incorporate themselves into a new group of cells. This in vitro behavior is maintained throughout the entire life of the culture (Fig. 5-19).

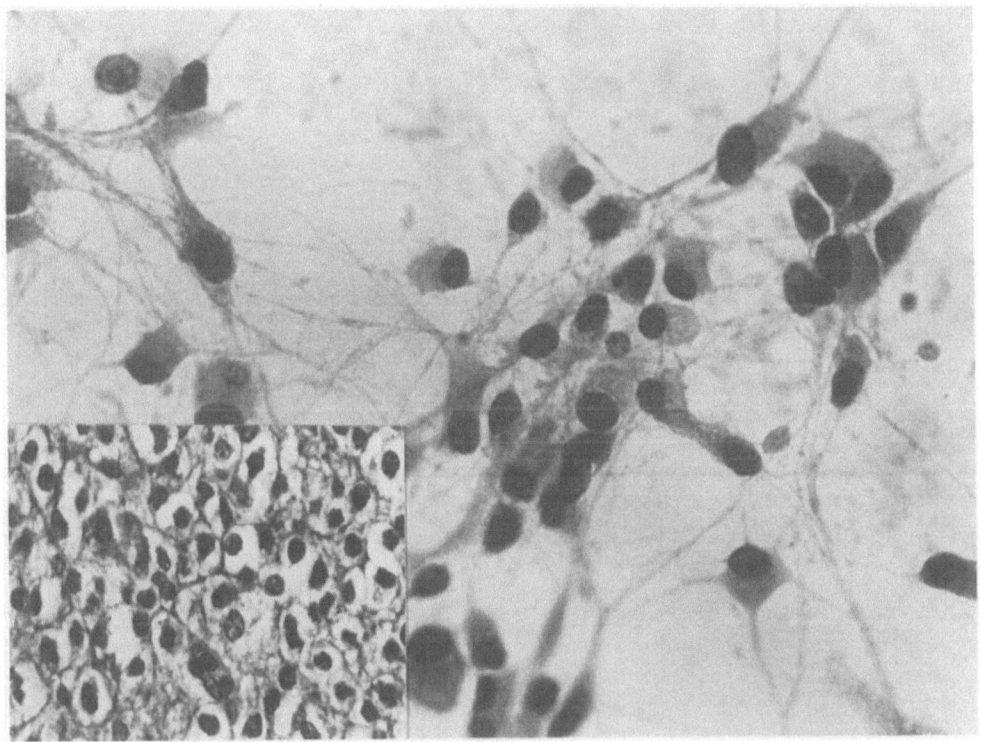

Fig. 5-18. Oligodendroglioma after six days of culture. The migrating cells are small, contain a round hyperchromatic nucleus, sometimes in an eccentric location. The cytoplasm is scanty and endowed with short, fine, diverging processes. The cells show a tendency to adopt a reticular association. (H&E, ×400.) *Inset:* Histologic preparation of the original tumor (H&E, ×200).

The described pattern is common to all the classic forms of oligodendroglioma and is independent of the mitotic activity. The eosinophilic oligodendrogliomas show a similar slow migration by cells, which by and large, retain the oligodendrocytic morphology, but have a plump eosinophilic cytoplasm. The association of neoplastic cells in small cell groups is also characteristic (Fig. 5-20). The cells display peculiar cytoplasmic features in this subtype of oligodendroglioma; these features do not appear to be degenerative, as they are maintained unaltered throughout the life of the culture. Because of this, it does not appear probable that the cytoplasmic appearance is dependent on the development of autophagic activity.[88] In this variety of oligodendroglioma, Kepes[50] demonstrated by ultrastructure, glial fibrils positive with GFAP.

A mixed tumor studied in the authors' laboratories showed a dual cell population, (i.e., oligodendroglial and astrocytic elements). A greater percentage of the usual mixture as described by Kersting[53] existed in this tumor. Both cell populations remained present throughout the entire life of the culture, although they grew in separate explants. This observation confirms the existence of mixed gliomas, although the nature of the biologic phenomenon remains to be elucidated. Two possibilities may be considered: a mixed tumor is made of elements derived from two entirely separate cells of origin, or the tumor is the outcome of the transformation of one mature cell into another.

The in vitro pattern of oligodendrogliomas is characterized by the slow migration

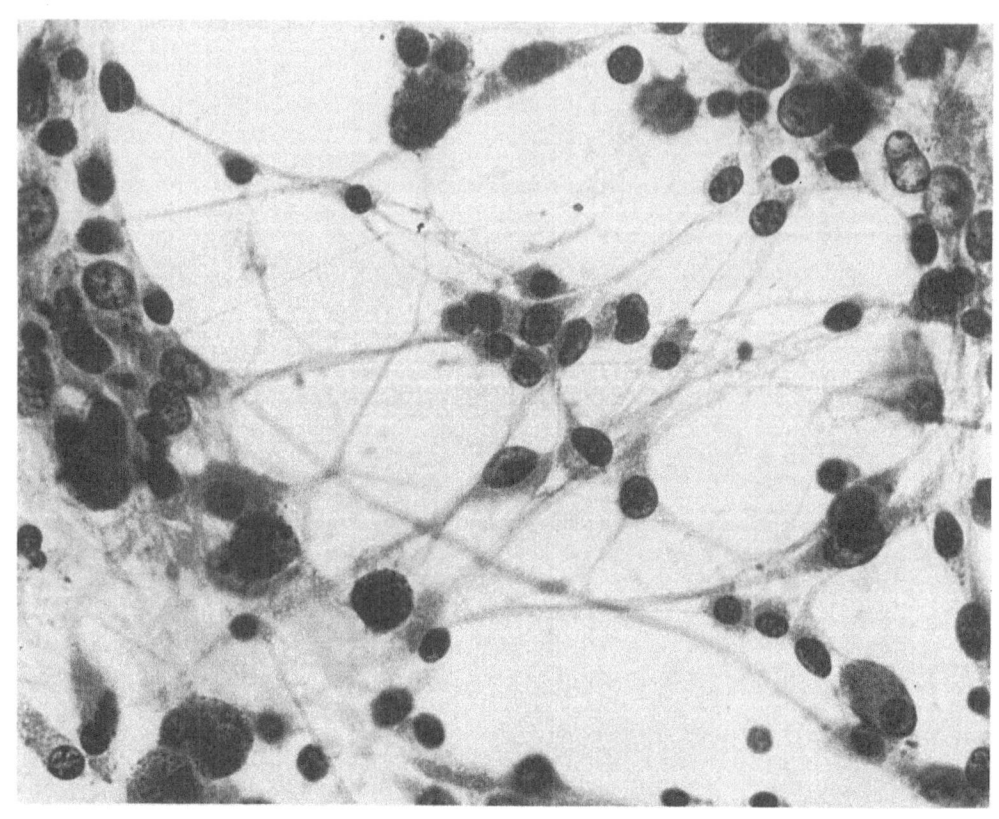
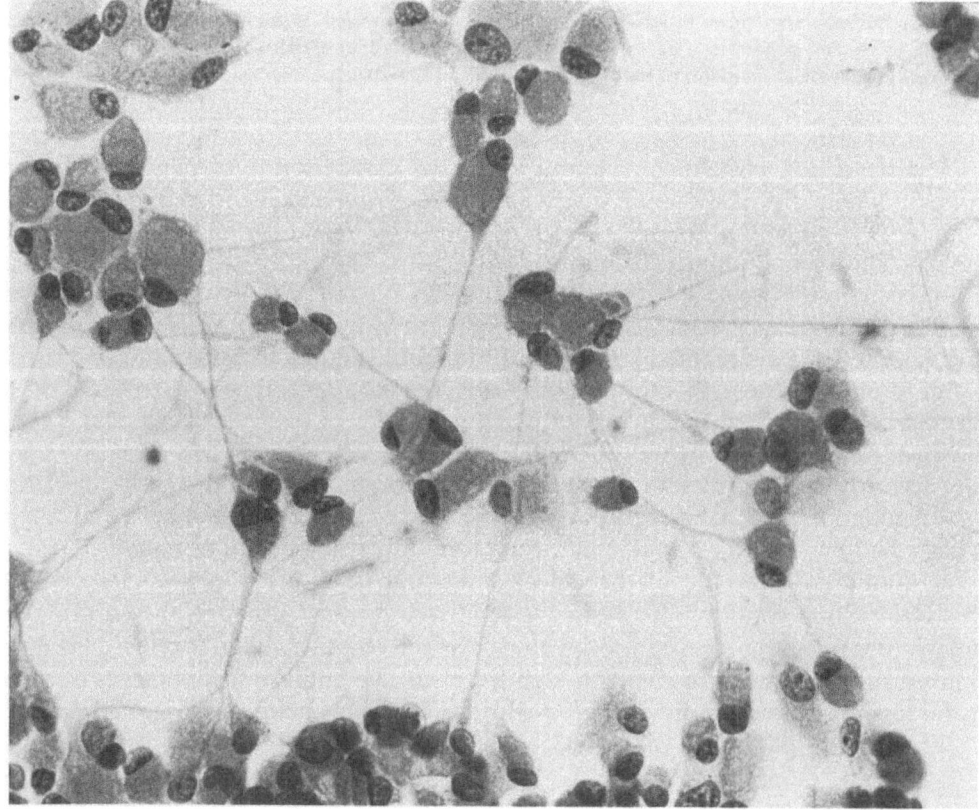

of cells with classical oligodendrocytic morphology. This migration is associated in the reticular pattern with vacuoles and with frequent formation of small cellular groups. This pattern is constant regardless of the proliferative activity of the tumor and is maintained in the unusual forms mentioned previously. The pattern is characteristic of the other gliomas of reticular pattern (astrocytomas, glioblastomas, and medulloblastomas) and much more so with regard to the mechanocytic or epithelial groups.

MEDULLOBLASTOMA

The well-known clinical and morphologic features of the medulloblastoma contrast with the failure to determine with certainty the cell of origin of this tumor. The application of methods, such as silver impregnation, enzyme and immunohistochemistry, electron microscopy, and experimental oncogenesis have not produced very illuminating results. The most constant feature of the medulloblastoma continues to be the lack of differentiation of its cells, and the paucity of cytoplasmic organelles, which in many instances are among the most valuable features for a histologic diagnosis.

In tissue cultures, expectations have not been met with the expected results, mainly because reasons for failures in establishing a tissue culture for this type of tumor are very numerous. As in the rest of the undifferentiated small cell tumors, the medulloblastoma cells are not very viable; most cells die in the explant before migrating and before in vitro proliferation begin. Frequently, as a result, the mesenchymal cells take over in many attempted cultures of medulloblastoma.

Important publications in this field are those of Kredel;[1] Russell and Bland;[84] Palacios;[75] Liss;[59] and Lumsdem,[60] as well as those from the Bonn group.[39,45,46,51–53] These publications defend two opposing viewpoints. Lumsden[86] and Scharenberg and Liss[86] defend a neuroblastic origin for medulloblastoma on the basis of two observations: (1) the migration of small groups of cells with round, hyperchromatic nuclei and invisible cytoplasm, that remain at the periphery of the explant in a seeding fashion, according to Batzdorf,[3] (2) the protrusion of radial neurites observed before cellular migration begins; this feature is comparable to a similar one frequently observed in neuroblastomas. The development of neurites in medulloblastomas is a late occurrence evidently requiring in some cases, up to one month to develop. Silver impregnation by the Bodian method is necessary in order to demonstrate the neurites, as they may be invisible in the standard H&E preparation.[60]

Gullotta and Kersting[45] believe in a mesenchymal origin of medulloblastoma based on the features of the migrated cells they observed in their cultures. Gullotta and Kost[46] reported that in only one out of 50 tumors studied in culture, they observed a behavior comparable to that described by Lumsden (Fig. 5-21). In all the other 49 tumors, there was growth of stellate cells with an oval-shaped, hypochromatic nucleus that suggested a mesenchymal derivation. These cells were constantly arranged according to a reticular pattern (Fig. 5-22).

Fig. 5-19. Oligodendroglioma after 24 days of culture. The cell morphology changes only slightly and the association patterns are retained. Small areolar spaces contain small groups of neoplastic cells (H&E, ×400).

Fig. 5-20. Eosinophilic oligodendroglioma after 12 days of culture. All the features retained in these cells and their association patterns are typical of those seen in classical oligodendrogliomas. The cells show abundant eosinophilic cytoplasm, which is characteristic for this variant of oligodendroglioma (H&E, ×400).

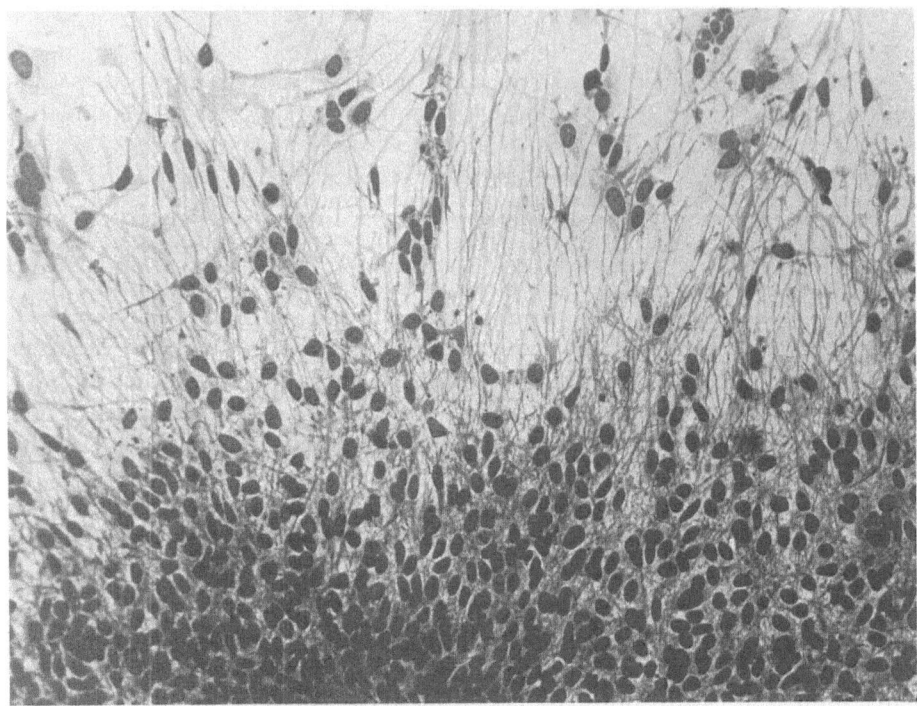

Fig. 5-21. Medulloblastoma after eight days of culture. The migrating cells in this case are elongated, bipolar, or sometimes stellate. The cell processes are argentophilic and form a dense plexus similar to that seen in neuroblastomas. (Bodian, ×40) (Reproduced with permission from *Pathologica* [*Genoa*] 72:27–34, 1980).

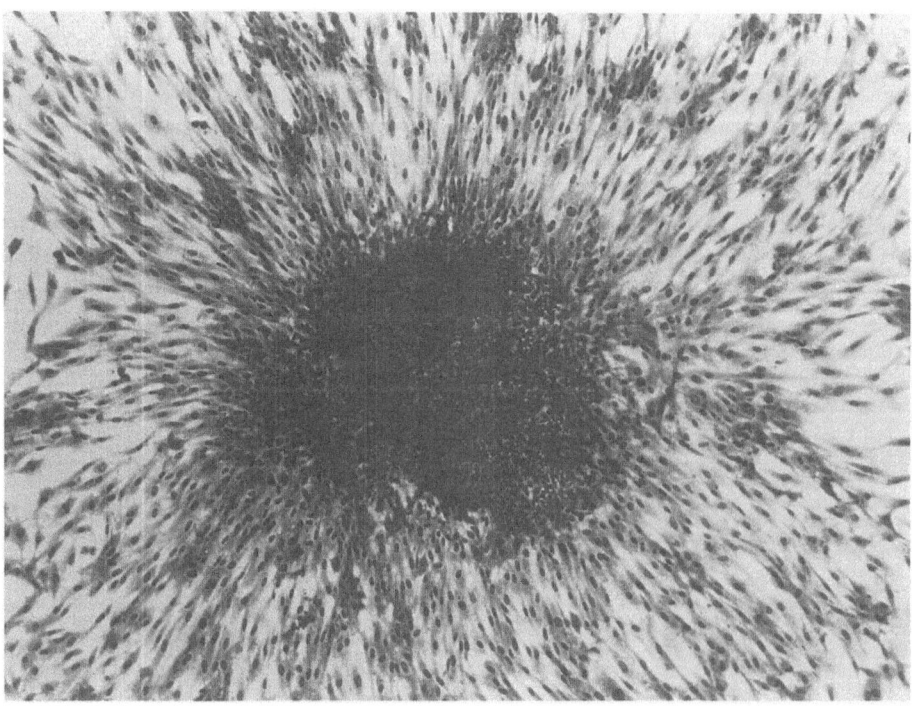

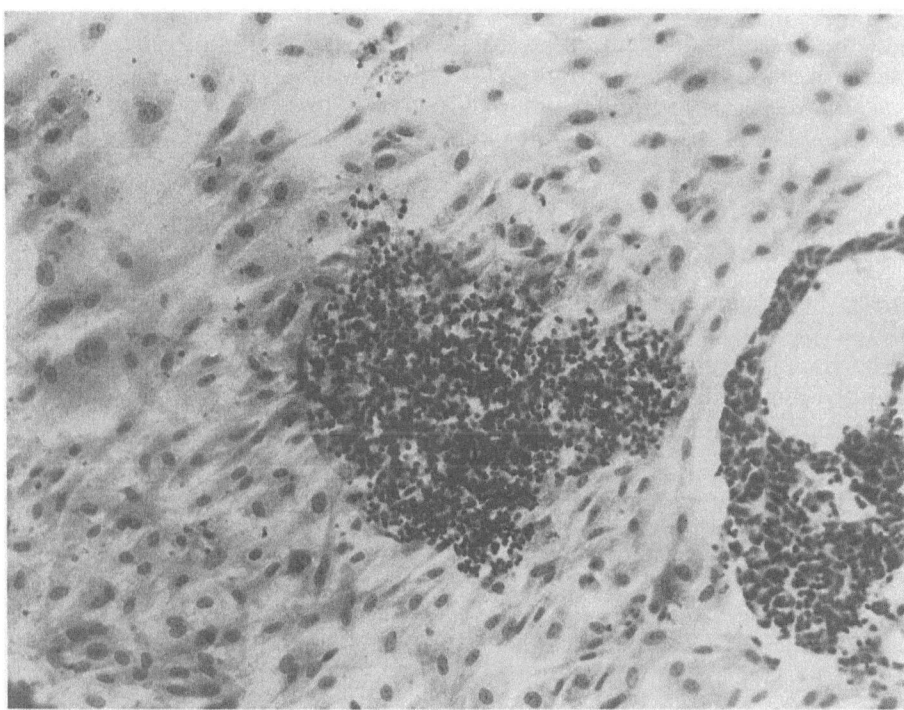

Fig. 5-23. Medulloblastoma after ten days of culture. The cellular proliferation originates from a group of elements having flat, elongated, endothelial-like appearance. A few neuroectodermic cells without apparent proliferative activity are seen in the vicinity of the explant. (H&E, ×40.) (Reproduced with permission from *Pathologica* [Genoa] 72:27–34, 1980).

The author has had unsatisfactory results in his attempts to grow medulloblastoma. In the few in which the cells grew, non-neoplastic mesenchymal elements took over the culture. In only two of the cases were the characteristic groups of small cells seen as described by others (Fig. 5-23). Based on the analysis of the literature and his own results, the author is skeptical about the applications of tissue culture to the analysis of medulloblastoma.

The suggestion by Lumsden to apply the Bodian method for the demonstration of neurites is somewhat surprising, because neurites in extracranial neuroblastomas are always visible with H&E. Gullotta and Kost[46] reported only one case among many in which there were elements of neuroblastoma; this had been previously demonstrated by del Rio-Hortega[20] and subsequently by others. The Lumsden series includes only five cases, and Scharenberg and Liss do not mention the number of cases they studied. As a result, their opinions cannot be generalized. A neuroblastic origin ascribed uniformly to all medulloblastomas does not explain the predictable localization of this tumor in the cerebellum, or the tumor's biologic behavior, which is different from other neuroblastomas', including those of the cerebral hemispheres.[22] The mesenchymal theory is con-

Fig. 5-22. Medulloblastoma after seven days of culture. Intense proliferation of fusiform cells that are disposed in a radial fashion. There is no similarity with the image shown in Fig. 5-21. (Bodian, ×16.) (Reproduced with permission from *Pathologica* [Genoa] 72:27–34, 1980).

trary to a basic postulate concerning growth of sarcomas in culture, (i.e., the preservation of the general, structural features regardless of the site of origin).

The applications of tissue culture to the diagnosis of medulloblastomas are minimal; they include the hope of finding synaptic structures that develop after long periods—a feature that has been interpreted as an expression of rematuration.[80]

Tumors of Epithelial Pattern

In this heterogeneous group, there are tumors as dissimilar from one another as the choroid plexus papillomas, craniopharyngiomas, brain metastases, and ependymomas. The tissue culture methods provide only a few bits of information that are not obtainable through routine techniques. The growth patterns are of interest, however, especially in the identification of subtypes of ependymomas.

TUMORS OF THE CHOROID PLEXUS

The application of tissue culture to the diagnosis of these tumors is limited compared to other techniques, because the in vitro behavior of choroid plexus tumors is similar

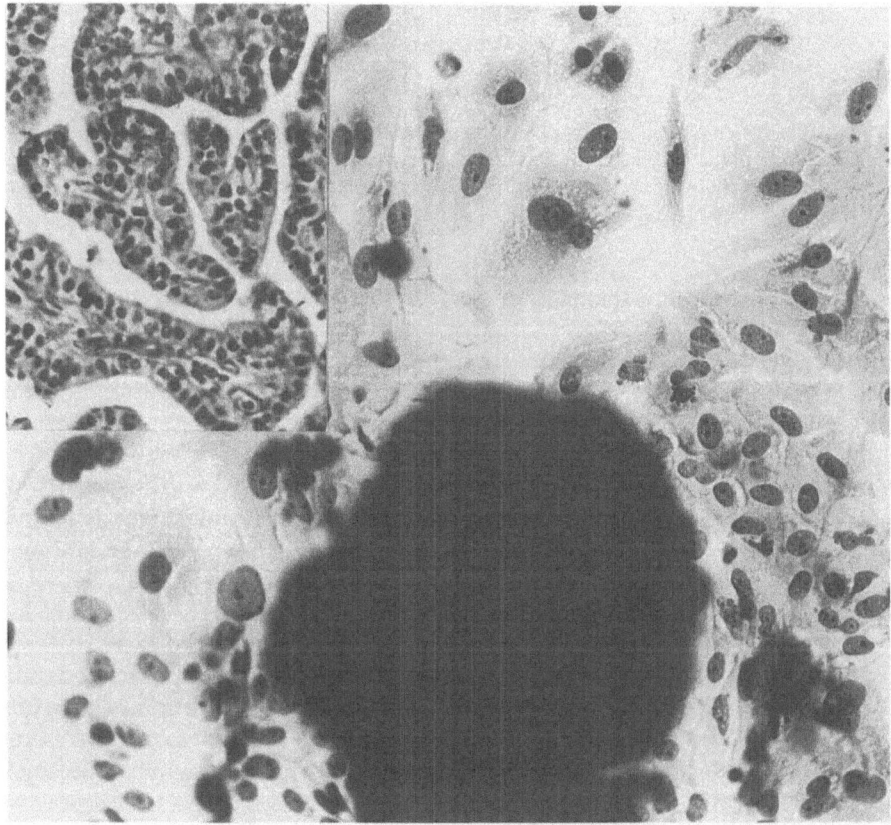

Fig. 5-24. Choroid plexus papilloma of the fourth ventricle after six days of culture. Polygonal flat cells arranged in a mosaic fashion migrate from the explant. The nuclear pleomorphism is characteristic in spite of the cellular isomorphism and the benign biologic behavior of the tumor. (H&E, ×200.) *Inset:* Histologic preparation of the original tumor (H&E, ×100).

to that of the entire group; there are no features that are characteristic for each neoplasm. Because of this, it is impossible to distinguish between the growth of choroid plexus tumor and that of epithelial metastases. The benign or malignant character of the tumor cannot be determined by tissue culture. The optimal application of tissue culture methods to this group of tumors resides in the ability to differentiate between choroid plexus papillomas and papillary ependymomas.

Cultures of benign choroid plexus papillomas grow in accordance with a pure epithelial pattern in which cells abandon the explant and adapt themselves to the glass slide in a short period of time. They maintain cohesion among them; the cells are polygonal and the nucleus is slightly pleomorphic even in completely benign tumors. On occasion multiple nuclei in a single cell may be seen; this lacks a prognostic significance.[51] The cytoplasm is abundant and eosinophilic, surrounded by a well-differentiated plasma membrane through which the cells adhere to one another forming a continuous and compact mosaic. In this manner, the explant is surrounded by an epithelial halo lacking the dense edge typical of the craniopharyngioma. The lack of intercellular fibrils in choroid plexus papilloma is significant and constitutes one of the most important features in the differentiation with ependymoma (Fig. 5-24).

In the only case of malignant choroid plexus papilloma the authors have studied,[57] the growth pattern was similar to that of the benign variety, but the nuclear pleomorphism was much more apparent (Fig. 5-25).

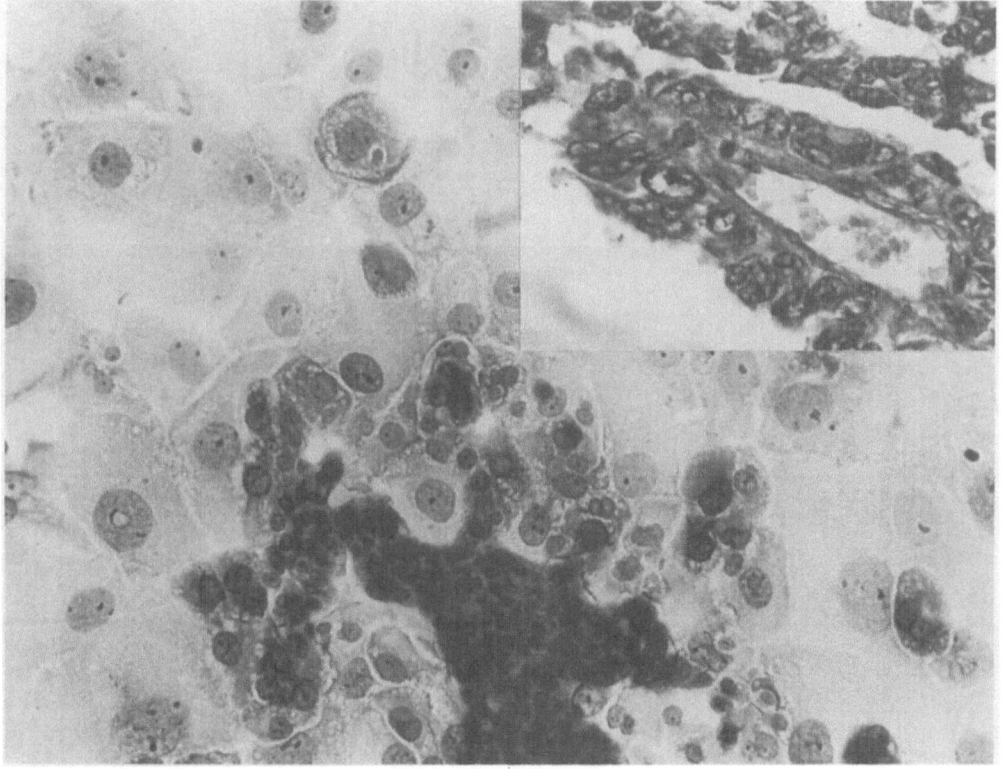

Fig. 5-25. Carcinoma of the choroid plexus after 12 days of culture. The cells entirely surround the explant (lower part of the field). These cells are polygonal, large, and contain nuclei with markedly pleomorphic features. (H&E, ×400). *Inset:* Histologic image of the original tumor (H&E, ×125).

CRANIOPHARYNGIOMA

The existing literature on tissue culture of craniopharyngioma is scarce,[13,35,51] but in all series one feature is constant: the rapid and precocious growth pattern of this tumor is remarkable when compared with the slow development of the in vivo process. Two to three days after starting the culture, there is a halo around the original explant in which the polygonally shaped cells, slightly elongated and intimately apposed to one another, form a continuous mosaic on the crystal. Within a few days this mosaic grows eccentrically and a dense edge develops; this edge is made up of cells tightly apposed against one another that form a dense ring. Here, the nuclei are more hyperchromatic and larger than those in the choroid plexus papilloma. Moreover, degenerative vacuoles are readily visible in the cytoplasm. This image of a central explant, surrounded by an epithelial continuous mosaic, which in turn is surrounded by a dense edge, is characteristic of craniopharyngioma[51] (Figs. 5-26 and 5-27).

In the late stages there appears in the interior of the mosaic, round eosinophilic epithelial structures, either without nucleus or with a basophilic central round structure. These are the in vitro equivalents of the keratin balls. It is common to find cells with cytoplasmic granules of keratohyaline (eleidin), whose presence can be demonstrated by means of the Astrablau. Craniopharyngioma has been defined by the application

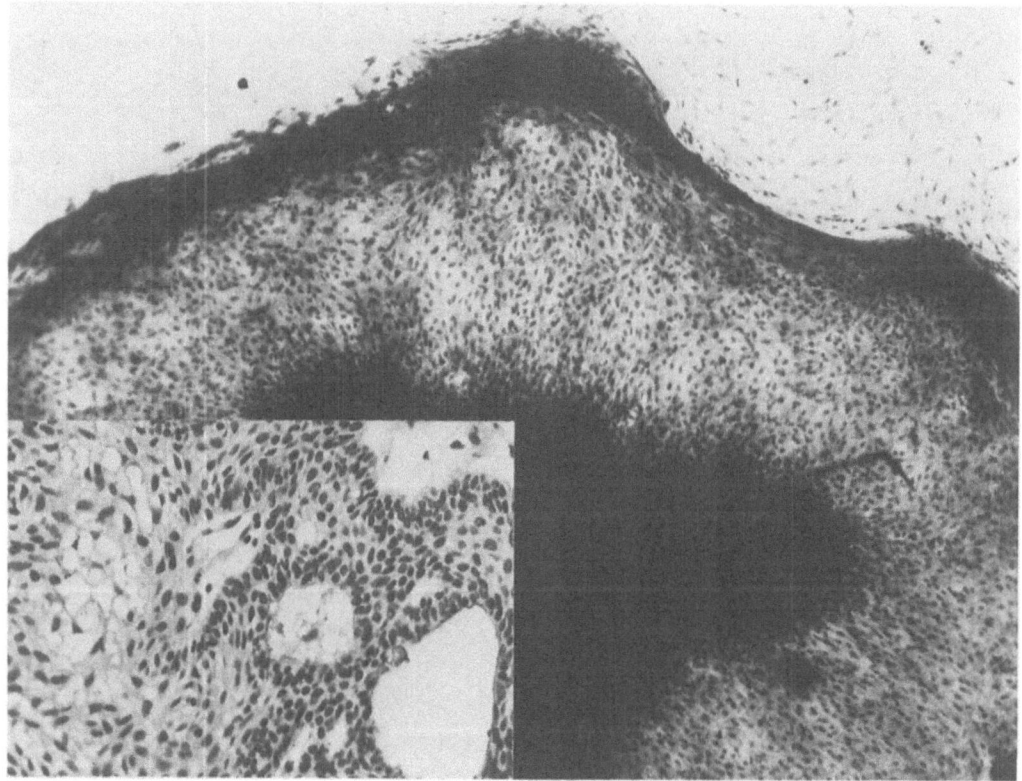

Fig. 5-26. Craniopharyngioma after 6 days in culture. Characteristically, the explant shows three concentric layers. The explant can be identified in the center. Next, there is a halo of epithelial growth continous with a peripherally placed layer of closely apposed cells. (H&E, ×40). *Inset:* Histologic preparation of the original tumor (H&E, ×125).

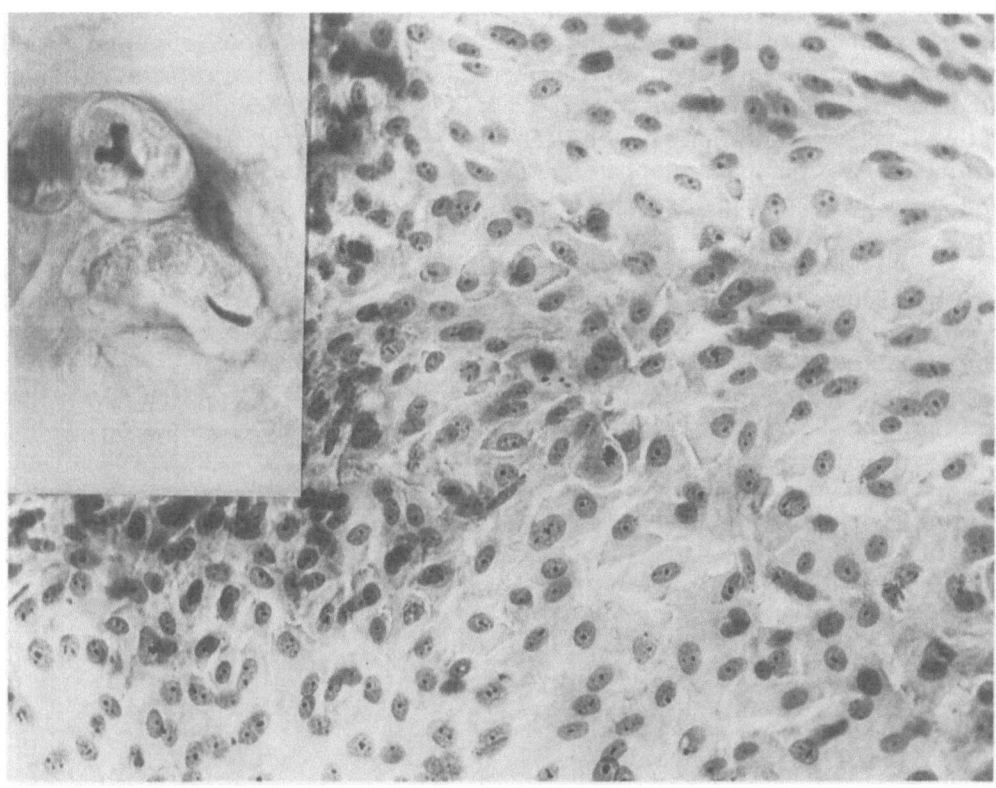

Fig. 5-27. Craniopharyngioma after 15 days of culture. These cells are polygonal, contain a vesicular nucleus, and a prominent nucleolus. The association pattern is typical for epithelium and the appearance of a mosaic is obvious. (H&E, ×200.) *Inset:* A few cells in the culture show keratinization, with marked cytoplasmic eosinophilia and nuclear pyknosis (H&E, ×1,000).

to the culture of histochemical and ultrastructural methods.[35] In the late phases of the culture, there are free intercellular spaces signifying degeneration of the culture and lacking any specific significance. Calcareous spherules, described by Cobb and Wright[13] are fragments of the explanted material that slid to the periphery of the explant and are probably unrelated to the activity of the tumor cells.

The craniopharyngioma behaves in vitro as a purely epithelial tumor of squamous cell type, and the analysis of this behavior does not support the suggestion that the craniopharyngioma is a mixed glial-epithelial tumor.[58] The astrocytes growing in some craniopharyngioma explants are probably derived from the scar surrounding the tumor.

CEREBRAL METASTASES

In spite of their rapid growth, the percent of failures among attempted cultures of brain metastases is close to 30%.[51] Lumsden[60] attempted unsuccessfully to culture metastatic cells isolated from the cerebrospinal fluid.

Explants of carcinomatous metastases grow according to the purely epithelial pattern, (i.e., polygonal cells that are closely apposed to one another). The nuclei maintain the atypical features of carcinoma cells with chromatin distributed in dense blocks and mixed with prominent nucleoli. The features of the cytoplasm vary according to the original tumor, but usually the cytoplasm is basophilic. Focal eosinophilic changes in metastases of squamous carcinomas are rarely seen. Carcinomatous cells grow eccentrically in irregular fashion but form the habitual halo around the explants. They end up detaching themselves from the free edge of growth and then disintegrate. Because of this, there is never a dense peripheral halo or a *crazy pavement* pattern. This differentiates metastases from the craniopharyngiomas and ependymomas. Explants of carcinomatous metastases are indistinguishable from the tumors of the choroid plexus (Fig. 5-28).

Tissue cultures of metastases from melanomas have served to demonstrate the capacity of these tumors to redifferentiate in vitro,[29,44] a concept that was doubted by some authors. The cultures of primitive melanomas, whether encephalic or choroidal[51,79] or metastatic melanomas,[60] lack the pure epithelial pattern of carcinomatous metastases. Instead, they harbor a mixture of fusiform-shaped cells having epithelial-like features and macrophages. Surprisingly, even in tumors that are either barely melanotic or amelanotic, the in vitro production of pigment is abundant. The melanin appears in all three cell types. This is a constant phenomenon that has been observed both in the primary brain melanomas and in metastases from cutaneous melanomas.

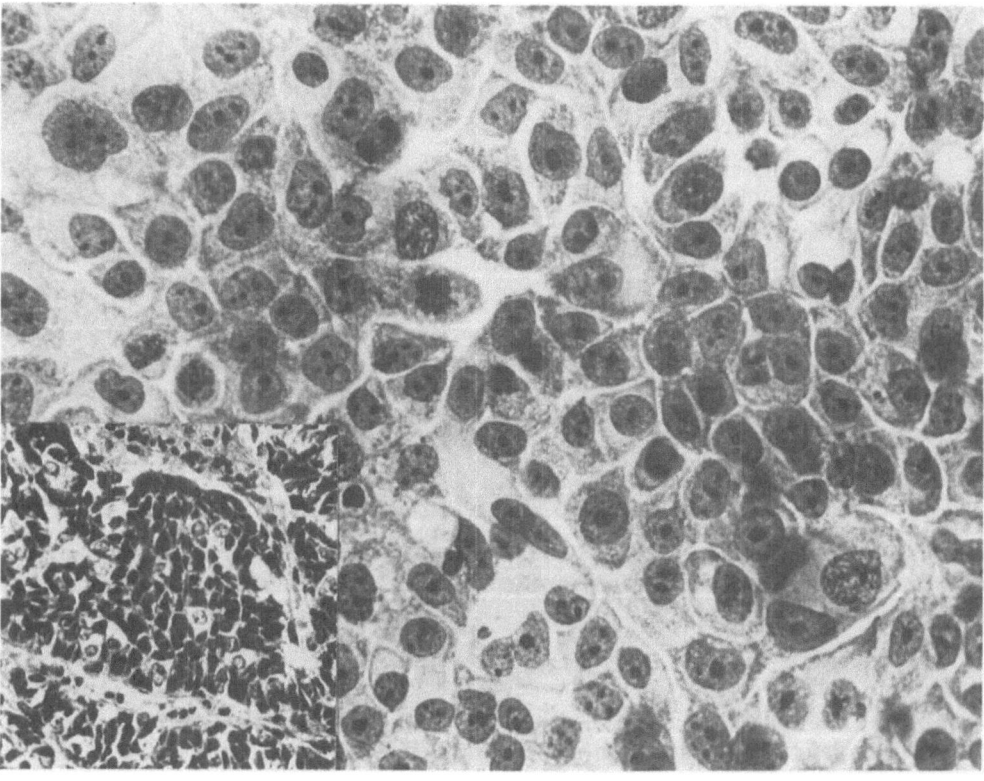

Fig. 5-28. Cerebral metastasis of a lung cancer after 15 days of culture. Large cells growing in a closely associated pattern reminiscent of a mosaic. The cytoplasmic features are well defined and the nuclei are large and endowed with one or more prominent nucleoli (H&E, ×200). *Inset:* Histologic image of the original tumor (×100).

EPENDYMOMA

The difficulties in diagnosing ependymomas are based on two factors: there are three different types of ependymomas: cellular, epithelial, and papillary—and there are variable degrees of differentiation. Epithelial ependymomas must be differentiated from neuroepitheliomas, medulloepitheliomas, and carcinomatous metastases; cellular ependymomas must be differentiated from medulloblastomas and glioblastomas, and finally, papillary ependymomas must be differentiated from choroid plexus tumors and from carcinomatous metastases with papillary differentiation.

The tissue culture has been utilized for the above purpose by Batzdorf and Pockress,[4] Liss,[59] Kersting,[51,53] Wilson,[94] Batzdorf,[3] Lumsden,[60,61] Scharenberg and Liss,[86] Vraa-Jensen, et al,[90] Haynes, et al,[49] and Casentini, et al.[12] On the bases of their observations, a reliable pattern of growth has been described that identifies these tumors.

The migrating cells in the explants are initially long, and bipolar, and have a round or oval-shaped nucleus surrounded by scanty perikaryon endowed with elongated, thin and thick processes. Slowly, the cells become more stubby and adopt a polygonal perikaryon containing one or various nuclei that are frequently eccentric. The cytoplasmic processes are scanty and short. These cytological features are not as characteristic as the association patterns among cells, of which there are three variants.

The most characteristic type is a cellular epithelial-like mosaic that surrounds the explant completely. At high magnification, the mosaic is formed by cells with clearly identifiable cytoplasm containing an eccentric round nucleus; these cells are firmly adherent to one another. Abundant and long, thin fibers that correspond to cytoplasmic processes from the proliferating cells are visible in the interstices. This association, of epithelium and fibrils described by Batzdorf and Pockress[4] under the term crazy pavement, has also been observed by Kersting,[51] Lumsden[60] Vraa-Jensen et al.,[90] and Casentini, et al.[12] (Fig. 5-29).

In other instances, the cells form tongues of an approximate triangular shape that collectively give a star-like aspect to the explant. Within the tongues, the image is similar to the mixed pattern previously described, (i.e., somewhat more elongated cells arranged in a radial pattern, and cells that maintain the mixture with the intercellular fibrils)[12,60] (Fig. 5-30).

The third type is the most irregular one, and its initial growth pattern is similar to that of the astrocytomas. Cells initially appearing bipolar slowly yield room to other cellular elements having a star-like shape. On day 18–20 of the culture, plaques having an epithelial aspect begin to form; these plaques are initially made of a few cells that slowly increase in number. In these plaques there is no reticular association and the crazy pavement pattern with intercellular fibrils promptly develops. Occasionally the image is less refined, and one sees an irregular pavement that lacks intercellular fibrils (Fig. 5-31).

Tissue cultures of ependymomas have growth patterns unique to themselves; there is a tendency to form peculiar epithelial associations not observed in other types of gliomas or in intracranial epithelial neoplasms. This pattern is the result of a mixture of the reticular pattern of an astrocytoma, oligodendroglioma with the purely epithelial pattern of tumors originating from the choroid plexus, craniopharyngioma, and metastatic tumors. There is no relationship between the three pavement types and the three subtypes of ependymoma. Any pavement type can appear in any kind of ependymoma.

The presence of small microexplants has been regarded in some publications as a reflection of the dissemination of primitive explants of larger size. The small microex-

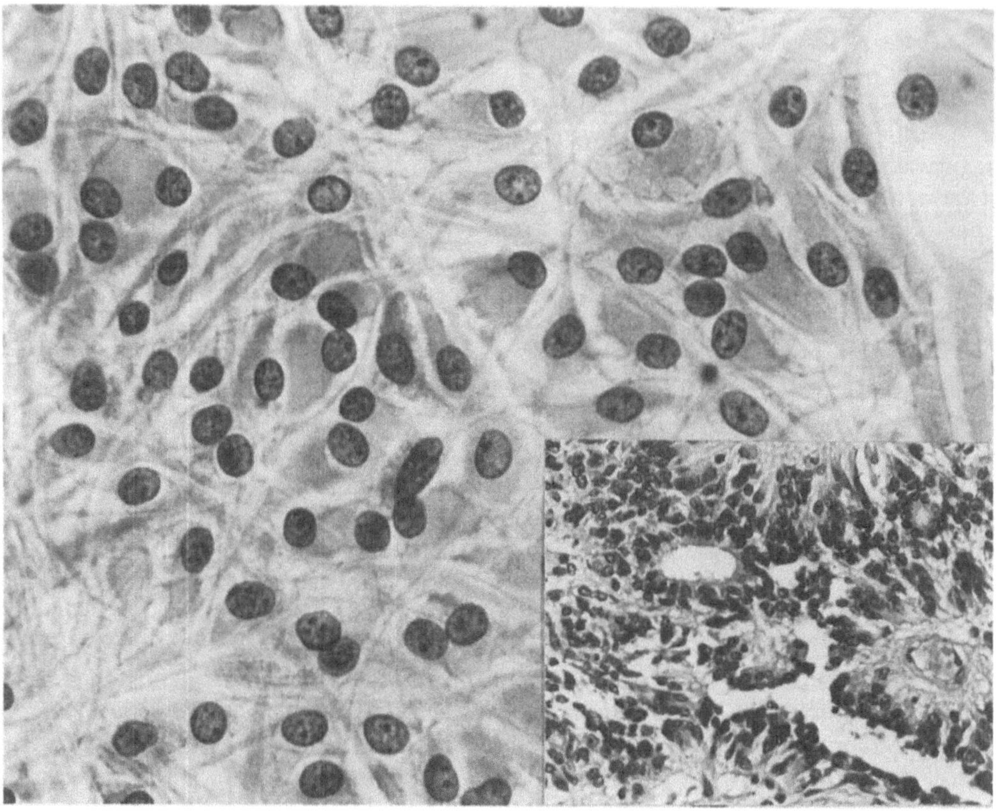

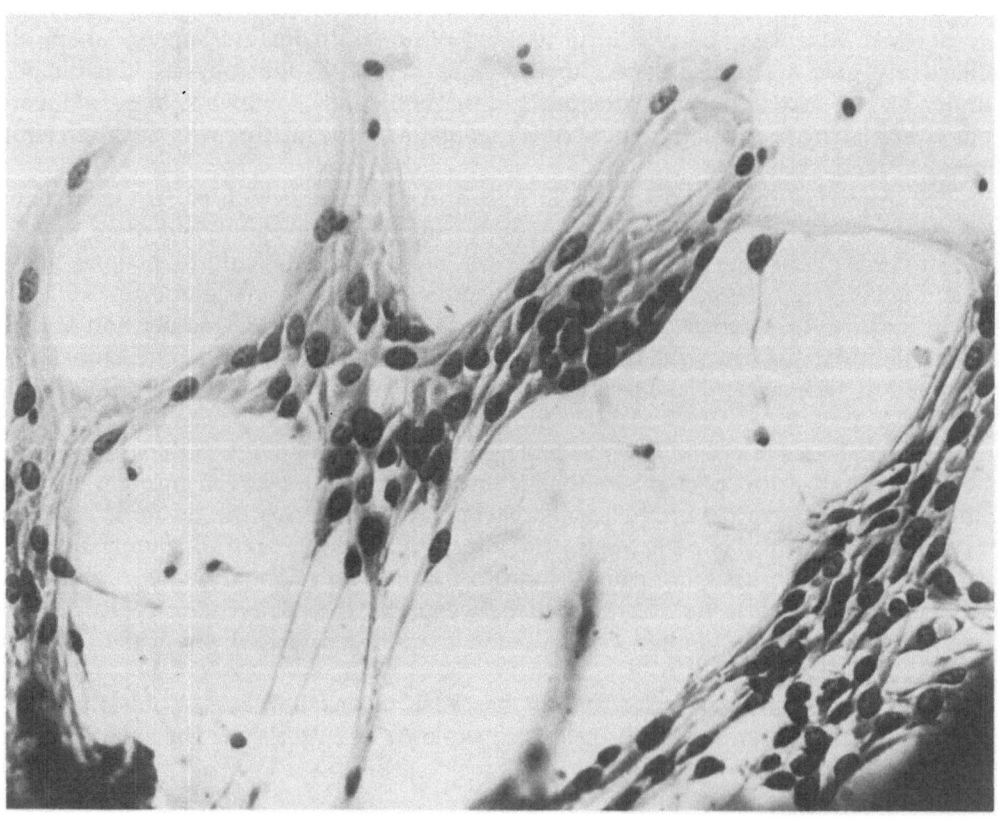

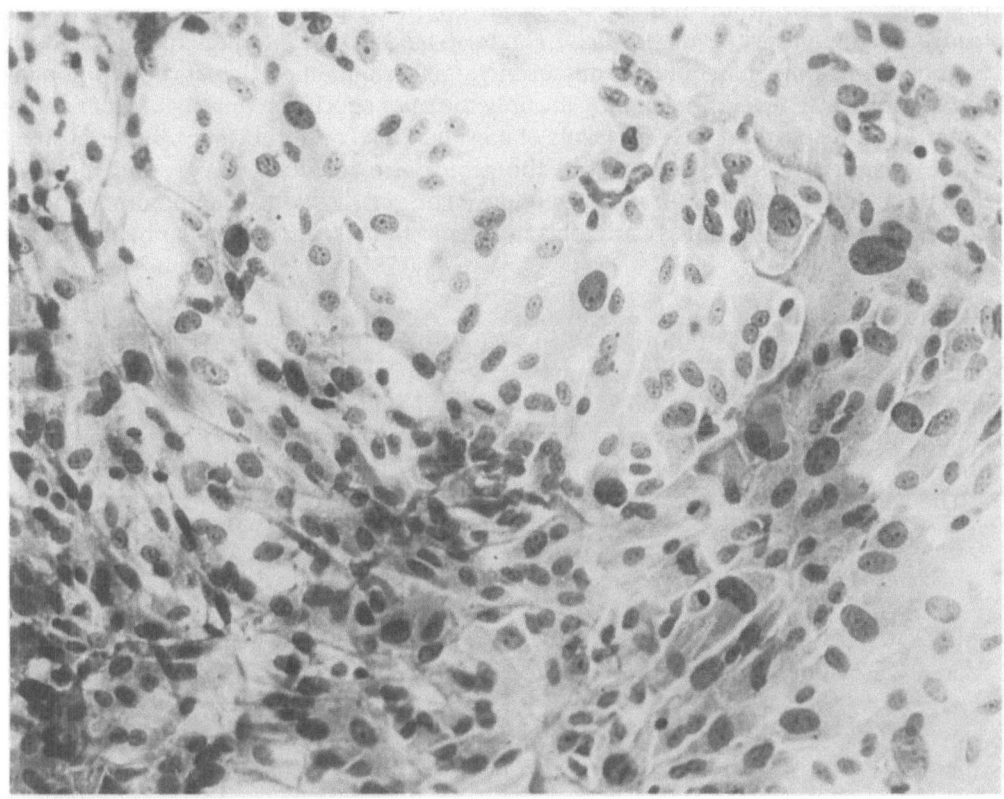

Fig. 5-31. Ependymoma of the fourth ventricle after 21 days of culture. The cells grew initially in fairly independent patterns. Slowly, the cells group themselves to form these wide epithelial plaques. The interstitial processes or fibers, although scarse, are visible in the lower part of the field. (H&E, ×200).

plants have been described with the term ''seeding,'' and they have been likened to the spinal fluid dissemination frequently seen in ependymomas. In agreement with Casentini, et al,[12] the authors believe that small microexplants are the result of technical artifacts; since they have been observed in other tumor types, both gliomatous and extraneural, they seem to lack specificity.

Tumors with a Mechanocytic Pattern

In this group, there are diverse tumors that have a growth pattern in common at the expense of independent cells, fusiform-shaped or, less frequently, star-shaped.

Fig. 5-29. Ependymoma of the fourth ventricle after 12 days in culture. The cells are polygonal, the cytoplasm is abundant, and the nucleus is eccentric. They appear to have an epithelial arrangement; yet, numerous thin and elongated cells processes traverse the field in various directions. (H&E, ×400) *Inset:* Histologic image of the original tumor (H&E, ×125).

Fig. 5-30. Ependymoma of the cerebral hemisphere after 12 days of culture. The cells migrate forming triangularly shaped arms. The cells processes characteristic of ependymomas are visible here as fibers. (H&E, ×200).

These cells do not group themselves in an epithelial pattern, but occasionally form plaques having a reticular disposition. The term *mechanocytic* is frequently applied with a restrictive meaning to neoplasms of mesenchymal origin, in particular those originating from fibroblasts. The term mechanocytic only means a specific in vitro behavior common to tumors of diverse origins. Neoplasms of mesenchymal or fibroblastic origin (mesoblastic) are included in this category, but the group also includes benign and malignant schwannomas (in spite of their neuroectodermal origin), as well as meningiomas (whose origin remains to be elucidated), angioblastic meningiomas, and cerebellar hemangioblastomas.

MENINGIOMA

No other intracranial tumor grows in tissue culture with the speed and the precocity of meningiomas. Most probably as a result, the bibliography on this type of growth is more abundant than that on other tumors. Among the pioneering in vitro studies of meningiomas are those of Kredel,[56] Buckley and Eisenhardt,[9] Bland and Russell,[6] and Murray.[69]

The cells of a meningioma culture migrate as early as 12–24 hours after the explant

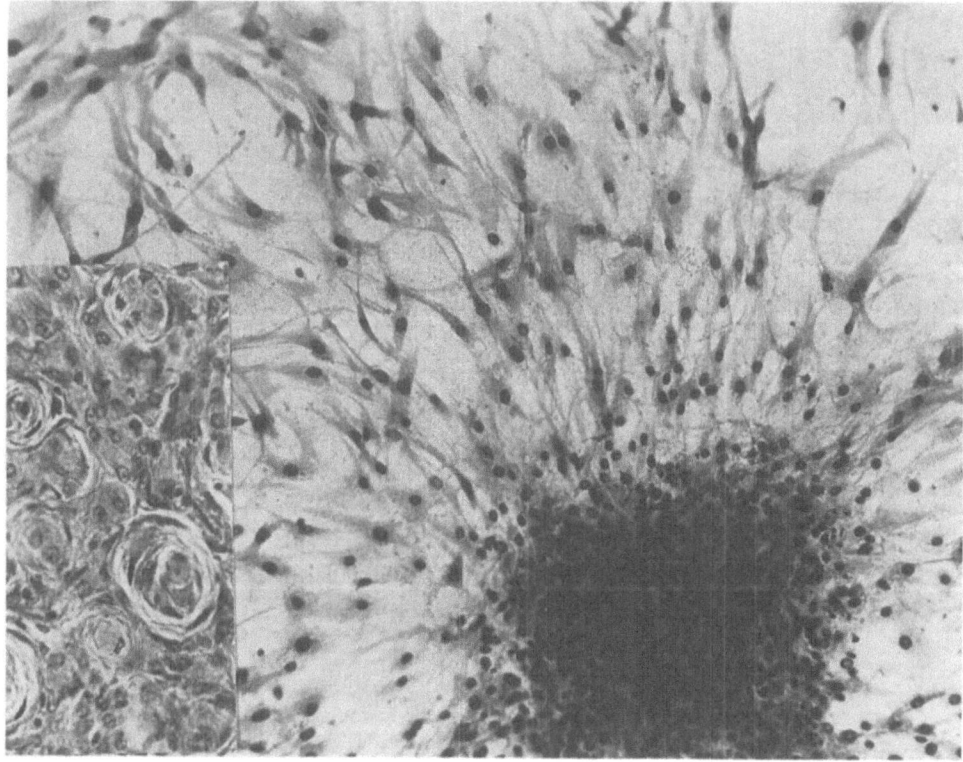

Fig. 5-32. Meningioma after 3 days of culture. The cells migrate from the explant precociously and in independent fashion. These elements have an oval or round nucleus and an elongated cytoplasm with bipolar shape. The cells usually adopt a radial pattern. (H&E, ×100.) *Inset:* Histologic preparation of the original tumor. (H&E, ×200).

is started. In the initial stages the cells are elongated, bipolar, and possess 1–3 nuclei and an eosinophilic, straight or slightly curved, ribbon-like cytoplasm, that may have two divergent processes. The association among cells is radially arranged, and is maintained for a long time. This morphology is described as type I[66] (Fig. 5-32).

Meningioma cells slowly give rise to other elements also of an elongated shape, but with more abundant cytoplasm. From the ends of these cytoplasmic processes originate smaller ones that are sometimes bifid. The nucleus is larger, clearer than in the previous stage, and the nuclear membrane is distinct and full of dense chromatin clumps. These cells can exist isolated or they may be apposed to one another, but without forming a mesothelial mosaic. These cells have been described as type II,[66] and they are the result of the transformation of the type I cells. This transformation takes place as the cells migrate away from the explant (Fig. 5-33). Coincident with the appearance of these cells, or slightly later, there appear in the culture other cells having a larger size and nuclear characteristics similar to those described previously, i.e., dense chromatin clumps. The cytoplasm is abundant, flat, and stellar; these new types of cells are related to one another through the ends of the cytoplasmic processes that form a reticular plexus similar to that described in gliomas (Fig. 5-34). Soon there appears a fourth type of cell, i.e., the type III of Morley.[66] This cell is large, the largest

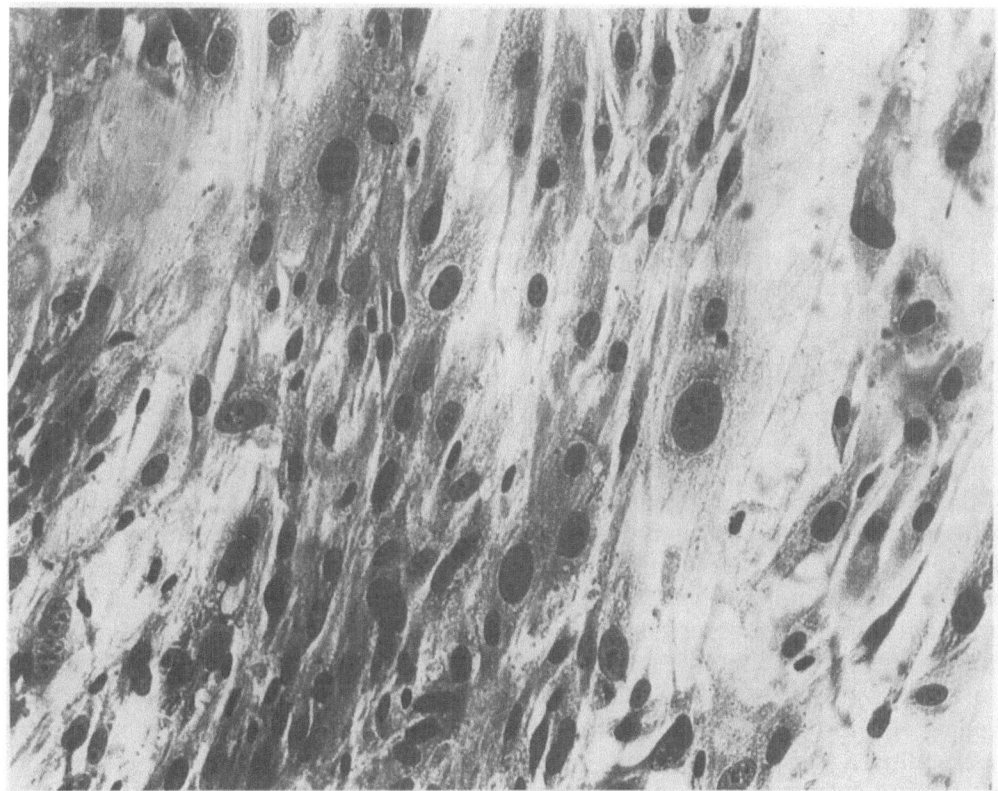

Fig. 5-33. Meningioma after 9 days of culture. Within a short period of time the cells develop abundant cytoplasm. The nucleus is oval and contains characteristic chromatin clumps. There is a preliminary tendency to the formation of cellular plaques. (H&E, ×200).

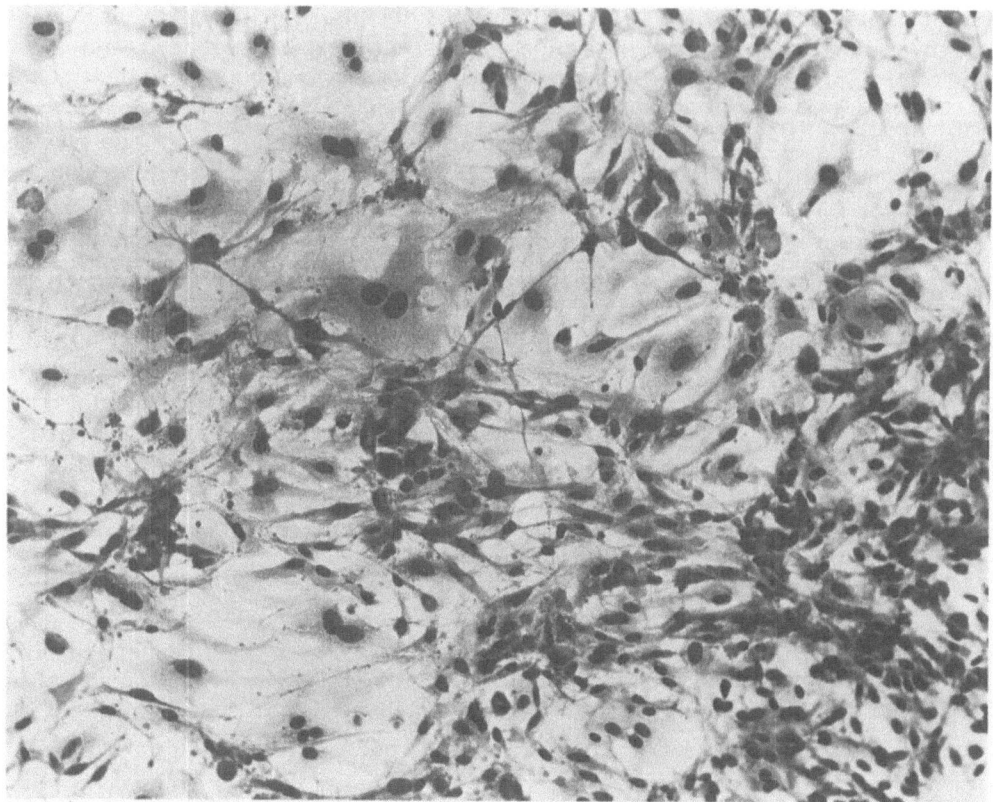

Fig. 5-34. Meningioma after 12 days of culture. An example of the busy cellular pattern frequently seen in mengioma explants. After retaining a bipolar shape next to the explant, the cells soon become polygonal at the most peripheral locations. A few of them are binucleated. (H&E, ×100).

of all of the meningiomas cell types, and possesses a single or double nucleus which sometimes is lobulated or cleaved, containing characteristic dense chromatin clumps. The cytoplasm is typically flat (Fig. 5-35).

The three cell types described above dominate during the period of stabilization of the culture and are arranged with respect to one another according to a predictable pattern, giving rise to a fairly typical image. The resultant structural pattern is centered by 1–3 of the large cells, limited by large fusiform or stellate cells that form a dense barrier, contrasting with the transparency of the cytoplasm of the central cell. This structural arrangement is repeated throughout and provides the culture with an alveolar appearance.

The reproducibility of the primary structures in tissue cultures is expressed in the meningioma through the formation of whorls. Kersting and Lennartz,[55] utilizing monolayer cultures after trypsinization, showed that these whorls are formed constantly. After a few days, a layer of stellate cells develops, forming a plexus that is each time denser than the previous one, ultimately covering the entire crystal. Whorls begin to appear at the sites of cell accumulation. The mechanism of formation of whorls studied through time-lapse cinematography appears to reside either in the turn of one or more

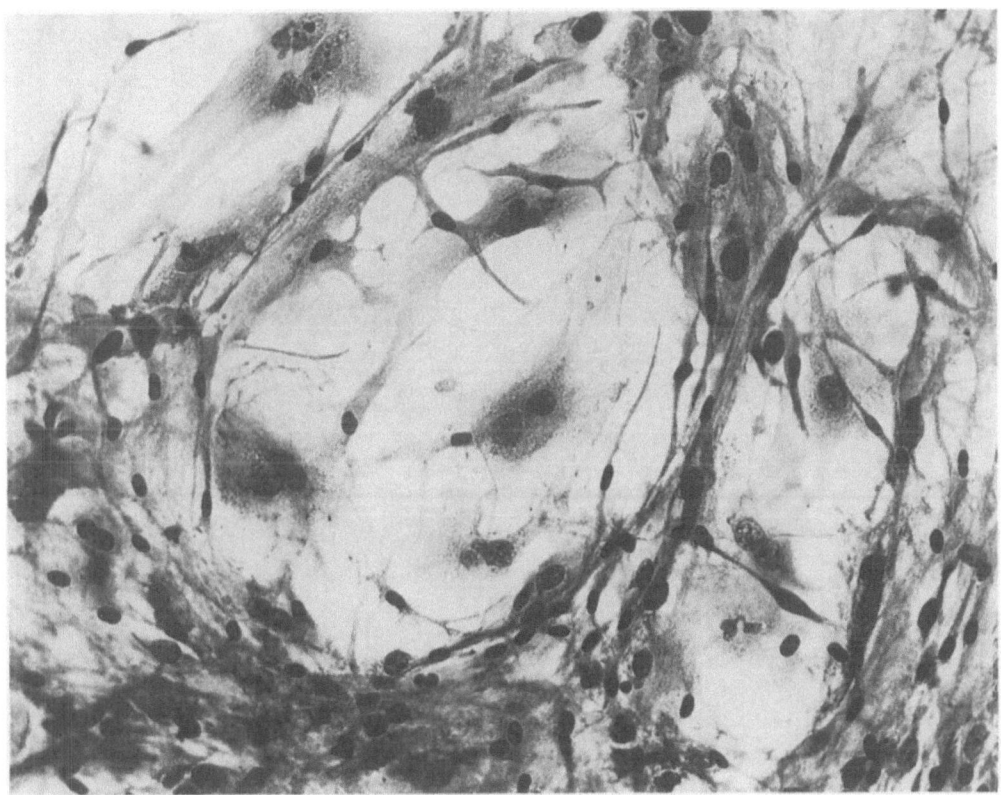

Fig. 5-35. Meningioma after 12 days of culture. Areolar structures: the center is occupied by two or three large cells, some of which are binucleated; smaller cells line the space. (H&E, ×200).

cells with relation to a theoretical central point;[78] or the apposition of two cells in the form of a cap. Cells disposed around a central one are surrounded by additional strata acquired without the requirement for a turn.[55] Possibly, both mechanisms coexist.

Although the formation of whorls dominates in monolayer cultures, whorls can also be obtained in explants.[74] If the explants are numerous and small, after an appropriate length of time, the glass surface will be covered by a layer of continuous cells having a similar appearance to that seen in monolayer; in this monolayer whorls are formed at the sites of cells aggregates (Fig. 5-36). At last, as is to be expected in cultures of rapid growth, multinucleated giant cells begin to appear in the final stages of the culture.

In summary, an accepted degree of specificity exists in the in vitro behavior of meningiomas; this rests not so much on a highly characteristic pattern, but rather on the composite aggregate of the features described above. The association pattern just described is applicable to all subtypes of meningioma (fibrous, vascular, and meningothelial); only a few differences in the predominance of one cell or another or the association among cells, exist in each subtype. Angioblastic meningiomas behave in culture according to a pattern that is similar to that described below for cerebellar hemangioblastomas (Fig. 5-37).

The ease with which meningioma cultures grow and the reliability of the growth

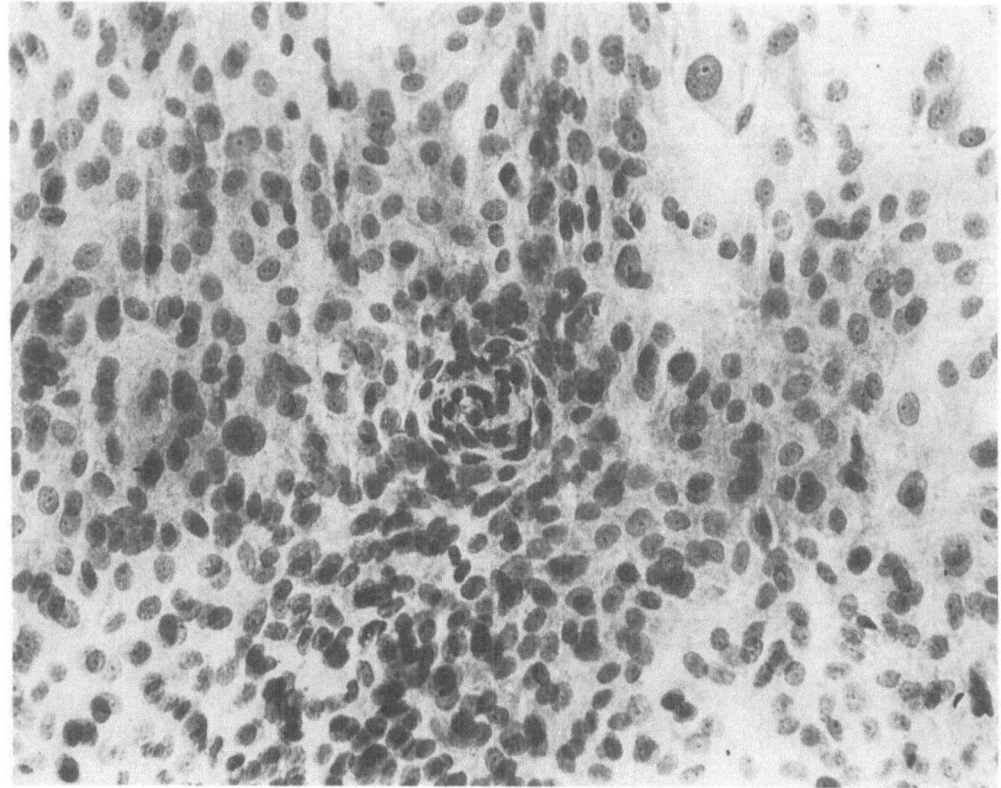

Fig. 5-36. Meningioma after 18 days of culture. Once the cells have covered entirely the glass surface. Whorls as the one shown here, can be frequently found and are constant in monolayer cultures, but only occasionally seen in explants. (H&E, ×200).

pattern as an indicator of the cell of origin contrast sharply with some truly overwhelming obstacles that reminds one of the limitations inherent to the methods of the tissue culture. Many of the following questions lack satisfactory answers at present.

The precocious growth of a tumor in tissue culture is not an indicator of biologic malignancy. Tumors with aggressive biologic behavior may grow slowly in culture. The growth pattern is a useful indicator of the cell of origin, but the early cell migration, the individual cell appearance , and the cellular disposition according to a radial pattern are the most useful features for identifying the cell of origin. Experienced observers may conclude that the tumor in tissue culture is a meningioma as soon as they observe the formation of tubes or pipes having the appearance described above; this is usually accompanied by a fast drop in pH in the culture medium.

The study of morphologic features of the proliferating migrating cell and the study of the pattern of the association pattern do not provide any clues as to the cell of origin of meningiomas. The growth pattern is different from that of fibroblastic tumors,[23] and it also lacks similarity with the cultures of mesotheliomas or synovial sarcomas.[1,2] We must be satisfied with the term "mesoblastic" to designate the growth pattern of meningiomas. This does not represent much advancement since the time of Bland and Russell[6] and Bland.[5]

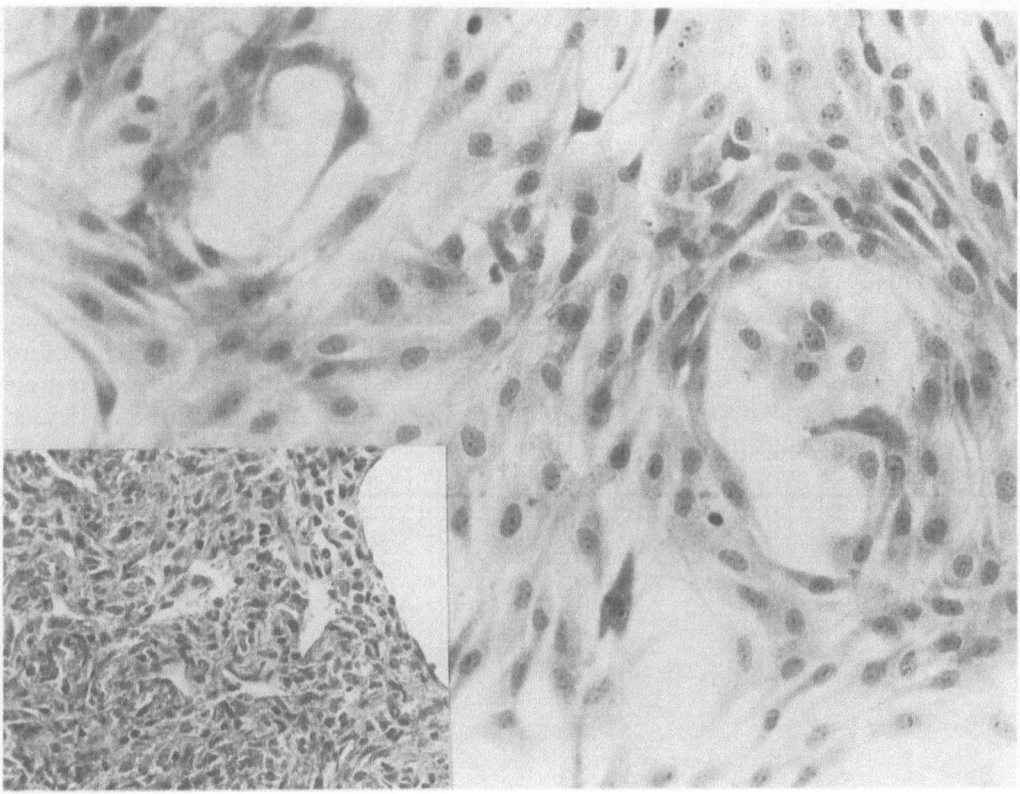

Fig. 5-37. Angioblastic meningioma. The gross pattern of this type of meningioma is similar to that of other meningiomas. The cells are bipolar, become progressively larger, and acquire more cytoplasm as seen in the circular structure to the right of the field. (H&E, ×200.) *Inset:* Histologic preparation of the original tumor (×100).

HEMANGIOBLASTOMA

Within the mesenchymal brain tumors, the main attraction in the application of tissue culture to the study of hemangioblastoma resides in the study of the cell(s) of origin. Unfortunately, tissue cultures have contributed little to answer this question. Few publications on this subject have appeared.[51,60,76] Pomerat's observations support the view that vascular structures form the fundamental component of the hemangioblastoma, but these opinions have not been confirmed by others. Kersting[51] interprets a growth of this tumor as being similar to that of a meningioma and proposes that the hemangioblastoma is a neoplasm derived from endothelium.

The images of tissue cultures are not too revealing; the patterns correspond to the mechanocytic growth of mesenchymal appearance resembling that of meningiomas in many cases, and specifically, the variant of angioblastic meningiomas. Individual cells have a fusiform shape that quickly transform into a stellate appearance, although each cell has short processes and abundant perikaryon. Within the period of stabilization, fusiform cells and star-like cells alternate in the growth halo. Occasionally, there is a large, round, flat cellular element containing a central nucleus that closely resembles a meningioma cell. The abundant perikaryon is similar to that of endothelial vascular or mesoblastic cells in tissue culture, but in the absence of studies with cell markers (e.g., factor VIII), one can only conjecture a vascular derivation. (Fig. 5-38).

In spite of the diverse appearance of the cells, the culture suggests that the cellular proliferation in hemangioblastoma is made at the expense of a single cell, which is capable of changing its shape frequently. The diverse images observed in this tumor may correspond to different developmental stages of a single cell.

SCHWANNOMA

Murray and Stout[68,69] compared the in vitro behavior of normal Schwann cells with that of neoplastic Schwann cells. Based on these observations, the authors described two cell types that they consider fibroblasts and Schwann cells, respectively. Kersting and Finkemayer[54] and Kersting[51] also found fusiform-shaped cells, but in their cultures there was a constant presence of macrophagic elements similar to those described previously by Weiss[91] in cultures of normal cells from peripheral nerve. Lumsden[60] demonstrated that these cells maintained in culture were capable of ingesting leprosy bacilli. Cravioto and Lockwood[18,19] described four cell types in schwannomas: fusiform cells, racket-shaped cells, cells shaped like a comet, and ameoboid cells. Of these, only the

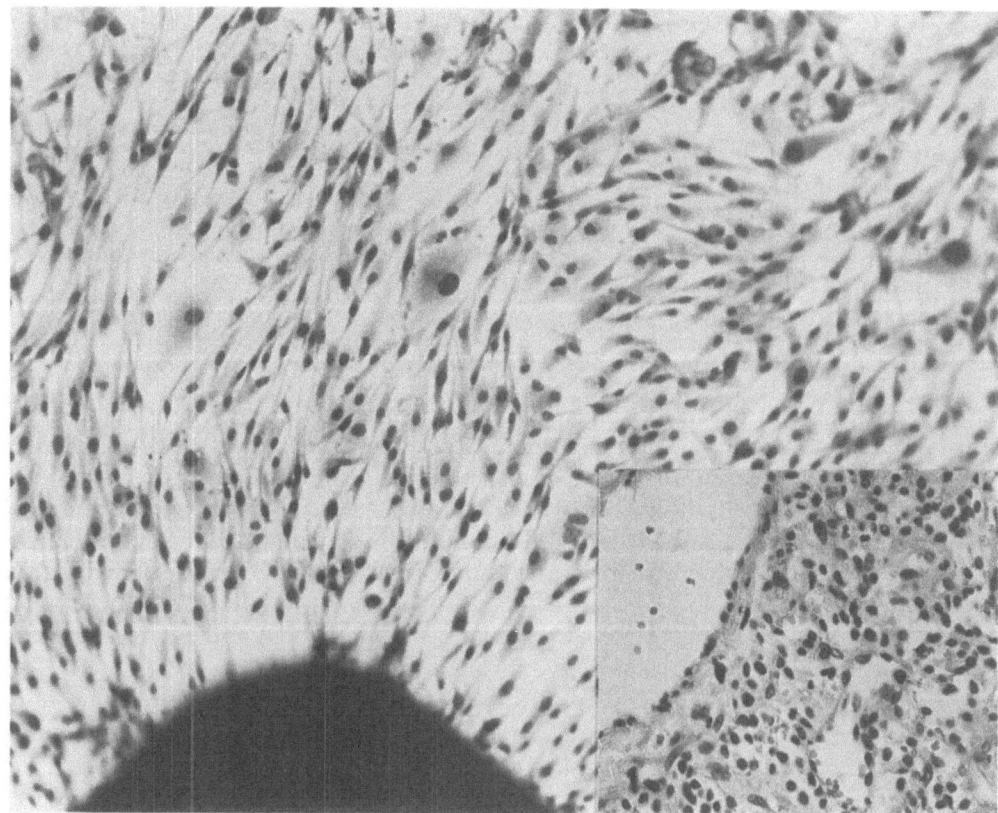

Fig. 5-38. Cerebellar hemangioblastoma after 12 days of culture. Most cells are bipolar and are arranged in a radial pattern. There are occasional larger cells occupying areolar spaces. There are close similarities with the growth patterns of mengiomas, e.g. Fig. 5-32, 5-35, and 5-37, (H&E, ×100). *Inset:* Histologic preparation of original tumor. (H&E, ×100).

latter one failed to appear in the cultures of normal peripheral nerve. According to Cravioto and Lockwood, only the fusiform cells and the ameoboid cells are authentically of schwannian derivation. The coexistence of fusiform cells and macrophages has been confirmed experimentally.[32,81] Thust, et al[88] interpret the macrophages as being accompanying cells, while Escalona-Zapata and Diez-Nau[23,27] believe that these are of Schwann derivation. The pure fusiform cell population of the cases reported by Mennell and Bucheler[65] is explained by the high malignancy rate of the drug-induced tumors and is comparable to the observations reported in malignant human schwannomas.

Four cell types can be identified in tissue cultures of schwannomas: (1) fusiform cells having an oval nucleus and bipolar cytoplasm arranged radially. These do not form a plexus and appear in all schwannoma cultures, move slowly, and fulfill the mechanocytic criteria of Wilmer (Fig. 5-39); (2) stellate cells are slightly smaller than the previous ones and have 2–5 short processes. The nucleus is oval-shaped and the cytoplasm contains birefringent droplets easily visualized with phase contrast. These cells are less abundant than the fusiform ones, but sooner or later can be observed in all tissue cultures; (3) small macrophages, with round nucleus and dense cytoplasm containing numerous small vacuoles. These cells exist in haphazard arrangements and display slow movements; they are constant components of all cultures, corresponding

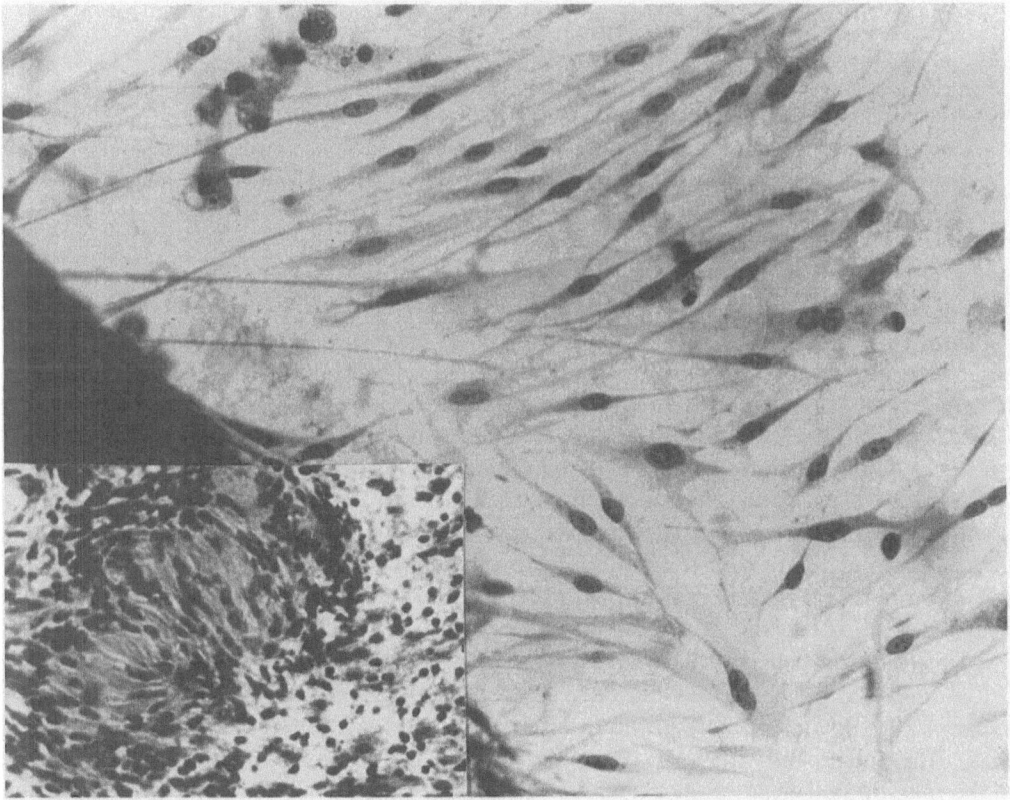

Fig. 5-39. Schwannoma of the cerebellopontine angle after 9 days of culture. Fusiform-shaped cells with long processes and oval nuclei predominate in this case. A group of macrophages is visible at the left upper corner. (H&E, ×200) *Inset:* Histologic image of the original tumor. (H&E, ×100).

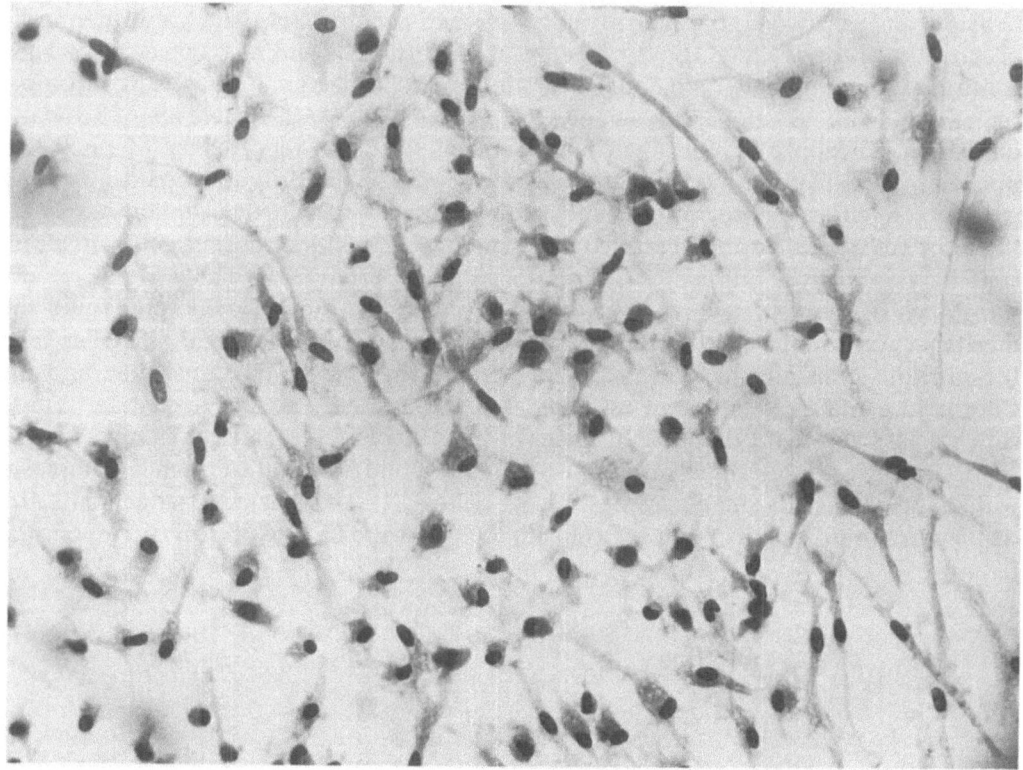

Fig. 5-40. Schwannoma of the cerebellopontine angle after 12 days of culture. Stellate cells and macrophages predominate in this case. There is a transition between the bipolar elements and the round macrophagic elements. (H&E, ×200).

to the ameoboid pattern of Wilmer (Fig. 5-40); and (4) multinucleated giant cells appear only occasionally.

During the development of the culture, one type of cell predominates, but there is no constant association pattern. In some cases, migration is begun by macrophages, which mix at the end with fusiform elements. In other instances, the beginning is mixed and at the end either fusiform patterns or macrophage predominate. Finally, in some cases the beginning is purely fusiform; this can be either maintained or can be switched to a predominant macrophagic cell. In any event, the two basic cells are obviously the fusiform cells and the macrophages and their simultaneous appearance during the stabilizing phase of the culture produces a pattern that is characteristic of schwannoma. The stellate cells appear to be an intermediate stage between the previous two.[23,27]

The fusiform cell may be the true equivalent in the culture of the Antoni type A cell. The macrophage is probably derived from the type A cell and is the predominant element at yellowish areas with abundant lipid, frequently seen in acoustic schwannomas. The stellate cells may represent the Antoni type B cell. The schwannian nature of the macrophage is suggested both by the tissue culture behavior and by its ultrastructural features, which are similar to those of Schwann cells.[92] The ability of the Schwann cell to ingest leprosy bacilli both in vivo[7] and in vitro[60] has been confirmed in tissue culture studies.

This in vitro behavior of schwannoma is constant and repetitive; it differs from any other tumor grown in culture and the behavior is maintained along the same pattern regardless of the site of origin of the tumor. There is no difference in the pattern observed in a tissue culture depending upon the area sampled in the tumor as being an area with predominant type A cell, type B cell, or macrophagic.

PERIPHERAL NERVE SARCOMA (MALIGNANT SCHWANNOMA)

The author studied two cases of malignant schwannoma in tissue culture: one was purely cellular and was removed from a patient with von Recklinghausen's neurofibromatosis. The second one was a mixed schwannoma with fusiform and epithelioid components. In both instances the growth was monotonous, composed of fusiform cells with an oval-shaped nucleus and bipolar cytoplasm that emerged promptly from the explant and adopted a typical radial growth pattern. This behavior remained unchanged free of a tendency to form a plexiform pattern, and it was typical to observe a bend at the distal end of the cytoplasm. Neither macrophages nor stellate cells appeared at any time. This pattern is similar to that which is typical of fibrosarcomas (Fig. 5-41).[23,25]

These findings may only have relative significance because the pattern lacks specificity. However, the observations are useful to arrive at the concept that schwannian sarcomas probably represent a fibroblastic evolution of the original cell in which all the other properties have been suppressed. According to this postulate, the malignant

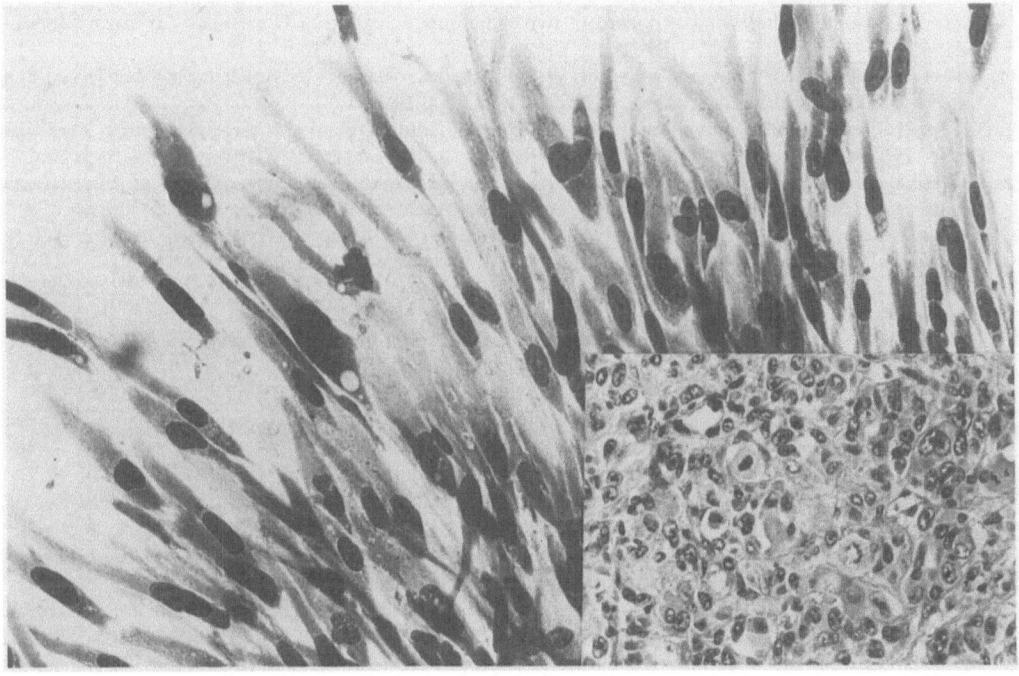

Fig. 5-41. Malignant schwannoma of posterior mediastinum after 9 days of culture. Despite the epithelial appearance of the original tumor, the migrating cells show a fibroblastic pattern. These cells are elongated, bipolar, exhibit marked nuclear pleomorphism, and occasional cytoplasmic vacuoles. (H&E, original magnification ×400.) *Inset:* Histologic image of the original tumor. (Original magnification ×200).

schwannoma would reflect the transformation of a Schwann cell into a perineural fibro-blast.

References

1. Alvarez-Fernandez E, Diez-Nau MD: Malignant fibrosarcomatous mesothelioma and benign pleural fibroma (localized fibrous mesothelioma) and tissue culture. A comparison of the *in vitro* pattern of growth in relation to the cell of origin. *Cancer* 43:1658–1663, 1979
2. Alvarez-Fernandez E, Escalona-Zapata J: Monophasic mesenchymal synovial sarcoma. Its identification by tissue culture. *Cancer* 47:628–635, 1981
3. Batzdorf U: Seeding of brain tumors in tissue culture. *Surg Forum* 18:458–460, 1967
4. Batzdorf U, Pockress SM: Architectural features of ependymomas in tissue culture. *J Neuropathol Exp Neurol* 27:333–347, 1968
5. Bland JOW: The growth of human meningiomata in culture compared with that of certain human tissues. *Arch Exp Zellforsch* 22:369–371, 1939
6. Bland JOW, Russell DS: Histological types of meningiomata and comparison of their behaviour in tissue culture with that of certain normal human tissues. *J Pathol Bacteriol* 47:291–309, 1938
7. Bradley WG: *Disorders of Peripheral Nerves*. Oxford, Blackwell, 1974
8. Buckley RC: Tissue culture studies of glioblastoma multiforme. *Am J Pathol* 5:467–472, 1929
9. Buckley WG, Eisenhardt L: Study of a meningioma in supravital preparations, tissue culture and paraffin sections. *Am J Pathol* 5:659–664, 1929
10. Burdman JA, Goldstein MN: Long-term tissue culture of neuroblastomas. III. *In vitro* studies of a nerve growth stimulating factor in sera of children with neuroblastoma. *J Natl Cancer Inst* 33:123–133, 1964
11. Canti RG, Bland JOW, Russell DS: Tissue culture of gliomata. Cinematographic demonstration. *Res Publ Assoc Nerv Ment Dis* 16:1–24, 1935
12. Casentini L, Gullotta F, Mohrer U: Clinical and morphological investigations on ependymomas and their cultures. *Neurochirurgia* 24:51–56, 1981
13. Cobb JP, Wright JC: Studies on a craniopharyngioma in tissue culture. I. Growth characteristics and alterations produced following exposure to two radiomimetic agents. *J Neuropathol Exp Neurol* 18:563–568, 1959
14. Costero I: Pathology of glial neoplasms, in, W.S. Fields P.C. Sharkey, (eds): *The Biology and Treatment of Intracranial Tumors*, Springfield, Illinois, Charles C Thomas, 1962
15. Costero I, Pomerat CM: Cultivation of neurons from the adult cerebral and cerebellar cortex. *Am J Anat* 89:405–467, 1951
16. Costero I, Pomerat CM: Cellular prototypes of central gliomata. (Proceedings of the 2nd International Congress on Neuropathology, London.) Excerpta Med (Amsterdam) 1:273–277, 1955
17. Costero I, Pomerat CM, Barroso-Moguel R, et al: Tumors of the human nervous system in tissue culture; analysis of fibroblastic activity in meningiomas. *J Natl Cancer Inst* 15:1341–1365, 1955
18. Cravioto H, Lockwood R: The behavior of normal peripheral nerve in tissue culture. *Ztchr Zellforsch* 90:186–201, 1968
19. Cravioto H, Lockwood R: The behavior of acoustic neurinoma *in vitro*. *Acta Neuropathol (Berlin)* 12:141–157, 1969
20. del Rio-Hortega P: Neuroblastomas. *Bol Acad Nac Med Buenos Aires* 1:352–379, 1940
21. Dereymacker A, Brucher JM, De Somer P, et al: La culture des tumeurs cerebrales humanes. Premiers resultats personelles. *Acta Neurol Psychiatr (Belgium)* 9:772–777, 1958
22. Escalona-Zapata J: Neuroblastische Tumoren der Grosshirnhemispheren. *Zbl Neurochir* 33:35–44, 1972
23. Escalona-Zapata J: Cytology and growth patterns of fibrosarcomas and related tumors, in Escalona-Zapata, J., Ozzello, L. (eds): *Tissue Culture in the Study of Tumors, Pathol Res Pract* 165:32–38, 1979
24. Escalona-Zapata J: Uncommon oligodendrogliomas. *Acta Neuropathol (Berlin) (Suppl)* 7:94–96, 1981
25. Escalona-Zapata J: Tissue culture in the study of tumors. *Pathologica (Genova)* 73:117–153, 1981
26. Escalona-Zapata J, Alvarez-Fernandez E, Llorca-Escuin F: The fibroblastic nature of dermatofibrosarcoma protuberans. A tissue culture and ultrastructural study. *Virchows Arch A (Pathol Anat)* 391:165–175, 1981
27. Escalona-Zapata J, Diez-Nau MD: The nature of macrophages (foam cells) in neurinomas. Tissue culture study. *Acta Neuropathol (Berlin)* 44:71–75, 1978
28. Escalona-Zapata J, Diez-Nau MD: The astrocytic nature of glioblastoma demonstrated by tissue culture. *Acta Neuropathol (Berl)* 44:71–75, 1981
29. Escalona-Zapata J, Diez-Nau MD: Distinctive growth patterns between cerebral and cerebellar astrocytomas. A tissue culture study. *Histopathology* 5:639–650, 1981

30. Escalona-Zapata J, Diez-Nau MD: Estudio de los astrocitomas y sus derivados por medio del cultivo de tejidos. *Patologia* (Madrid) 16:23–45, 1983
31. Escalona-Zapata J, Ozzello L: Tissue culture in the study of tumors. *Pathol Res Pract* 165:32–38, 1979
32. Fornatto L, Schiffer D: *In vitro* culture observations on neurinoma induced experimentally in the rat by ethilnitrosourea. *Acta Neuropathol* (Berlin) 20:199–206, 1972
33. Fu YS, Chen ATL, Kay S, et al: Is subependymoma (subependymal glomerate astrocytoma) an astrocytoma or ependymoma? *Cancer* 34:1992–1994, 1974
34. Gaszo L, Afra D, Muller W: Supratentorial recurrences of gliomas. Tissue culture studies with astrocytomas and oligodendrogliomas. *Acta Neuropathol* (Berlin) 44:135–139, 1978
35. Genth J, Gullotta F, Puig-Serra J: Elektronoptische und enzymhistochemische Vergleichuntersuchungen an Kraniopharyngiomen und ihren Gewebekulturen. *Acta Neuropathol* (Berlin) 28:331–341, 1974
36. Goldstein MN, Burdman JA, Journey LJ: Long-term tissue culture of neuroblastomas. Morphological evidence for differentiation and maturation. *J Natl Cancer Inst* 32:165–200, 1964
37. Goldstein MN: Neuroblastoma cells in tissue culture. *J Pediatr Surg* 3:166–167, 1968
38. Gullotta F: La genesi formale de la fibra de Rosenthal. *Acta Neurol* (Napoli) 20:704–711, 1965
39. Gullotta F: *Das Sogenannte Meduloblastom*. Berlin, Springer, 1967
40. Gullotta F: General remarks on brain tumors *in vitro*, in Escalona-Zapata, J. (ed): *Tissue Culture in the Study of Tumors*, Pathologica (Genova) 73:128–129, 1981
41. Gullotta F, Cervos-Navarro J, Puig-Serra J: Istologia, ultrastruttura e comportamento *in vitro* di un ganglioglioma cerebrale. *Acta Neurol* (Napoli) 25:188–196, 1970
42. Gullotta F, Fliedner E: Spongioblastomas, astrocytomas and Rosenthal fibers. Ultrastructural, tissue culture and enzyme histochemical investigations. *Acta Neuropathol* (Berlin) 22:68–78, 1972
43. Gullotta F, Fliedner E, Wullenweber W, et al: Tissue culture, electron microscopic and enzyme histochemical investigations on a sympathetic ganglioneuroblastoma. *Acta Neuropatol* (Berl) 24:107–116, 1973
44. Gullotta F, Kersting G: Coltura *in vitro* di tumori cerebrali in fantili. *Acta Neuol* (Napoli) 25:585–587, 1970
45. Gullotta F, Kersting G: The ultrastructure of medulloblastoma in tissue culture. *Virchows Arch A (Pathol Anat)* 356:111–118, 1972
46. Gullotta F, Kost HG: *In vitro* studies of so-called medulloblastomas. *Pathologica* (Genova) 72:27–34, 1980
47. Gullota F, Kreutzberg G: Das Gliom des Opticus. Morphologische und histochemische Untersuchungen am Schnittpraparat und der Gewebekultur. *Acta Neuropathol* (Berlin) 2:413–424, 1963
48. Harrison RG: Observations on the living developing nerve fiber. *Anat Rec* 1:116–118, 1907
49. Haynes LW, Davis BE, Mitchell J, et al: Cell proliferation in explant cultures of malignant gliomas. *Acta Neuropathol* (Berlin) 42:87–90, 1978
50. Kepes JJ: Astrocytic differentiation of neoplastic oligodendrocytes. In *9th International Congress on Neuropathology*, Vienna, 1982, 158. (Abstract.)
51. Kersting G: *Die Gewebszuchtung Menschlicher Hirngeschwülste*. Berlin, Springer, 1961
52. Kersting G: Die Gewebszuchtung der Medulloblastome. *Acta Neuropathol.* (Berlin) 8:100–105, 1967
53. Kersting G: Tissue culture of human gliomas, in Krayenbuhl-Maspes-Sweet (eds): *Progress Neurol Surgery*, Vol. 2. Chicago, Karger, Basel; and Year Book, 1968, 165–202.
54. Kersting G, Finkemayer H: Das Wachstum menschlicher Neurinomgewebes *in vitro*. *Zbl Neurochir* 18:2–11, 1958
55. Kersting G, Lennartz H: *In vitro* cultures of human meningioma tissues. *J Neuropathol Exp Neurol* 16:507–513, 1957
56. Kredel FE: Intracranial tumors in tissue culture. *Arch Surg* 18:2008–2018, 1929
57. Lacruz C, Salinero E, Peraita P, et al: Carcinoma de los plexos coroideos. Estudio con cultivo de tejidos. *Patologia* (Madrid) 14:137–142, 1981
58. Landolt AM: Die Ultrastruktur des Kraniopharyngioms. Schweiz *Arch Neurol Neurochir Psychiatry* 111:313–328, 1972
59. Liss L: Morphology of nervous system tumors *in vitro*, in *Proceedings of the 6th International Congress on Neuropathology*, Vol. 2. Stuttgart, G. Thieme, 1962, 247–254.
60. Lumsden CE: The study by tissue culture of tumors of the nervous system, in 3rd Edition E Russell-Rubinstein, (ed): *Pathology of Tumors of the Nervous System*, London, E Arnold, 1971.
61. Lumsden CE: Tissue culture of brain tumors, in *Vinken-Bruyn: Handbook of Clinical Neurology*, Vol. 17/II. North Holland Publ. Co., Amsterdam, 1974, 42–103.
62. Lumsden CE, Pomerat CM: Normal oligodendrocytes in tissue culture. *Exp Cell Res* 2:103–114, 1951
63. Manoury R, Vedrenne C, Arnoult J, et al: Culture *in vitro* du tissue glial normal et neoplasique. Croissance, cytologie, ultrastructure. *Neurochirurgie* 18:101–120, 1972
64. Manuelidis EE: Long-term lines of tissue cultures of intracranial tumors. *J Neurosurg* 22:368–373, 1965

65. Mennell HD, Bucheler J: Experimentally induced malignant neurinomas as transplantable tumors. Morphology and *in vitro* behavior. *Acta Neuropathol* (Berlin) 27:153–161, 1974
66. Morley TP: The morphology of meningiomas grown *in vitro*. *J Neuropathol Exp Neurol* 17:635–643, 1958
67. Murray KJ, Chou SN, Douglas D: Topographical anatomy of human cerebral and cerebellar astrocytomas *in vitro Surg Neurol* 6:337–340, 1976
68. Murray MR, Stout AP: Schwann cell versus fibroblast as the origin of the specific nerve sheath tumors. Observations upon normal nerve sheaths and neurilemmomas *in vitro*. *Am J Pathol* 16:41–60, 1940
69. Murray MR, Stout AP: Demonstration of the formation of reticulin by Schwannian tumor cells *in vitro*. *Am J Pathol* 18:585–593, 1942
70. Murray MR, Stout AP: Distinctive characteristics of the sympathicoblastoma cultivated *in vitro*. A method for prompt diagnosis. *Am J Pathol* 23:429–441, 1947
71. Murray MR, Stout AP: A sympathetic ganglioneuroma cultivated *in vitro*. *Cancer* 1:242–247, 1948
72. Nakamura Y, Becker LE: Subependymal giant-cell tumor: Astrocytic or neuronal? *Acta Neuropathol* (Berlin) 60:271–277, 1983
73. Neumann J: Zur typisiering del Oligodendrogliome Grad I bis III in der Gewebekultur. *Neurochirurgia* 23:143–146, 1980
74. Ovary E, Bencze Y: Meningioma Organizaton in tissue culture. In *Proceedings of the 4th International Congressional Congress on Neuropathology*. Excerpta Med., Amsterdam, 1965, 916–922
75. Palacios O: Neuroblastoma in der Gewebekultur, in *Proceedings of the 4th International Congress on Neuropathology, Vol. 2*. Stuttgart, G. Thieme, 1962, pp. 255–259.
76. Pomerat CM: Dynamic neuropathology. *J Neuropathol Exp Neurol* 14:28–38, 1955
77. Pomerat CM, Crue BL, Kasten F: Observations on the cytology of an oligodendroglioma cultivated *in vitro*. *J of the Natl Cancer Inst* 33:517–533, 1964
78. Pomerat CM: Todd EM, Goldblatt D: Activity of meningioma whorls *in vitro*, in WS Fields and PC Sharkey (eds): *The Biology and Treatment of Intracranial Tumors*, Springfield, Illinois Charles C Thomas, 1962
79. Reese AB, Ehrlich G: The culture of uveal melanomas. *Am J Ophthalmol* 46:163–176, 1958
80. Rubinstein LJ: *In vivo* and *in vitro* studies of neoplastic neuroepithelial differentiation, in *8th International Congress on Neuropathology* Washington, D.C., 1978, 576. (Abstract.)
81. Rubinstein LJ, Conley FK, Herman MM: Studies on experimental nerve sheath tumors maintained in tissue and organ culture system. I. Light microscopy observations. *Acta Neuropathol* (Berlin) 34:277–291, 1976
82. Rubinstein LJ, Herman MM: Studies on the differentiation of human and experimental gliomas in organ culture systems. *Rec Res Cancer Res* 51:35–51, 1975
83. Rubinstein LJ, Herman MM, Foley VL: *In vitro* characteristics of human glioblastomas maintained in organ culture system. Light microscopy observations. *Am J Pathol* 71:61–80, 1973
84. Russell DS, Bland JOW: A study of gliomas by the method of tissue culture. *J Pathol Bacteriol* 36:273–283, 1933
85. Russell DS, Bland JOW: Further notes on the tissue culture of gliomas with special reference to Bailey's spongioblastoma. *J Pathol Bacteriol* 39:375–380, 1934
86. Scharenberg K, Liss L: *Neuroectodermal Tumors of the Central and Peripheral Nervous System*. Baltimore, Williams & Wilkins, 1969
87. Sipe JC, Herman MM, Rubinstein LJ: Electron microscopic observations on human glioblastomas and astrocytomas maintained in organ culture systems. *Am J Pathol* 73:589–606, 1973
88. Takei Y, Mirra SS, Miles ML: Eosinophilic granular cells in oligodendrogliomas. An ultrastructural study. *Cancer* 38:1968–1976, 1976
89. Thust R, Warzok R, Batka H: Die Morphologie experimenteller Tumoren des Nervensystems *in vitro*. I. Transplazentar induzierte Tumoren des Nervus trigeminus der Ratte. *Arch Geschwulstforsch* 40:300–307, 1972
90. Vraa-Jensen J, Herman MM, Rubinstein LJ, et al: *In vitro* characteristics of a fourth ventricle ependymoma maintained in organ culture system. Light and electron microscopic observations. *Neuropathol Appl Neurobiol* 2:349–364, 1976
91. Weiss P: *In vitro* transformation of spindle cells neural origin into macrophages. *Anat Rec* 88:205–221, 1944
92. Weller RO, Cervos-Navarro J: *Pathology of Peripheral Nerves*. Boston, Butterworths, 1977
93. Willmer EN: Morphological problems of cell type, shape and identification, in Willmer (ed): *Cells and Tissue in Culture, Vol. 1*. Academic Press, Orlando, Florida 1965 pp. 143–176
94. Wilson CB, Barker M, Slagel DE: Tumors of the central nervous system in monolayer culture. *Arch Neurol* 15:275–282, 1966

6

Brain Biopsy

J. H. Garcia
J. Cervós-Navarro

Introduction

Because of ethical implications, a decision to biopsy the brain must be considered carefully by the patient (if capable of making the decision), the next of kin, the neurologist, the surgeon, and the pathologist. A careful appraisal must be made as to whether the purpose of the biopsy is diagnostic, as in the case of organic dementia, or therapeutic. Persistent deficits or death as a complication of brain biopsies are extremely unlikely (less than 1.0%), but the probability of arriving at a conclusive diagnosis through a brain biopsy is not high, especially when the evaluation is done only with the light microscope. In some patients, the brain may be biopsied during the early stages of a disease, (i.e., when the lesion is difficult to recognize by light microscopy alone). Moreover, expectations for therapeutic benefits in the cases where the diagnosis is feasible are relatively low.[103]

One of the reasons for biopsying the brain of children, in particular, is to aid in genetic counseling; establishing the diagnosis of a neurologic disorder may be important to the parents and unborn siblings. The percentage of brain biopsies yielding positive results in children with neurodegenerative diseases has been estimated at 15%–20%. However, techniques other than brain biopsy are available for the diagnosis of most neurodegenerative disorders. In this group, only Alexander's disease and Canavan's spongy degeneration must be diagnosed by brain biopsy.[93]

A brain biopsy may be unnecessary in cases in which the microscopic evaluation of either a skin biopsy or circulating lymphocytes is sufficient to diagnose a neurologic disorder. Ceroid neuronal lipofuscinosis, generalized glycogenosis, Tangier's disease, and some leukodystrophies, among others, can be identified through these less invasive methods.[28]

In appropriately selected instances, brain biopsy is the indicated procedure both to confirm the diagnosis of *viral encephalitis* and to isolate (by inoculation or serologic methods) the causative organism. This is especially true of presumptive cases of *herpes simplex encephalitis*, a disease that may be amenable to being treated successfully with chemotherapeutic agents such as adenine arabinoside.[104]

In addition to the analysis of structural changes to be described, a definitive diagnosis from brain biopsy often requres biochemical, histochemical, and microbiologic evaluation of the tissue sample. For this reason, diagnostic brain biopsies are best done in hospitals where clinicians, pathologists, biochemists, microbiologists, and virologists cooperate closely.

In this chapter, the interpretation of microscopic abnormalities observed in meningeal and brain biopsies is discussed. Sometimes brain fragments that are examined microscopically are obtained as the indirect result of surgical procedures, such as lobectomies to relieve increased intracranial pressure or seizures. Occasionally, brain tissue may be obtained during craniotomy performed to place an intraventricular catheter.

Cerebral tissues surgically obtained for diagnostic analysis may reveal structural deviations from the normal, attributable to one or more of the following:

1. Aging results in vascular changes, an increased amount of collagen deposited under the arachnoidal membrane (Fig. 6–1), abundant *corpora amylacea* (Fig. 6–2), intracellular accumulation of lipofuscin, neuritic or senile plaques, and neurofibrillary tangles.[152,153]

2. Acute ischemic effects (i.e., less than a few hours old) are secondary to the hemostatic measures that must precede tissue excision. These effects can be exaggerated by delayed fixation, desiccation, immersion in hypotonic solutions, and brief fixation.[44,83] These changes must be distinguished from ischemic alterations that precede the surgical intervention by several hours.

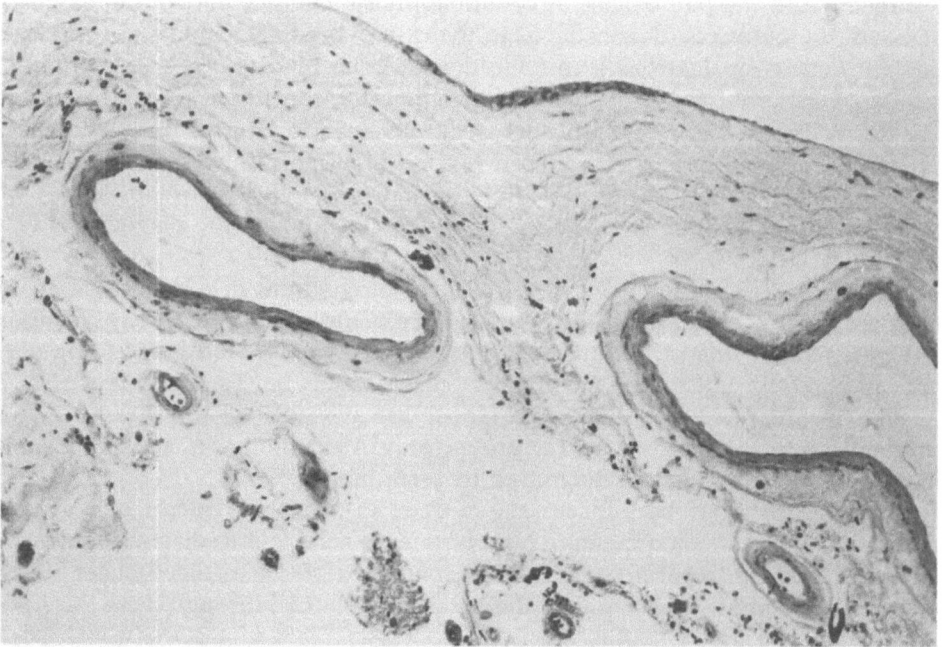

Fig. 6-1. Arachnoidal membrane (superior temporal gyrus). The sample shows collagen deposition under the arachnoid and in the adventitia of subarachnoid blood vessels in an 83-year-old patient (×63).

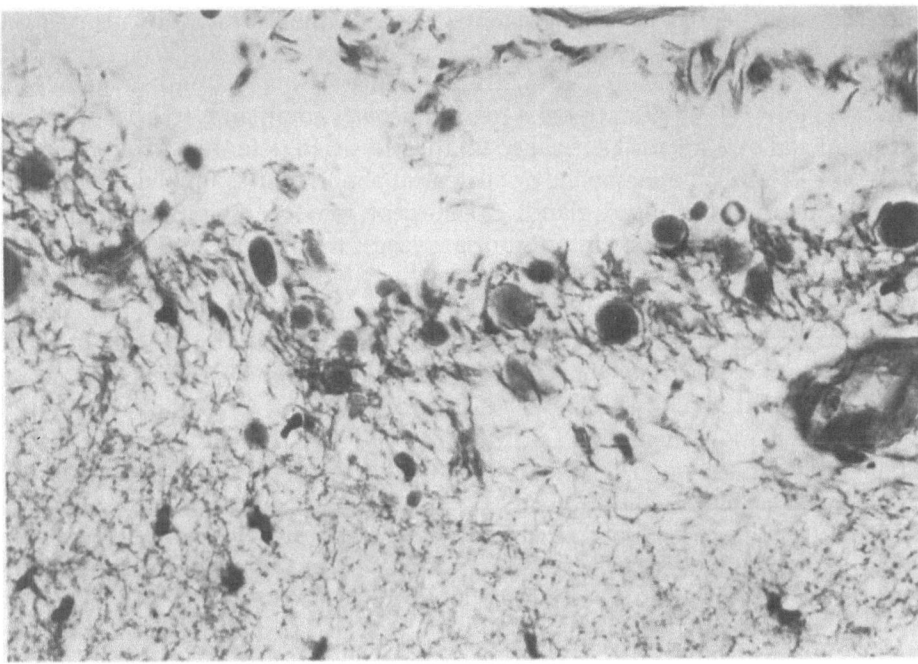

Fig. 6-2. Corpora amylacea in the subpial portion of the cerebral cortex of a 67-year-old patient. They appear as round or cylindrical bodies, sometimes containing concentric rings and a darker center; these bodies range widely in diameter and are strongly PAS-positive (×160).

3. Mechanical distortion may be induced by the procedures necessary for cutting, holding, sucking, or slicing the tissue samples by either the surgeon or the pathologist.
4. Inadequate tissue processing reflects the consequence of delaying fixation, using fixatives having an unsatisfactory composition, or applying improper methods for tissue processing, cutting, and staining.

The consequences of structural deviations 2, 3, and 4 listed above are generally designated artifacts to signify that they are the result of manipulation. Some common artifacts in neural tissues are illustrated and discussed in separate chapters.

5. The effects of disease may be broadly classified into:
   (a) vascular-circulatory disorders, such as congestion, edema, ischemia, and hemorrhage;
   (b) infections and inflammations;
   (c) neoplastic growths;
   (d) diseases affecting primarily myelin sheaths;
   (e) toxic-metabolic disorders;
   (f) congenital/developmental defects;
   (g) effects of immunologic abnormalities; and
   (h) miscellaneous disorders of uncertain origin, sometimes designated "degenerative."

These categories do not encompass all possibilities nor are they exclusive of one another; thus, severe circulatory changes accompany most brain infections and neoplasms. Moreover, some infectious agents, such as the papova viruses, can induce not only inflammation but also extensive demyelination.

The usual sequence leading to a diagnosis, based on anatomic evidence, might proceed as follows: (1) a patient with a neuromuscular complaint, (e.g., a seizure disorder), is examined by a medical specialist; (2) the physician determines that the symptom is a reflection of probable metabolic or structural abnormalities involving either neuromuscular tissues or the pituitary gland; (3) a surgeon removes a biopsy from the intracranial or intraspinal contents, or in appropriate cases, from peripheral nerves or skeletal muscles; (4) analysis of the structural abnormalities by microscopic examination places the disorder in the category of inflammation, as an example, with abundant intranuclear inclusion bodies. The diagnosis is nearly complete once it is determined that the inclusion body is composed of particles whose features are compatible with those of *herpes simplex virus* (HSV); (5) and finally, serologic evidence or immunocytochemical staining determines that the microorganism (HSV) is the cause of the neurologic disease. The information contained in this chapter deals mainly with step #4: the recognition and interpretation of microscopic abnormalities.

Most brain biopsies include a fragment of cerebral (or cerebellar) parenchyma and overlying leptomeninges. Structural alterations involving dura mater, leptomeninges, blood vessels, gray matter, and white matter are discussed separately.

Dura Mater

The dura mater (hard or thick meninges) is a thick collagenous membrane that is firmly attached intracranially to the endostium; in the spinal canal, the dura is normally separated from the vertebrae by a wide epidural space containing loose adipose tissue that is especially abundant in the lower thoracic and lumbar regions. The presence of branches of the meningeal arteries usually permit the microscopic identification of the outer surface of the intracranial dura. The inner surface is lined by a monolayer of dural border cells[118] that are not easily recognized by light microscopy.

Hemorrhages

Bleeding in the intracranial epidural space is a lesion of the younger age groups. The hemorrhage is almost always traumatic in origin, and the blood clot is excised surgically, most frequently, during the acute stage (i.e., a few hours after the injury). Fragments of dura mater or skull are seldom resected with an epidural hemorrhage. Nontraumatic and cryptic causes of symptomatic intracranial epidural bleeding (e.g., neoplasms or angiomatous malformations) are extremely rare.

Pieces of intracranial dura mater are removed surgically in most instances together with blood or fluid accumulating in the potential space existing between the dura and the arachnoid, that is the subdural space. Typically, blood collected in this space becomes attached within a few hours to the inner dural surface. Here, an outer membrane of the subdural hemorrhage begins to form quickly, while an inner membrane eventually separates the hemorrhage from the arachnoidal membrane and causes the blood clot to remain attached to the inner dural surface. Both the outer and inner membranes of a subdural hemorrhage are made of fibrin and fibroblasts that become activated under the stimulus of various peptides originating from circulating cells. The development of these subdural membranes (i.e., the organization of the hematoma) follows a relatively predictable pattern that, in most instances, allows an approximate microscopic estimate of the age of the hemorrhage. Capillary growth and extravasation of white blood cells can be seen after 3–4 days, next to the outer membrane. The development of the inner membrane is delayed by several days, compared to that of the outer membrane. Chronic subdural hemorrhages are lined by fibrous membranes containing few erythrocytes and abundant hemosiderin-laden macrophages. It is common to see, even in very old hematomas, collections of intact erythrocytes in the midst of abundant granulation tissue. Most subdural hemorrhages are of traumatic origin, but occasionally, the microscopic evaluation of these clots uncovers either neoplastic growths (usually metastatic) or vascular anomalies as the associated causative factors.

Suppurative bacterial infections localized in the intracranial subdural space, (i.e., subdural empyemas) are usually the result of penetrating traumatic head injuries.

Leptomeninges

The normal constituents of the human adult leptomeninges (thin or soft meninges) include an arachnoidal membrane composed of aggregates or arachnoidal (or meningothelial) cells, occasionally found surrounding a psammoma body and resting on a well-defined basement membrane, which is normally in physical contact with the innermost layer of the dura (Fig. 6–3).[56] Children less than 6 years of age have a multilayered arachnoid membrane that does not contain psammoma bodies (Fig. 6–4). The leptomeningeal interstitium, or subarachnoid space, contains cerebrospinal fluid (CSF) bathing

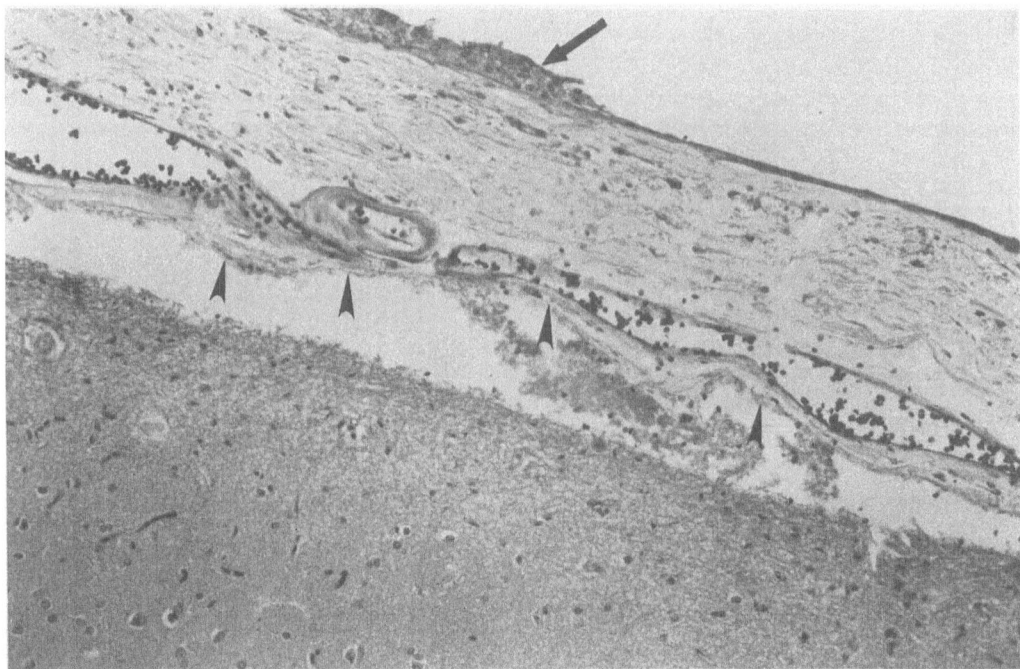

Fig. 6-3. Arachnoidal cells (arrow) and deposits of collagen in the leptomeninx of a 69-year-old patient. The pia (arrowheads) is artificially detached from the brain surface, (×63).

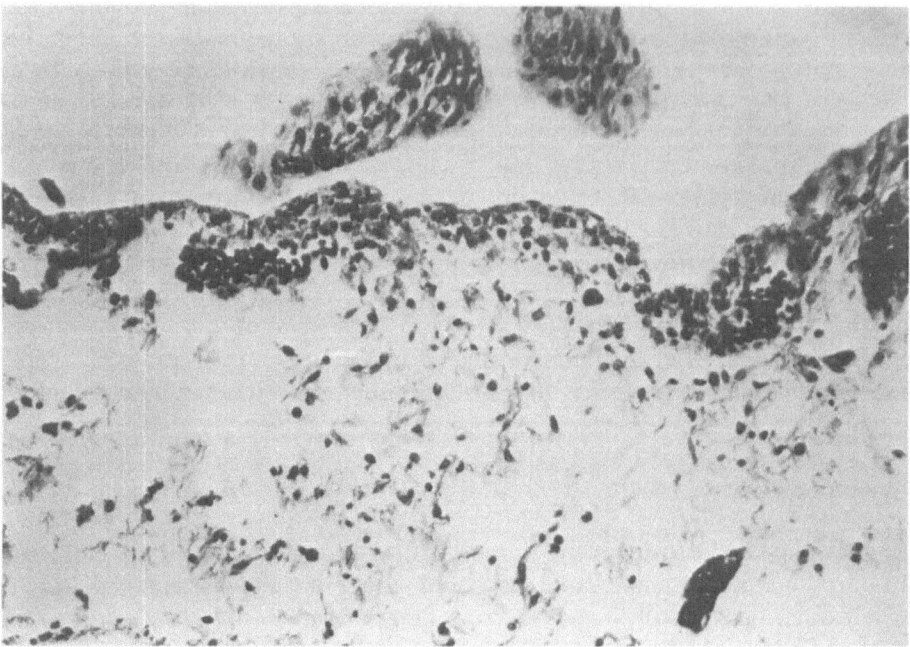

Fig. 6-4. The arachnoid in this sample from a full-term newborn is multilayered and the subarachnoid space contains more cells than are seen in the normal adult (×160).

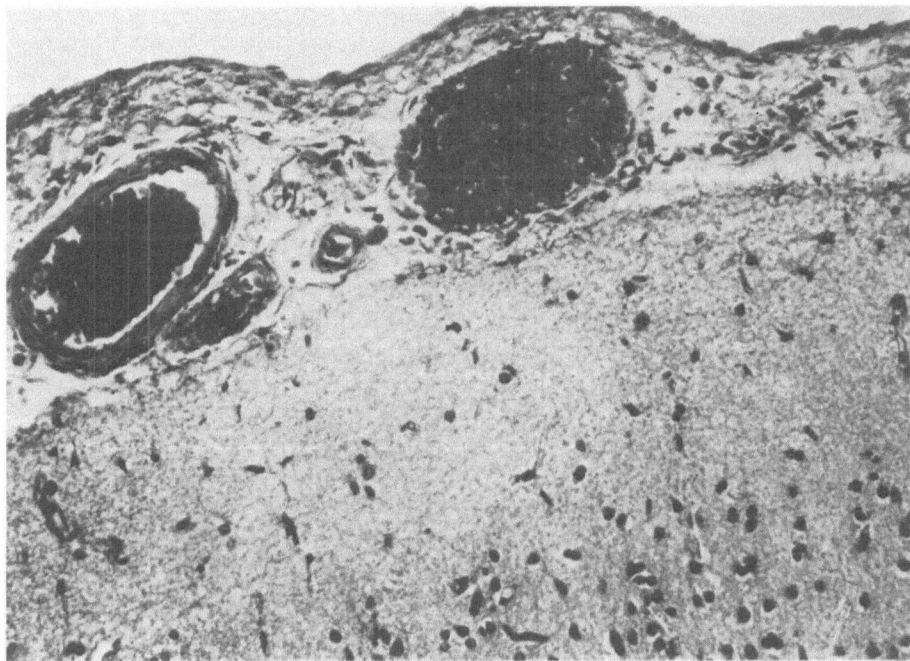

Fig. 6-5. Cerebral cortex (67-year-old patient). The arachnoid is at the top. The subpial portion of the cortex, normally devoid of readily visible neurons, is the molecular layer. A few mononuclear cells are visible in the subarachnoid space (×40).

the adventitial surface of the large arteries, veins, and dural sinuses. Collagen fibers and occasional mononuclear cells, presumably derived from the arachnoid, are normally present in the subarachnoid space (Fig. 6–5), but their numbers and proportions differ according to age. The pia is a porous basement membrane that probably allows direct communication between the subarachnoid space and the brain extracellular space (ECS); an occasional leptomeningeal or arachnoidal cell abuts the pia.[14] Structural changes in human leptomeninges attributable to aging include: increase in the amount of collagen fibers and fibroblasts, particularly under the arachnoid, and a greater thickness of collagenous fibers in the tunica adventitia of subarachnoid blood vessels (Fig. 6–6).

Inflammations

Suppurative leptomeningitis is manifested by collections of polymorphonuclear leukocytes, proteinaceous exudate, fibrin, and cellular debris in the subarachnoid space; purulent leptomeningitis is most frequently associated with the entry of pus-producing bacteria, such as *Diplococcus pneumoniae*, into the subarachnoid space. Circulating bacteria may gain access to the subarachnoid space through the choroid plexus, the arachnoidal capillaries, or the walls of arteries or veins normally present in the subarachnoid space. Suppurative inflammation of the leptomeninges is seldom seen in material surgically removed from the intracranial or intraspinal contents (Fig. 6–7). Brain biopsies that include fragments of leptomeninges from the basal cisterns occasionally reveal granulomatous inflammation (Fig. 6–8); the most frequent causes of this type of reaction are: (1) infections by tubercle bacillus, (2) fungal infections, (3) sarcoidosis, (4) foreign bodies introduced at previous craniotomies or by penetrating injuries, and (5) *Treponema pallidum*. Granulomatous inflammations of the leptomeninges caused by the tubercle bacillus

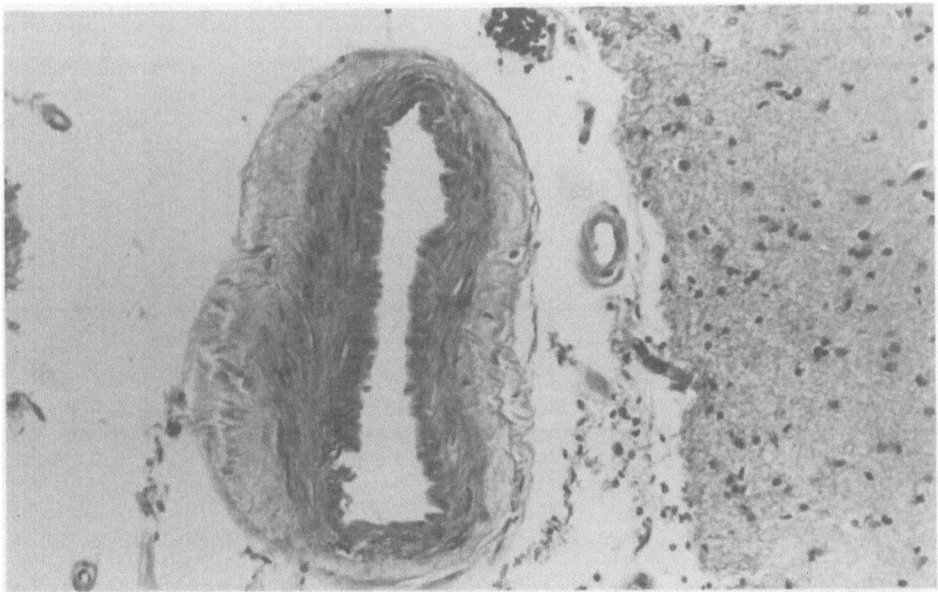

Fig. 6-6. Thickened tunica adventitia in a subarachnoid arterial branch from a 60-year-old patient who died with pulmonary cancer (×40).

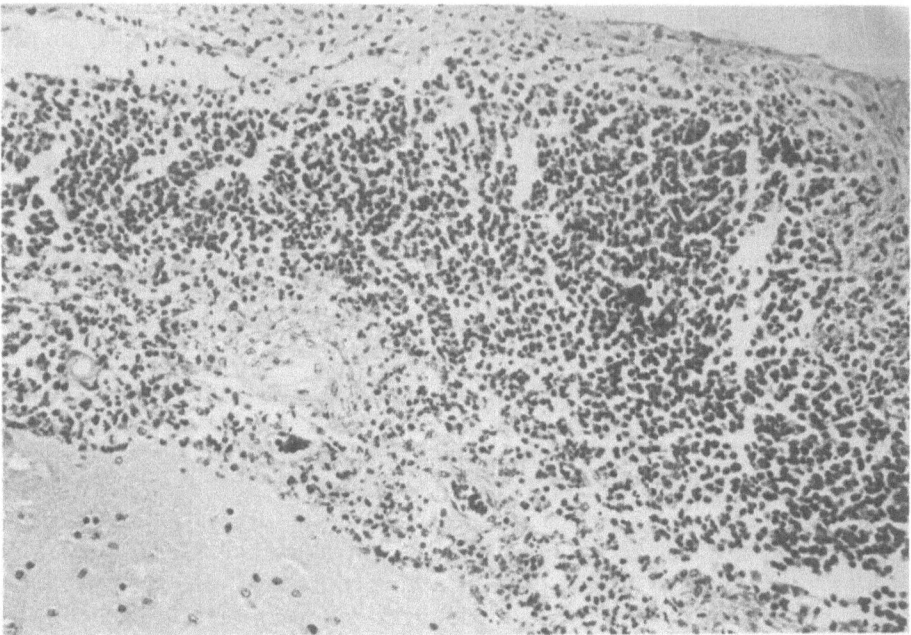

Fig. 6-7. Suppurative leptomeningitis: the arachnoid is at the top and cerebral cortex is partly visible at the left lower corner. Exudate made of fibrin, bacteria, polymorphonuclear leukocytes, and cellular debris fills the subarachnoid space (×64).

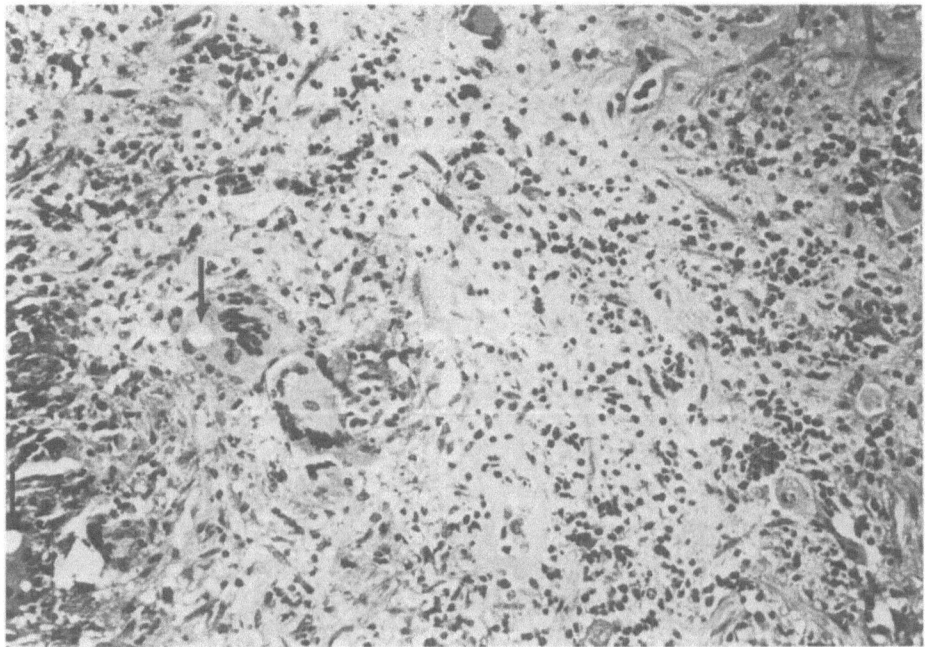

Fig. 6-8. Leptomeningeal granulomata in a case of infection produced by *Coccidioides immitis;* round spaces (arrow) in the multinucleated giant cells correspond to the sites occupied by the microorganism (×64).

or by fungi are not commonly associated with caseation necrosis. A conclusive diagnosis of either type of infection requires histologic demonstration of the microorganism, a task facilitated by the use of acid-fast and PAS-staining methods. Most granulomas in patients with sarcoidosis are not associated with caseation necrosis. By definition, microorganisms are not demonstrable in this condition; therefore, sarcoidosis is a diagnosis of exclusion. Sarcoidosis generally becomes manifest as a chronic pulmonary disease; however, in a few patients (1.5%) with sarcoidosis, the initial complaint indicates neurologic dysfunction.[87] Among the unique structural features of neurosarcoidosis is the perivascular nature of the granulomata, which sometimes obliterate the vascular lumen[67] (Fig. 6–9). Inflammatory lesions primarily localized to the brain parenchyma, (i.e., abscesses and microglial nodules), are discussed below under the heading of white matter inflammations.

Cysts

A cyst is a sac (normal or abnormal) containing liquid or semisolid material; most cysts are lined by a recognizable epithelium. Cystic lesions in the leptomeninges form three major categories and are described below.

1. Cystic lesions on the brain surface, which most commonly occur either in the middle or the posterior fossa of the skull, are called arachnoidal cysts. The relative prevalence of arachnoid cysts in the pediatric population and the absence of trauma or inflammation in most cases suggest a congenital origin.[65] In most instances, the arachnoidal cyst is a developmental defect that probably reflects anomalous splitting

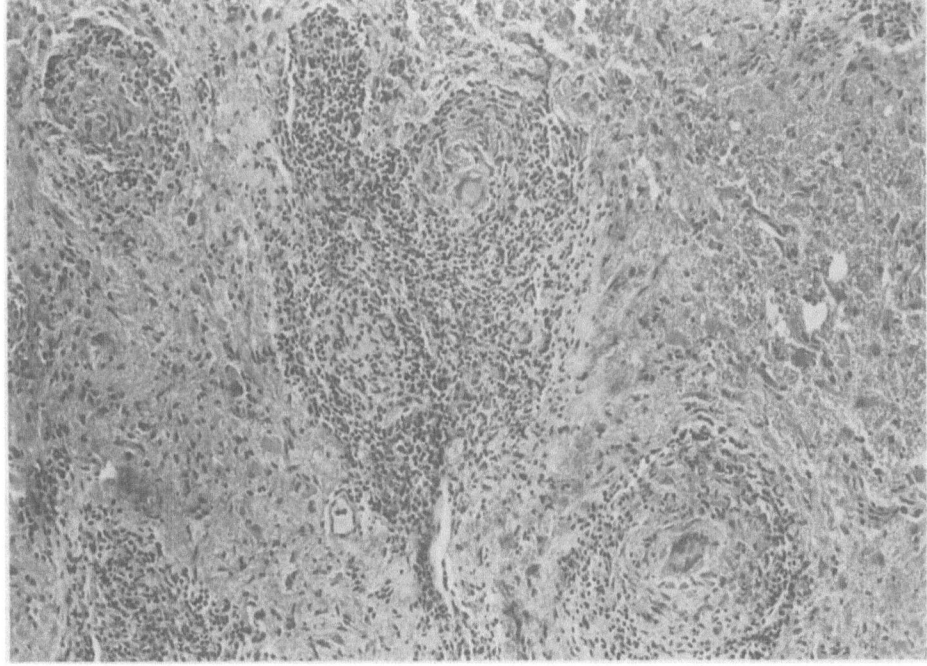

Fig. 6-9. Twenty-year-old woman with generalized sarcoidosis. Sample from midbrain showing at least four noncaseating granulomata, each surrounding a relatively large-caliber blood vessel (×63).

and duplication of the endomeninx during neural tube folding.[65] For this reason, this lesion could be more appropriately designated as an intra-arachnoid cyst.[138] The light and electron microscopic evaluations of these lesions usually show loose connective tissue and a monolayer lining of flattened cells displaying features of arachnoidal cells[86] that join with normal arachnoid at the margins of the cyst.[65] Moreover, the ultrastructural features of the lining cells are compatible with those found in secretory cells.[58] Approximately one-half of all arachnoid cysts are located in or near the sylvian fissure;[65] 12% of all arachnoid cysts occur in the suprasellar area,[121] and an equal percent may be found in the posterior fossa.[91]

2. A second variety of cyst usually found in the subarachnoid space is composed of lesions lined by one or more layers of epithelial cells. The nomenclature of these cysts is determined by the features of the lining epithelium. *Epidermoid* cysts are lined by squamous epithelium; *dermoid* cysts contain, in addition, skin appendages such as hair follicles and sebaceous glands. Dermoid cysts are frequently associated with dysraphic syndromes, especially those located in the posterior fossa and spinal canal. Epidermoid cysts, of which craniopharyngioma may be considered a variant, are not generally associated with bony defects and in most cases are isolated lesions. Intracranial epidermoid cysts arise from epithelial tissues that become displaced between the third and fifth weeks of gestation.[10] The areas most often involved are the cerebellopontine angle and the parasellar region; these cysts grow through the accumulation of normally dividing cells.[10]

Intraparenchymal brain cysts lined by a single cell layer have been designated "arachnoidal" to indicate their probable derivation from arachnoidal cells. The lining of these cysts and that of some ventricular and parenchymal cysts is similar, (i.e., it is composed of a monolayer). Hence, it has been suggested that all such lesions, regardless of location, in either subarachnoid or intraparenchymal sites, be designated "neuroepithelial" cysts to signify their possible neuroectodermal derivation.[136] Controversy on what constitutes the proper designation for these cysts stems from the difficulty in deciding whether the lining epithelium is derived from arachnoidal cells, ependymal cells, or (in the case of colloid cyst) respiratory epithelium.[54] Epithelial cysts have been found in the subarachnoid space in all compartments of the skull and spinal canal.[89]

The traditionally designated colloid paraphyseal cyst of the roof of the third ventricle constitutes still another variety of neuroepithelial cyst. Some authors suggest, on the basis of ultrastructural observations, that this cyst represents a derivation of epithelium from the respiratory tract.[72]

Cysts associated with the CNS are a miscellaneous group of lesions whose origin may be connected to cells of arachnoidal, systemic epithelial, or neuroepithelial origin. Because the lining is usually flattened, the origin of these cells is often difficult to determine in individual lesions. Some of the possible developmental origins for various CNS cysts have been discussed at length by Leech and Olafson.[89]

3. Subarachnoid and intraventricular lesions, having the gross appearance of a cyst, may represent the CNS infestation by either the cysticercus of *Taenia solium* or embryos of *Echinococcus granulosus*. Microscopic identification of the organism is essential for the diagnosis of cysticercosis and hydatid cyst, respectively.[33] The cysticercus can be readily identified by the characteristic scolex (Fig. 6-10), a task that may require multiple histologic preparations of the same block. When only the membranous structures are available for microscopic evaluation, the diagnosis is suggested by an easily visible concentric three-layered structure. The outermost layer consists of an unevenly scalloped eosinophilic membrane around an irregular collection of mononuclear cells.

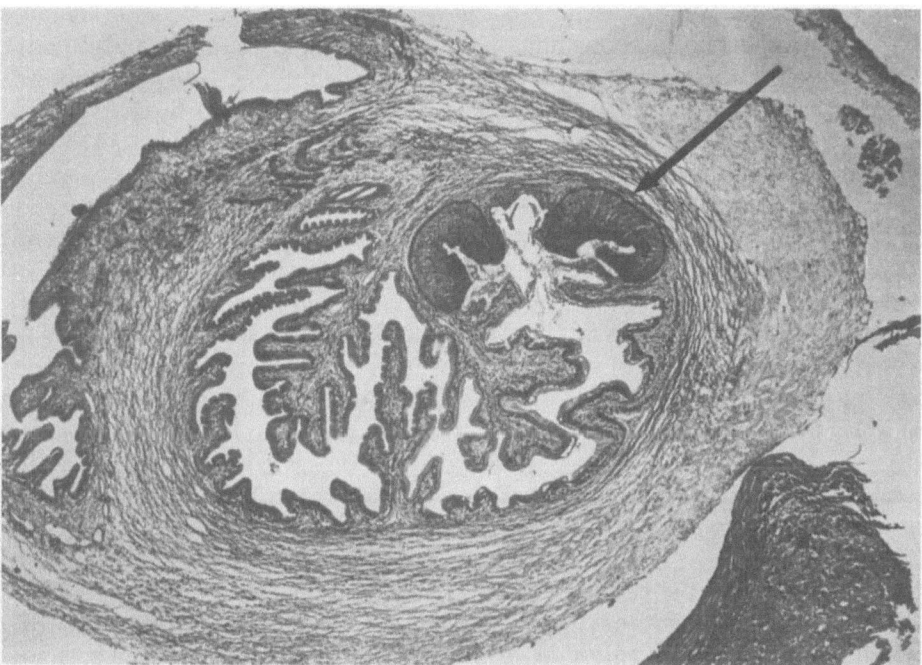

Fig. 6-10. Cysticercus removed from the subarachnoid space of a patient who complained of seizures and headaches. Scolex (arrow) is characteristic of *Taenia solium* (×16).

The innermost layer shows a villous appearance with numerous finger-like projections.[33] Cysticercosis is the most common parasitic disease of the CNS. The main clinical manifestations of neurocysticercosis are: seizures (usually focal), hydrocephalus, and an abrupt onset of focal neurologic deficits such as hemiparesis. These symptoms reflect the involvement of structures in various multiple sites where these parasites may lodge in the CNS. In decreasing frequency, neurocysticercosis may involve: the subarachnoid space, the cerebral ventricles (especially the fourth), and the brain parenchyma. Multiple intracranial calcifications (measuring 2–10 mm in diameter), as demonstrated by either computerized tomography or magnetic resonance imaging among patients with the symptoms previously mentioned, are characteristic of neurocysticercosis. These cysts may incite an intense inflammation that subsides following the death of the scolex; most organisms are said to die after a period of approximately 18 months.[98]

Other varieties of cystic lesions that may occur in or near the subarachnoid space include: epidermoid cysts, teratomas, craniopharyngiomas, and cysts of Rathke's pouch. These lesions are discussed and illustrated in the section dealing with parasellar tumors (Volume I).

Neoplastic invasion of the subarachnoid space is discussed in Volume I.

Blood Vessels: Arterial, Venous, and Capillary

Normal intracranial arteries, particularly the branches of internal carotid and basilar vessels, differ anatomically from extracranial arteries of comparable caliber. The intracranial and intradural arteries have (as seen in routine histologic preparations) a single, thin internal elastic layer, and only 3–4 layers of smooth muscle cells in the tunica media. Special digestion methods demonstrate elastic fibers in the media and adventitia of these arteries.[101] Systemic vessels of comparable caliber, by contrast, have a thicker tunica media and a prominent external elastic lamina. Cerebral capillaries also differ from extracranial ones by having nonfenestrated (or tight) endothelial junctions and a nearly complete circumferential ensheathment by astroglial processes. These features make brain capillaries impervious to the passage of circulating macromolecules (e.g., albumins and proteins) and form the anatomical basis for the blood-brain barrier. Extra-cerebral capillaries and brain capillaries located at specific sites such as the area postrema are fenestrated and allow free passage of macromolecules.

Abnormalities in the vessels supplying the brain that are detectable in surgically excised specimens include: (1) atherosclerosis; (2) aneurysms: saccular, "mycotic," and dissecting; (3) angiomatous malformations; (4) angiitis and (5) miscellaneous angiopathies.

Atherosclerosis

Atherosclerosis of the cervicocranial arteries tends to be particularly marked, and therefore, to become symptomatic at the sites of origin of the internal carotid, the intracranial segment of the vertebral vessels, the middle segment of the basilar artery, and the initial segment of the middle cerebral artery.[124] Atherogenesis, a process confined primarily to arteries, involves sub-endothelial or intimal thickening accompanied by focal deposition of plasma-derived lipids (cholesterol included), proliferation of smooth muscle fibers, intramural presence of circulating monocytes, and deposition of connective tissues (Fig. 6-11). In human samples, one of the cells to first show lipid deposits is the subintimal smooth muscle fiber.[53] The atherosclerotic process in the cerebral vessels is histologically the same as elsewhere in the body.[52] Atheromatous material surgically removed from the initial segment of the internal carotid artery, by means of an endarterectomy, frequently consists of the inner layers of the tunica media and the atherosclerotic ulcerated lesion that may be partly covered by fibrin and platelets. Thrombosis during the acute postoperative period and regrowth of the atheromatous plaques as a delayed event, have been verified in an autopsy study of 19 patients who underwent carotid endarterectory at various intervals before death.[40] Atherosclerosis in the cervicocranial vessels is usually most severe in the first 2.0 cm and on the posterior wall of the proximal internal carotid artery; disease in this area is usually heralded by a minor stroke or transient ischemic attack, attributed to either "low flow" or embolism to the intracranial or retinal vessels.[84]

Aneurysms

A saccular aneurysm is an ectatic deformity of an artery, localized to a segment of the vascular circumference. The walls of saccular aneurysms are composed of endothelium, thin tunica media containing few or no smooth muscle fibers, fragmented or absent elastic fibers, and thin adventitia[110,140] (Fig. 6-12). Saccular or "berry" aneurysms are more common at sites where the tunica media normally thins out to an interrupted layer of smooth muscle (i.e., branching sites).

Arterial dilatations developing at the site of localized bacterial infections in the

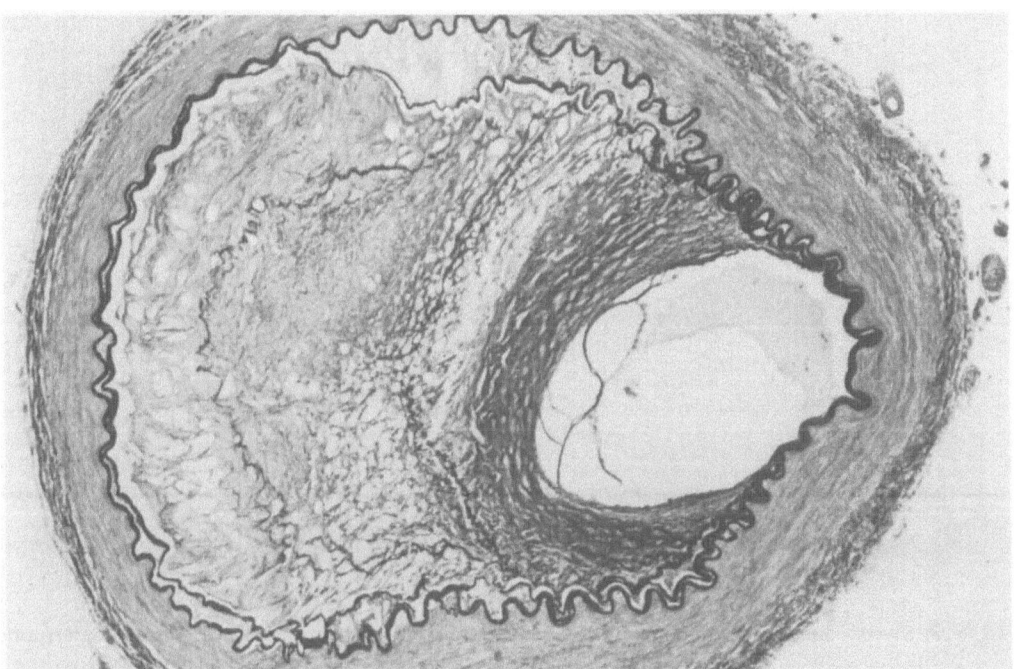

Fig. 6-11. Cross-section of anterior cerebral artery demonstrates marked luminal narrowing by an atheromatous plaque including "reduplication" of the internal elastic lamina (dark wavy fibers) (Verhoeff van Gieson, ×16).

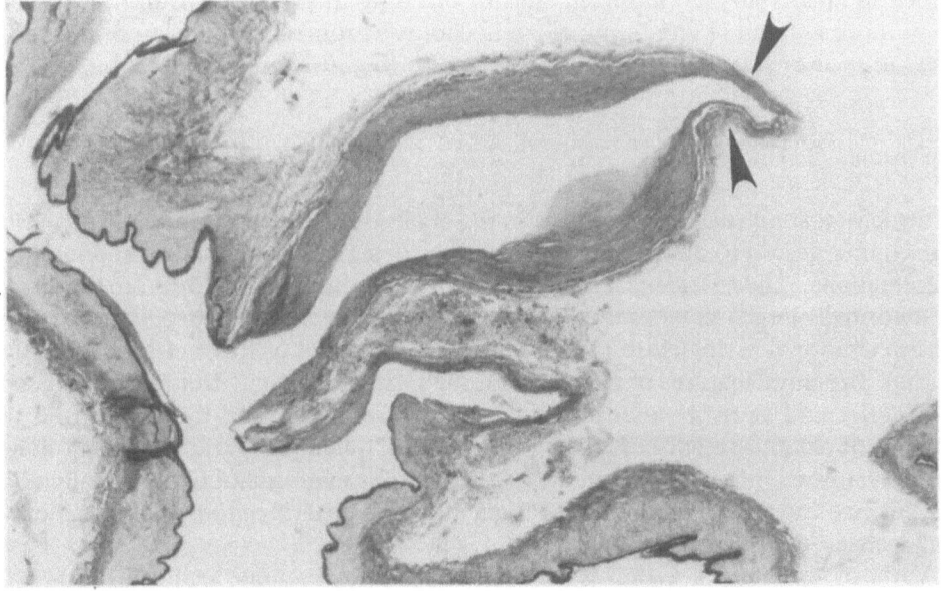

Fig. 6-12. Longitudinal section of basilar artery demonstrating a saccular aneurysm; elastic lamina and smooth muscle fibers are missing in the aneurysmal wall. The apex of the aneurysm (arrowheads) has an extremely thin wall (Verhoeff van Gieson, ×1).

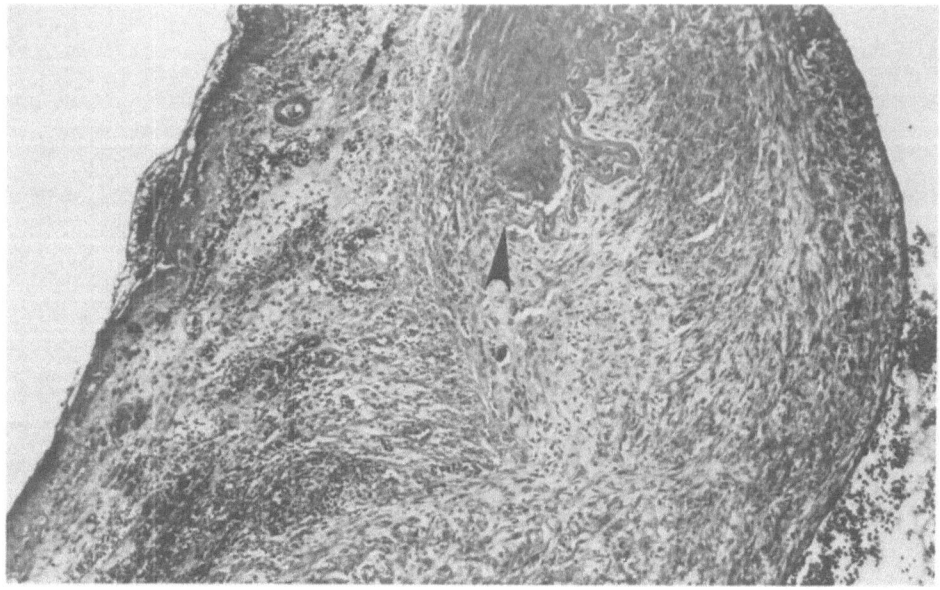

Fig. 6-13. Mycotic aneurysm. Cross-section of a segment of middle cerebral artery wall showing interruption of the tunica media (arrowhead) at the site of acute and chronic bacterial inflammation (×24).

vessel wall are inappropriately called "mycotic" aneurysms.[139] At these sites, light microscopy reveals segments of interrupted tunica media containing abundant polymorphonuclear or mononuclear leukocytes (Fig. 6-13). Dissecting aneurysms involve mostly the carotid and vertebral arteries,[11] but they may also occur in other intracranial vessels.[3] Dissecting aneurysms are localized sites of bleeding in the vessel wall having usually one or more luminal or extraluminal connections. Thrombotic occlusion of the vascular lumen at or near the site of bleeding is common (Fig. 6-14).

Angiomatous Malformations

Structural abnormalities of vessels in the skull, dura mater, leptomeninges, or brain parenchyma related to developmental faults are designated as vascular or angiomatous malformations. These lesions are recognized under the microscope on the basis of: the abnormally large caliber of the vascular channels, the multiplicity of vascular lumina, and the abnormal architecture of the walls, (i.e., absence of three clearly recognizable tunicae). Structural features of angiomatous malformations range from those of recognizable arteries and veins to vessels having alternatingly thick and thin hyalinized walls. Evidence of old and recent hemorrhage, segmental dilatations, and large irregular nodules of hyalinized intima are frequent.[99] Angiomatous malformations are usually divided into: varices, cavernous angiomas, venous angioma, arteriovenous malformation, and telangiectasis.

Varix of the vein of Galen is a variation of arteriovenous malformations (AVM) that involves the great vein of Galen; the abnormality often becomes symptomatic during childhood in the form of cardiac failure, progressive hydrocephalus, or seizures.[61] All varicous dilatations of the vein of Galen are connected to an arterial supply that

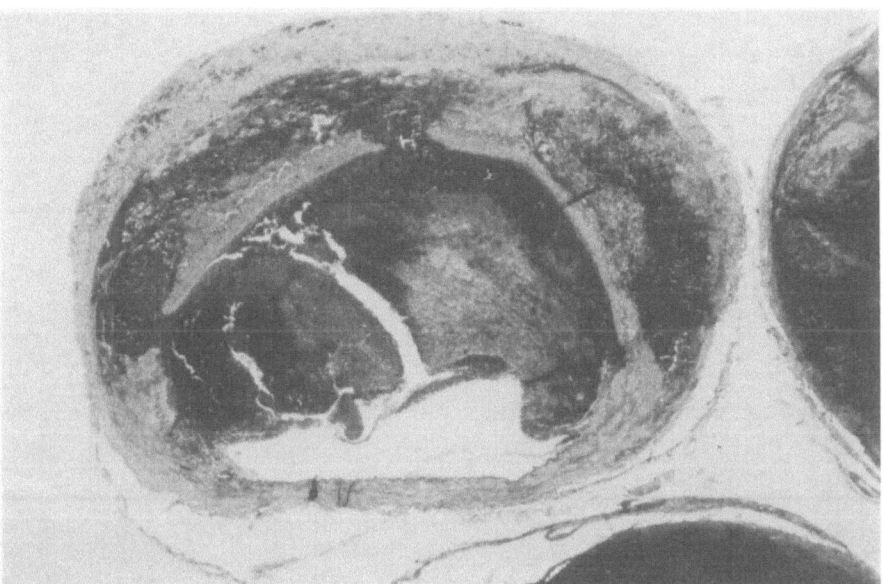

Fig. 6-14. Dissecting aneurysm. Cross-section of left vertebral artery showing intramural hemorrhage connected with the lumen at two sites. An organizing thrombus occludes partly the vascular lumen (×1).

usually originates from one of the posterior cerebral arteries.[71] Cavernous hemangiomas are closely clustered, thin-walled, large-caliber blood channels usually lacking intervening neural tissue, whose mural architecture is markedly altered by thick or thin stretches of tissues where the absence of elastic lamina and smooth muscle fibers is most conspicuous (Fig. 6-15). True cavernous angiomas tend to be located in the deeper portions of the brain, such as the thalamic nuclei. This is in contrast with the superficial location of most AVM's. Venous angiomas are composed of structures having their entire inflow originating from veins, the intervening brain tissue being normal.[100] These are among the least common of the angiomatous malformations and may require angiographic evaluation to demonstrate their sole venous connections.

Arteriovenous malformations (AVM) is the generic designation commonly applied to angiomatous malformations of the brain and spinal cord having abundant venous and arterial components. The histologic features are usually those of segmentally abnormal vessels having irregular walls with abundant collagen but without orderly tunica media or elastic lamina. Large calcium deposits are frequent. Abundant normal or scarred brain tissue, sometimes with evidence of old hemorrhages, may be interspersed with the abnormal vessels. Most AVM's are reflections of lesions arising at about 3 weeks of gestation in which an arrest in the capillary development results in a direct artery-to-vein communication.[141] The addition of more arterial contributions, repeated small hemorrhages and the occlusion of some of the channels may be responsible for the more common occurrence of neurologic symptoms (usually hemorrhage or seizures) in the second and third decades than in childhood.[141]

Telangiectases or capillary hemangiomas are abnormalities of monolayer, distal vessels lined by endothelium, and measuring up to 200 μm in caliber. They often occur in a cluster that measures up to 2.0 cm in diameter and are usually embedded in normal cerebral parenchyma (Fig. 6-16). The most common site of telangiectases is

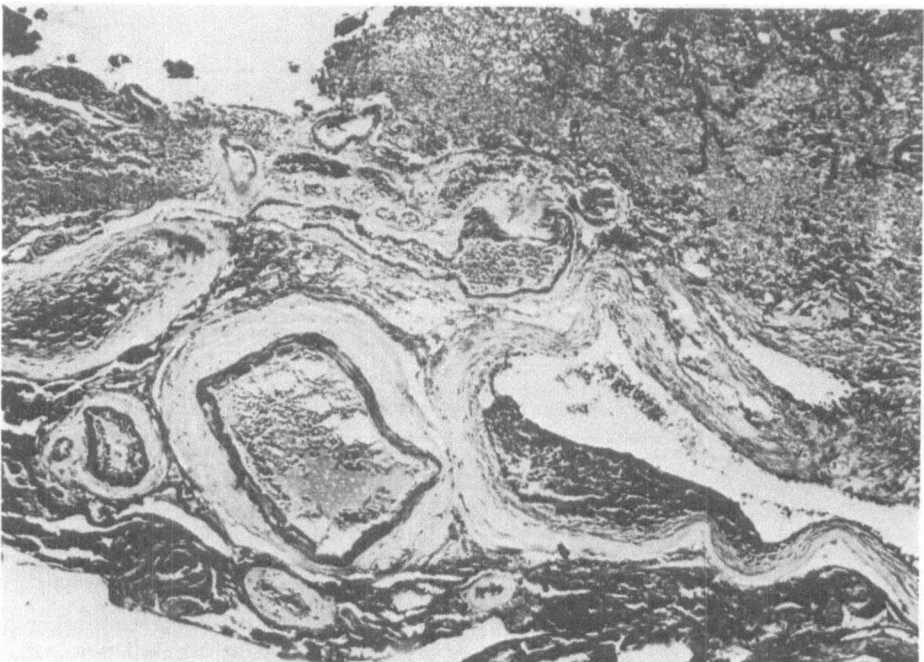

Fig. 6-15. Cavernous hemangioma. Large aggregate of blood vessels with thickened, hyalinized walls devoid of recognizable elastic fibers or smooth muscle cells (Trichrome, ×16).

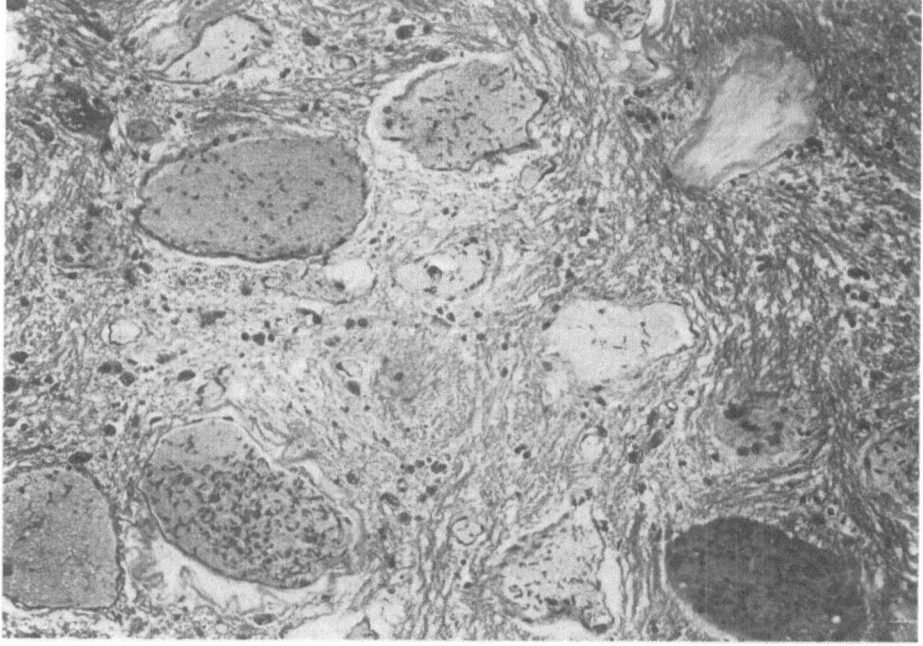

Fig. 6-16. Telangiectasis: a frequent, incidental finding in the base of the pons. The intervening brain parenchyma is normal (×40).

the base of the pons;[99,112] therefore, their surgical resection is seldom achieved. Neoplasms thought to be derived from angiomatous cells, either endothelial (i.e., hemangioblastoma) or pericytic (i.e., hemangiopericytoma) are discussed in Volume I. Malformations and neoplastic growths derived from adult arterial wall components are extremely rare. Some hemangioblastomas may be difficult to distinguish from capillary hemangiomas.

The Sturge-Weber syndrome (encephalotrigeminal angiomatosis) is a disorder characterized by port-wine stain, or nevus flammeus, of the face with angiomatosis of the ipsilateral cerebral leptomeninges and extensive calcification in the underlying cerebral cortex.[9] Presence of hemangiomas in the scalp or face, especially those located within the dermatome innervated by the first sensory trigeminal branch, correlates most consistently with the existence of abnormal cerebral blood vessels.[116]

Miscellaneous Angiopathies

Almost any systemic disease involving blood vessels in a diffuse manner, (e.g., lupus erythematosus, rheumatoid arthritis, and thrombotic thrombocytopenic purpura) may become manifest through the involvement of the central nervous system blood vessels.[139] However, a brain biopsy is not an appropriate diagnostic procedure for these patients, and consequently, most systemic angiopathies would not appear in brain biopsies. Systemic disorders characterized by vascular abnormalities are more commonly demonstrated in nerve biopsy than in brain biopsy, with the exception of systemic lupus erythematosus, lymphomatoid granulomatosis, thrombotic thrombocytopenic purpura, and cerebral amyloid angiopathy.

Arterioles in the central nervous system are almost exclusively intraparenchymal vessels that lack a continuous internal elastic lamella and have a tunica media thicker than that of veins. In contrast to systemic arterioles that have several layers of smooth muscle, brain arterioles are endowed with only 1–3 smooth muscle cell layers.[126] Brain arterioles are nutrient as well as distributive vessels. A common abnormality of brain arterioles is hyalinosis or replacement of the wall by glassy, eosinophilic, homogeneous, acellular material. The chemical, immunological composition and ultrastructure of hyalin closely resembles that of basement membranes.[163] Arteriolar hyalinosis is associated with aging, systemic arterial hypertension, and diabetes mellitus. In some patients, cerebral arteriolar hyalinosis may be accompanied by parenchymal changes in the perivascular areas. These lesions include widening of the perivascular space, myelin loss, vacuolation, and astrogliosis.[17] Arteriolar fibrinoid changes are more common in hypertensive than in normotensive individuals; hyalin and fibrinoid are not easily distinguished from one another on the basis of light-microscopic features alone. Small arteries and arterioles located at the basal ganglia and the brain stem can also show, in addition to arteriolarsclerosis, signs of atherosclerosis, (i.e., subintimal lipid deposits).

Arteriolar changes, secondary to long-standing systemic hypertension, are more readily seen in the basal ganglia, cerebellar white matter, and pontine base where small arteries and large arterioles are abundant. None of these tissues is likely to be biopsied; however, some of the subcortical arterioles may show muscular hypertrophy, hyalinization, and mural fibrin deposits, all of which are suggestive of hypertensive angiopathy.

Cerebral amyloid angiopathy has been associated with a syndrome of recurrent intraparenchymal hemorrhages in elderly, normotensive individuals.[123] The diagnosis of cerebral amyloid angiopathy, a condition which is usually not associated with systemic amyloidosis, is based on the demonstration of amyloid in the small arteries and arterioles of the leptomeninges, cerebral cortex, and subcortical white matter. Staining with H&E reveals glassy, homogeneous eosinophilic deposits, which after staining with congo red and examining with polarizing filters, have a green-yellow birefringence. Amyloid fluoresces after staining with thioflavin S and examination with ultraviolet light. Amyloid is formed of fibrils measuring about 9–9.5 nm in diameter.[57] Giant cell arteritis is a systemic disease that commonly becomes manifest through involvement of the superficial temporal artery; the disease process rarely affects the leptomeningeal and cerebral vessels.[164] The most typical changes are seen in the inner half of the tunica media of large caliber arteries. Necrosis and cellular inflammation composed of neutrophils, lymphocytes, macrophages, eosinophils, and multinucleated giant cells are typical. The longitudinal involvement of the artery is segmental. For this reason, multiple cross-sections of the vessel must be examined before reporting the biopsy.[115] The inflammatory changes (i.e., angiitis) of noninfectious conditions such as Wegener's granulomatosis and polyarteritis nodosa are usually demonstrable in blood vessels of spinal and cranial nerves; these conditions do not involve brain vessels. Abundant mineral salts deposits in the blood vessels and parenchyma of the cerebral cortex (which characteristically are intensively hematoxynophilic) may exist in association with a facial angiomatous nevus, as part of the syndrome of Sturge and Weber. Vascular mineralization may accompany dysfunction of parathyroid glands or calcium/iron salts deposits may be an expression of a hereditary idiopathic condition sometimes known as Fahr's disease.

Cerebral and Cerebellar Cortices

Only a small portion of a neuron is seen in the usual histologic preparation examined by light microscopy (Fig. 6-17); "neuronal soma" designates this cellular part, further divided into nucleus and perikaryon. The perikaryon is the portion of cytoplasm that surrounds the nucleus; this is in contrast with the dendrites and the axis cylinder that extend considerably from the parent cell.[118] In the case of the spinal motor neurons, many axons extend for a distance of several feet. The term neuropil (literally: nerve hair) designates aggregates of dendrites, axons, and glial processes diffusely interspersed among neurons. In hematoxylin and eosin (H&E) preparations, the neuropil is homogeneous, pale, and pink (Fig. 6-18). Identification of brain cells in light-microscopic preparations is usually based on the recognition of nuclear features that are characteristic of each cell type. Accurate identification of a cell, in light microscopy (H&E), is not always achieved because of intermediate and uncertain forms (Fig. 6-19). In the cerebellar cortex, the following special elements are recognized: external granule cells, Purkinje cells, basket cells, internal granule cells, and Bergmann glia (Fig. 6-20). Normally, the external granule-cell layer of the cerebellum disappears after the first year of life. Corpora amylacea (Fig. 6-2) are normal components of human brain and spinal cord, increasing with age;[122] they are more abundant in perivascular, subpial, and subependymal locations.

Dense microsphere (DM) is the designation suggested for a round, eosinophilic structure (average diameter about 5.0 μm) normally found in the neuropil of the human cerebral cortex. Ultrastructurally, DMs are made of a homogeneously electron-dense material, surrounded by a membrane. The significance of DM is presently unknown;

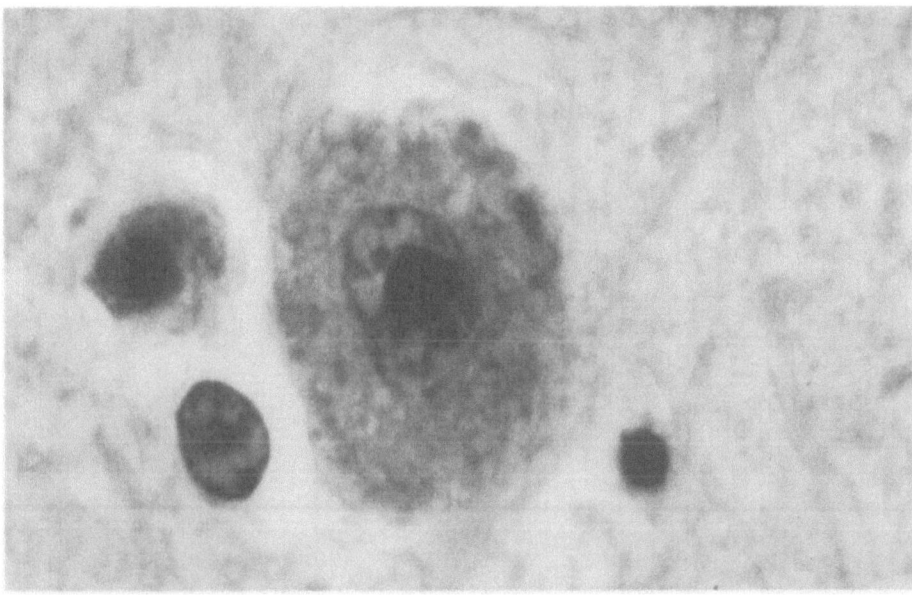

Fig. 6-17. Large pyramidal neuron from the motor cortex of an adult (56-year-old) who died with acute myelogenous leukemia. A large, prominent nucleolus is easily visible. Neurons, smaller than the one shown, may not be easily identified in this type of preparation (×100).

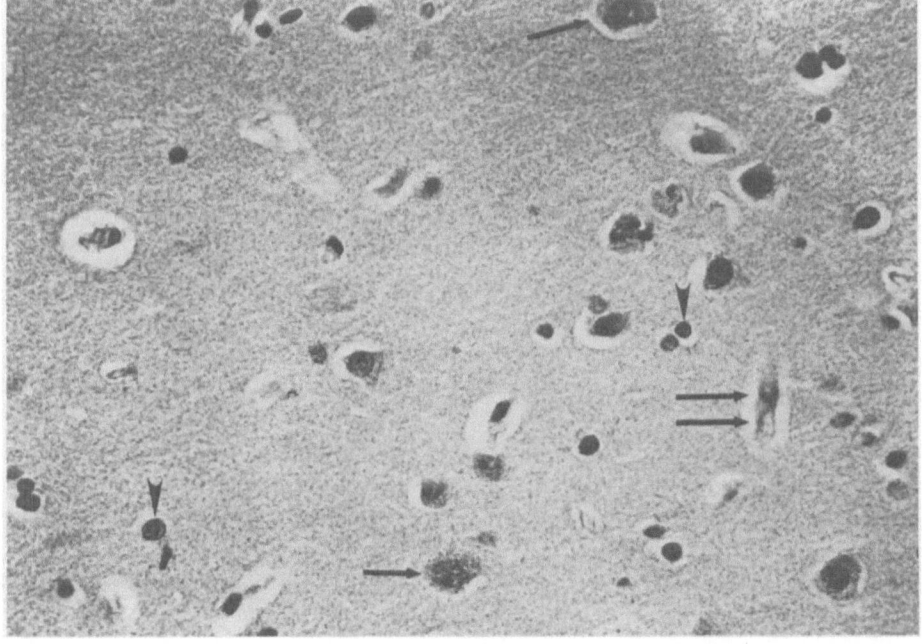

Fig. 6-18. Cerebral cortex from 67-year-old patient to demonstrate neurons (arrows), glial nuclei (arrowheads), and capillaries (double arrows). The areas where nuclei are not visible constitute the neuropil (×64).

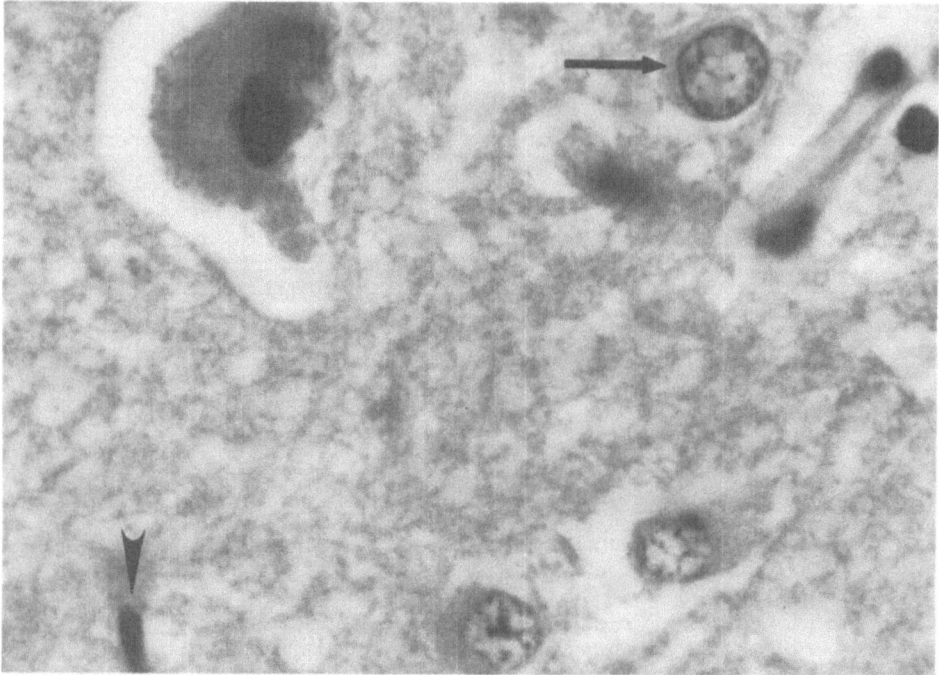

Fig. 6-19. Thirty-four-year-old leukemic patient who suffered an episode of cardiorespiratory arrest 10 days before death. Right parietal cortex showing shrunken neuron (left upper corner), swollen astrocyte (arrow), "rod cell" (arrowhead), and oligodendrocyte (right upper corner) (×100).

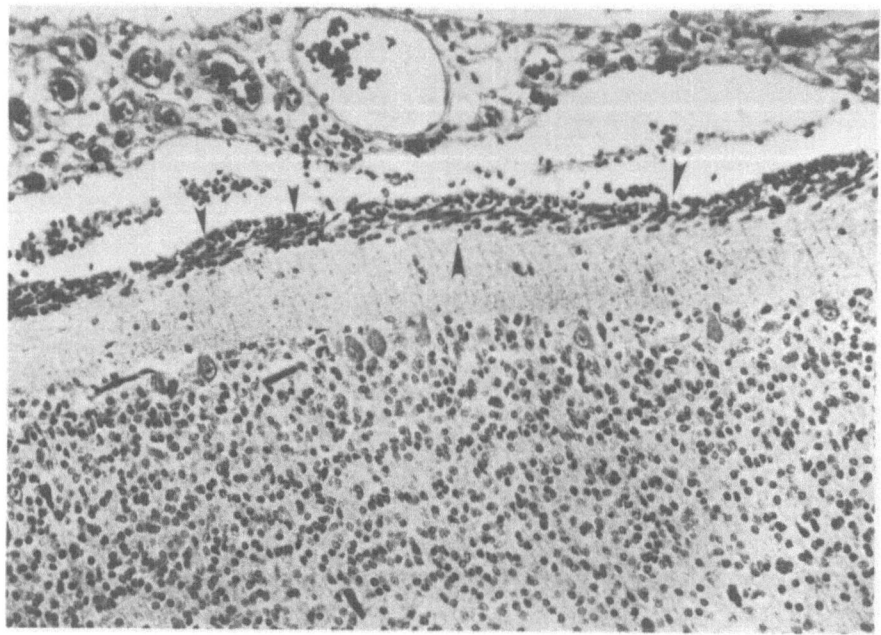

Fig. 6-20. Normal cerebellar cortex, full-term newborn; leptomeninges are visible at the top. The external granular cell layer (arrowheads) is visible beneath the pia and outside the molecular layer. Purkinje cell layer and internal granular cells are also visible (×64).

the frequency with which this structure is found in samples of cerebral cortex seems to be inversely related to age.[5]

Hirano body is the designation given to fusiform or cylindrically shaped, eosinophilic structures measuring up to 30 μm in length and about 10 μm in diameter; they are frequently present in the neuropil of the pyramidal cell layer (hippocampus) of elderly individuals. Hirano bodies appear to be either perikaryal or dendritic aggregates of paracrystalline structures. The number of Hirano bodies in human brain tissues appears to increase as a reflection of nonspecific neuronal "degeneration."[132]

The definition and significance of structural abnormalities affecting the neuronal soma are discussed with regard to diagnosis in human brain biopsies. All tissues removed at biopsy are subjected to two types of injury before fixation: acute ischemia, secondary to the hemostatic procedures; and mechanical trauma. The combined effects of some of these manipulations are referred to as "fixation artifacts," a designation implying incorrectly that the fixative may be the cause of alterations such as those illustrated in Fig. 6-21. Undesirable effects that may interfere with the microscopic evaluation of the sample can be minimized by prompt immersion of the sample in the fixative and minimal handling of the unfixed specimen. Some of the earliest changes observed in tissues totally deprived of circulation for several minutes include: clumping of nuclear chromatin, dilatation of rough endoplasmic reticulum and Golgi cisternae, and pallor of Nissl granules[47,50,155] (Figs. 6-22 A,C).

Changes in Neuronal Stainability and Neuronal Volume

One of the most common alterations affecting the stainability and volume of neuronal perikaryon has been designated "dark neuron." This abnormality has been variously

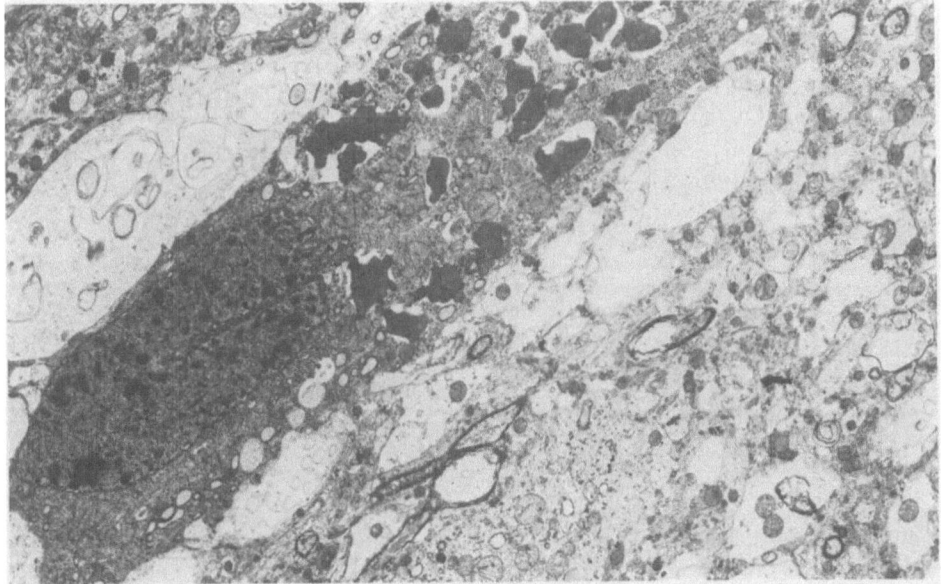

Fig. 6-21. Cerebral cortex from area traumatized during surgical removal; the development of dark neurons in this sample from a normal cat brain was attributed to the manipulation of unfixed tissue (×3,000).

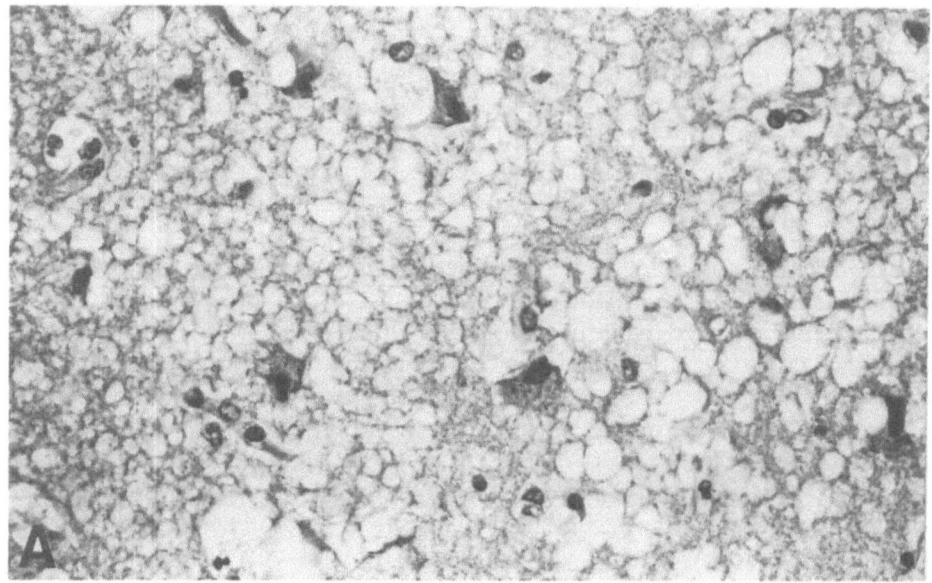

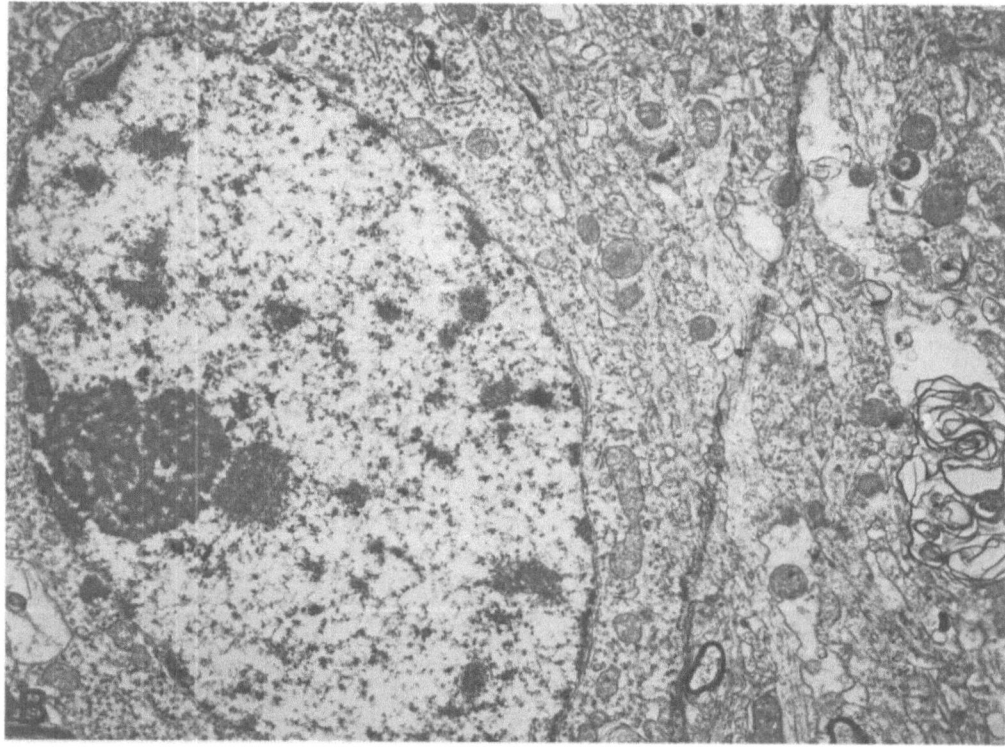

Fig. 6-22. (A) Cerebral cortex; patient had transient cardiac arrest, followed by permanent coma and death 10 days later. The significant difference (compared to the abnormality shown in Fig. 6.21) is the heterogeneous vacuolation of the neuropil (×63); (B&C) Cerebral cortex of cat subjected to complete ischemia of about 30 min. duration (without reperfusion). Clumping of chromatin granules, mitochrondrial swelling, and formation of vacuoles and myelin figures could be seen both in neurons and glial cells. (Original magnification ×4,000).

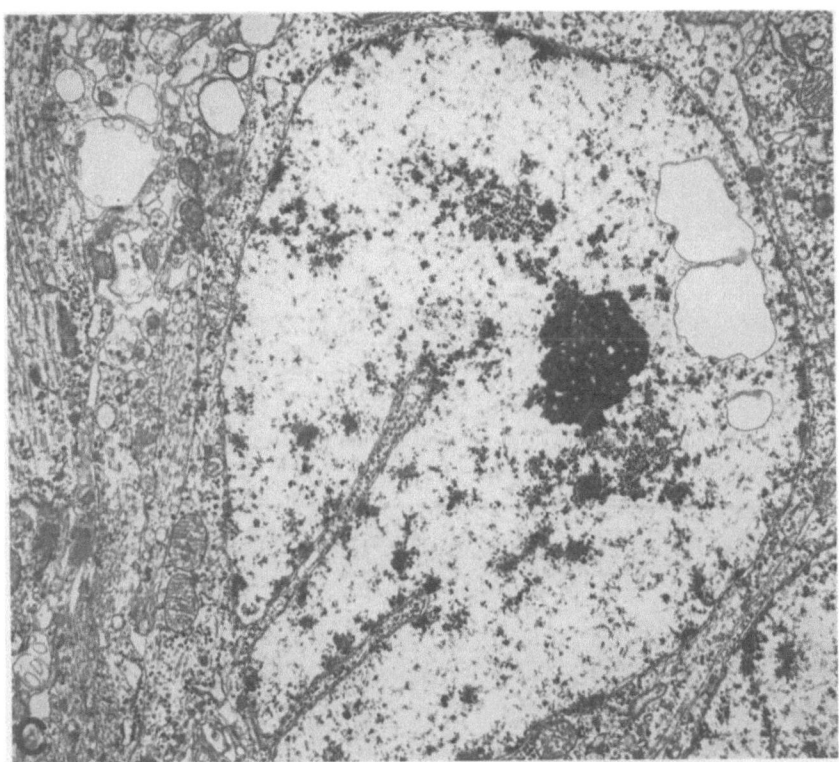

attributed to "artifact" (not further defined), hypoxia or ischemia. Unfortunately, many of these interpretations are not based on data derived from appropriately designed experiments. Thus, the significance of "dark neurons" in human neuropathology remains controversial.

Dark neurons (Figs. 6-23 A-C) are not seen in normal cerebral tissues, maintained at 37°C, and fixed *in situ* as late as 2 hours after death.[47,50] Dark neurons (Fig. 6-24), however, are readily seen in fragments of the cortex, obtained from normal animals, whose brain was biopsied in a manner similar to that used in human neurosurgical procedures, (i.e., under general barbiturate anesthesia and through a burr hole).[44] Dark neurons are also seen in tissues that are either partially or transiently ischemic;[45,82] these cells also appear in the brains of normal cats whose intracranial contents were exposed to the atmosphere for a short time.[77] Deafferentation,[22] as well as incomplete osmotic stabilization, may also induce the development of dark neurons.[113]

According to Cammermeyer,[19] in situ perfusion fixation of animal brain tissues by means of cardiovascular perfusion precludes the formation of dark neurons. He suggested that the trauma inflicted by the manipulation of incompletely fixed tissues was the mechanism responsible for the appearance of dark neurons in brains fixed by immersion. Significantly, in most normal animal brains, the cortical dark neuron is an isolated feature in the midst of an otherwise intact cortical ribbon. Markedly different are the dark neurons appearing in animal brains made ischemic several hours before in vivo fixation was applied to the organ. In this instance, the darkly stained neurons exist amidst numerous other alterations including deformities of neuronal perikaryon, vacuolation of neuropil, and hypertrophy of astrocytes[43] (Figs. 6-25, 6-26). In general, dark

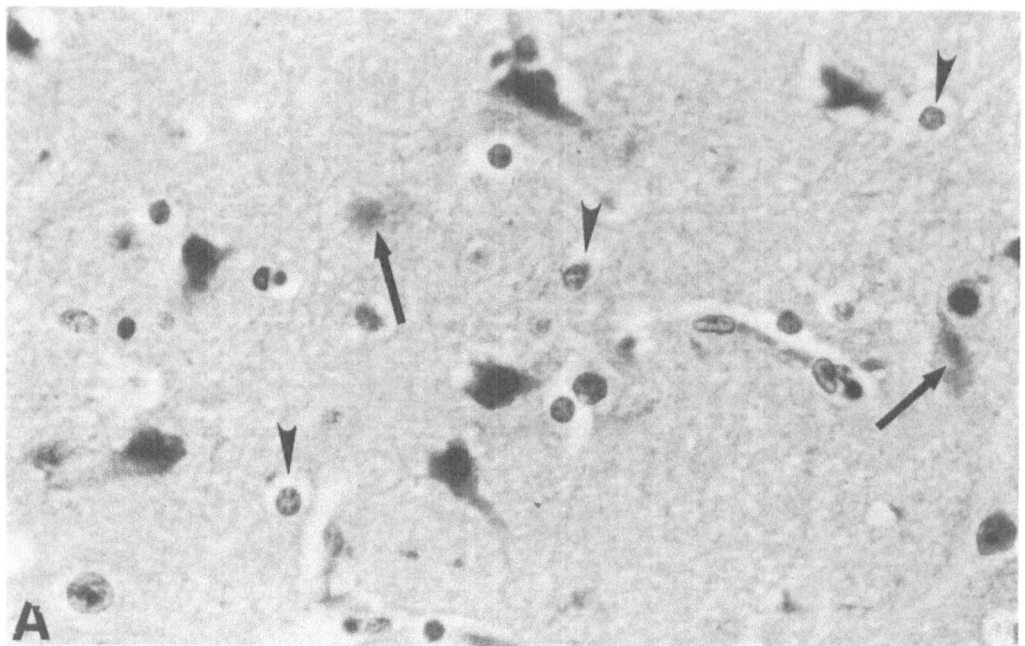

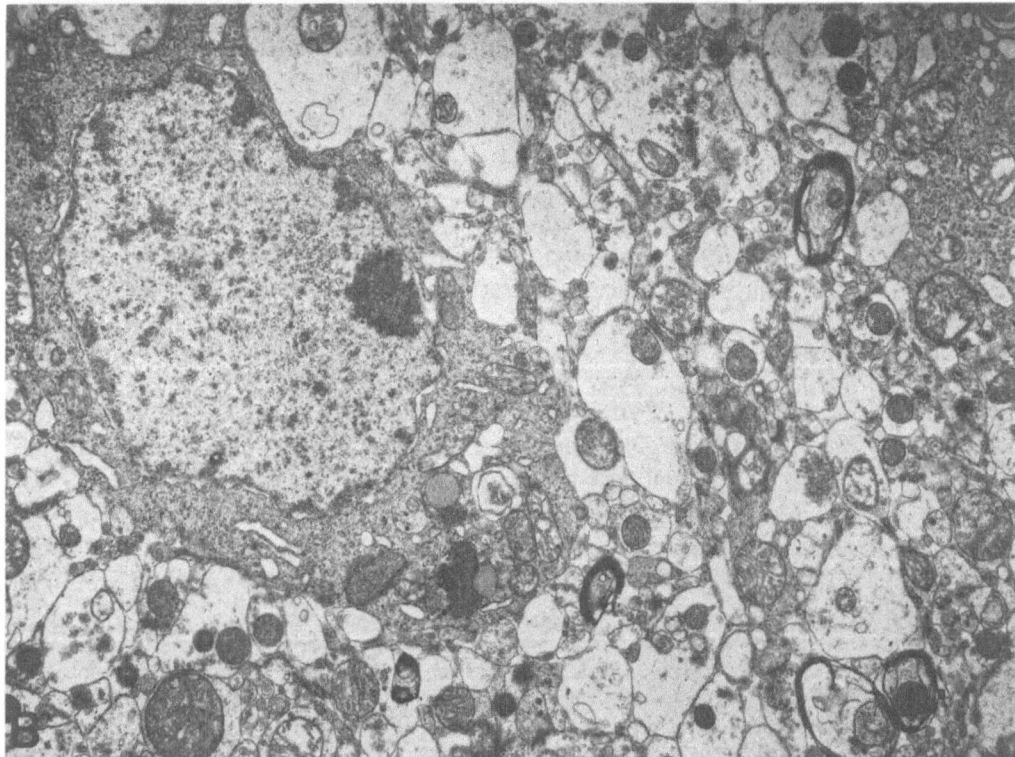

Fig. 6-23. (A) Human cerebral cortex; ischemia secondary to arterial occlusion occurring about 24 hours before sample was fixed. Most neurons are shrunken and angular, some are swollen (left lower corner), others are barely stainable (arrows), while astrocytes are progressively swollen and prominent (arrowheads) (×64); (B) Experimental brain infarction (about 4 hours old) showing neuronal shrinkage and characteristic heterogeneous vacuolation of neuropil. (Original magnification ×3,000); (C) Cerebral cortex from same animal and same area as in Fig. 6-23 *B*, to demonstrate massive swelling of astrocytic nucleus and cytoplasm in the face of minimal mitochondrial changes. (Original magnification ×4,500).

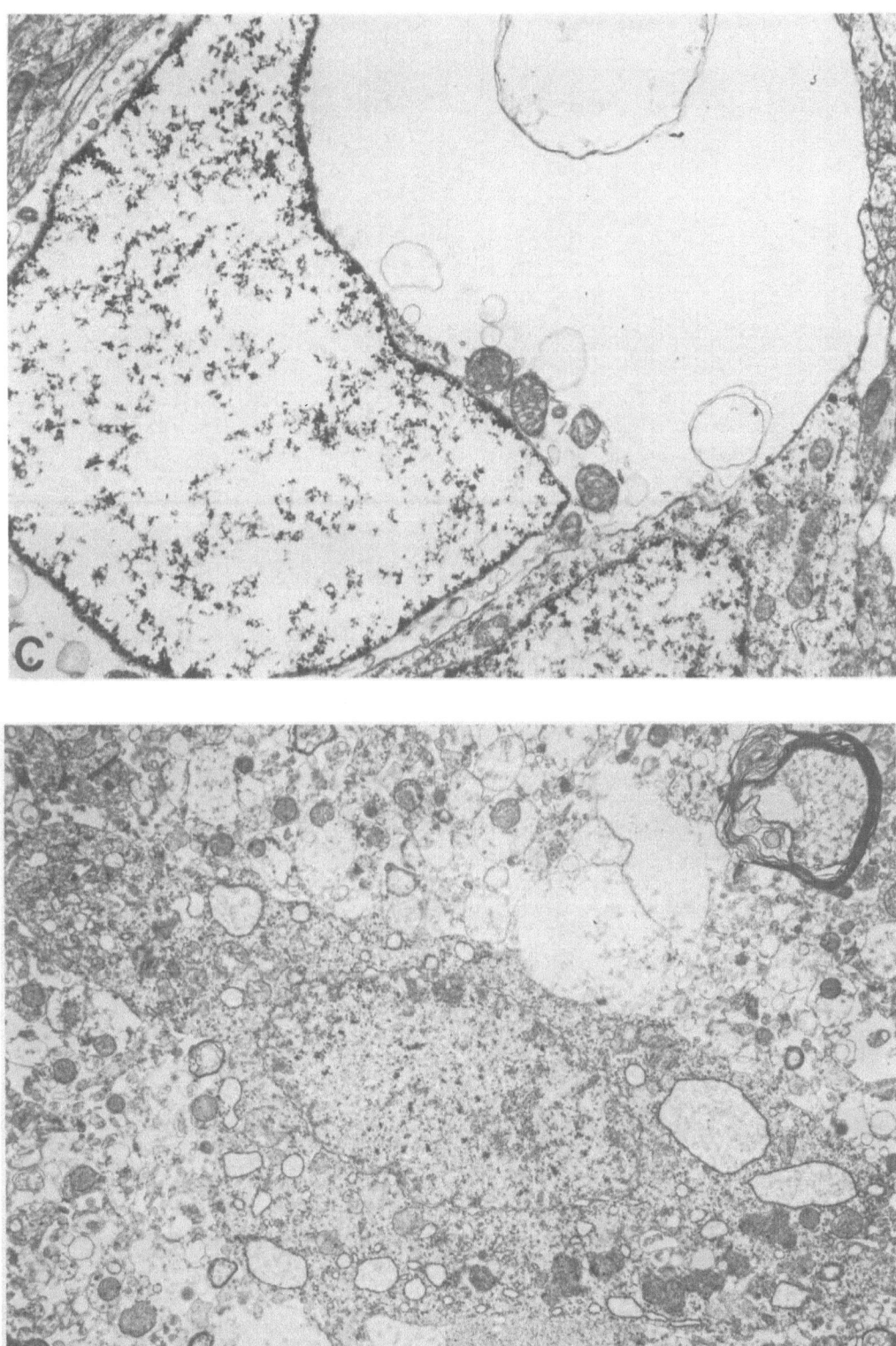

Fig. 6-24. Sample of normal cerebral cortex (cat) biopsied through a burr hole and fixed by immersion after a short delay; the neuron is shrunken and the endoplasmic reticulum cisternae are dilated. (Courtesy of Y. Kamijyo, M.D.) (Original magnification ×3,000).

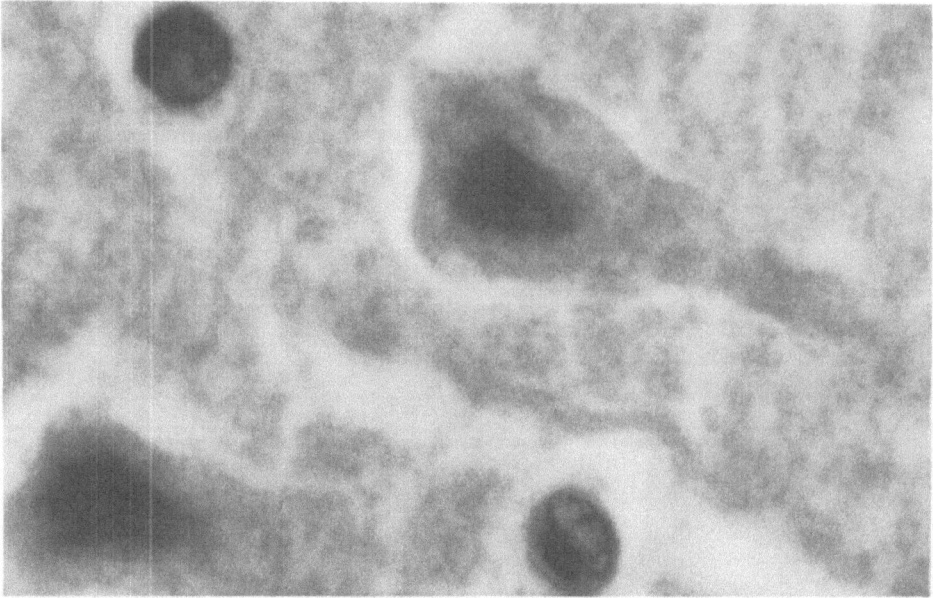

Fig. 6-25. "Red neurons." Pyramidal cells from hippocampus showing pyknotic nucleus and absence of cytoplasmic, hematoxynophilic substances; glial nuclei show slightly better preserved chromatin granules (×200).

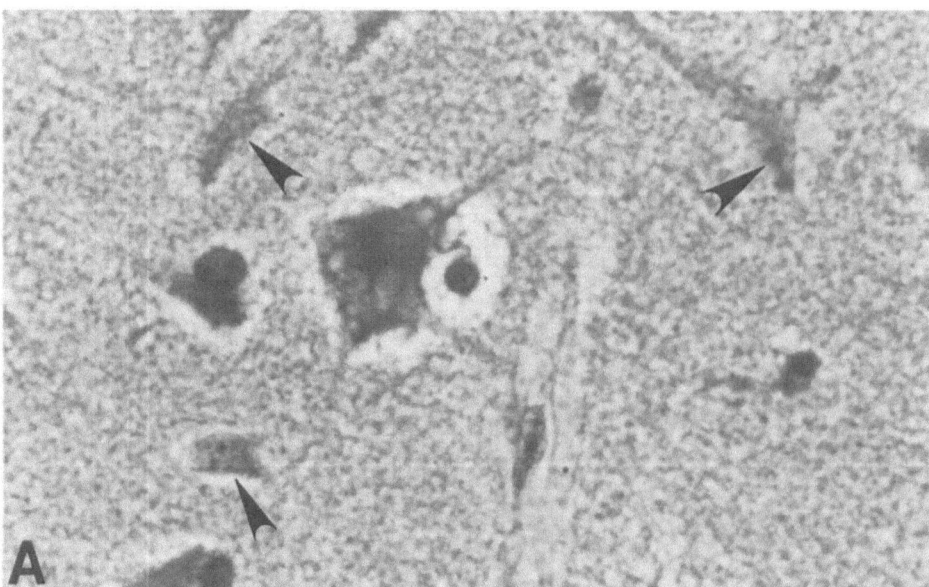

Fig. 6-26. (A) Cerebral cortex (cat) made partially ischemic several hours earlier by ligating an artery. Neuronal features are blurred giving rise to "ghost" cells (arrowheads), while the neuron in the center contains vacuoles and is now surrounded by a halo (×100). (B) Twenty-four-hour-old lesion secondary to MCA occlusion demonstrating swelling of astrocytic and dendritic processes and various stages of injury to neuronal perikaryon (×2,500). (C) Internal capsule from animal subjected to temporary arterial occlusion. The sponginess of the white matter corresponds in this instance to alterations in myelin sheaths (×3,000).

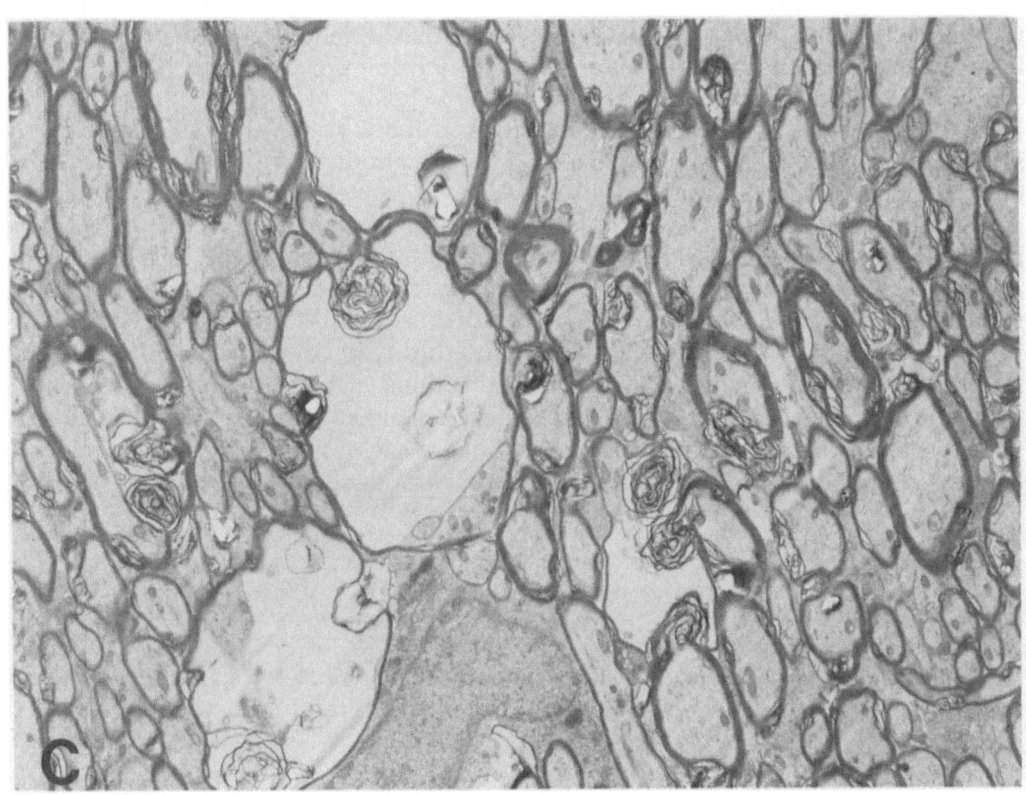

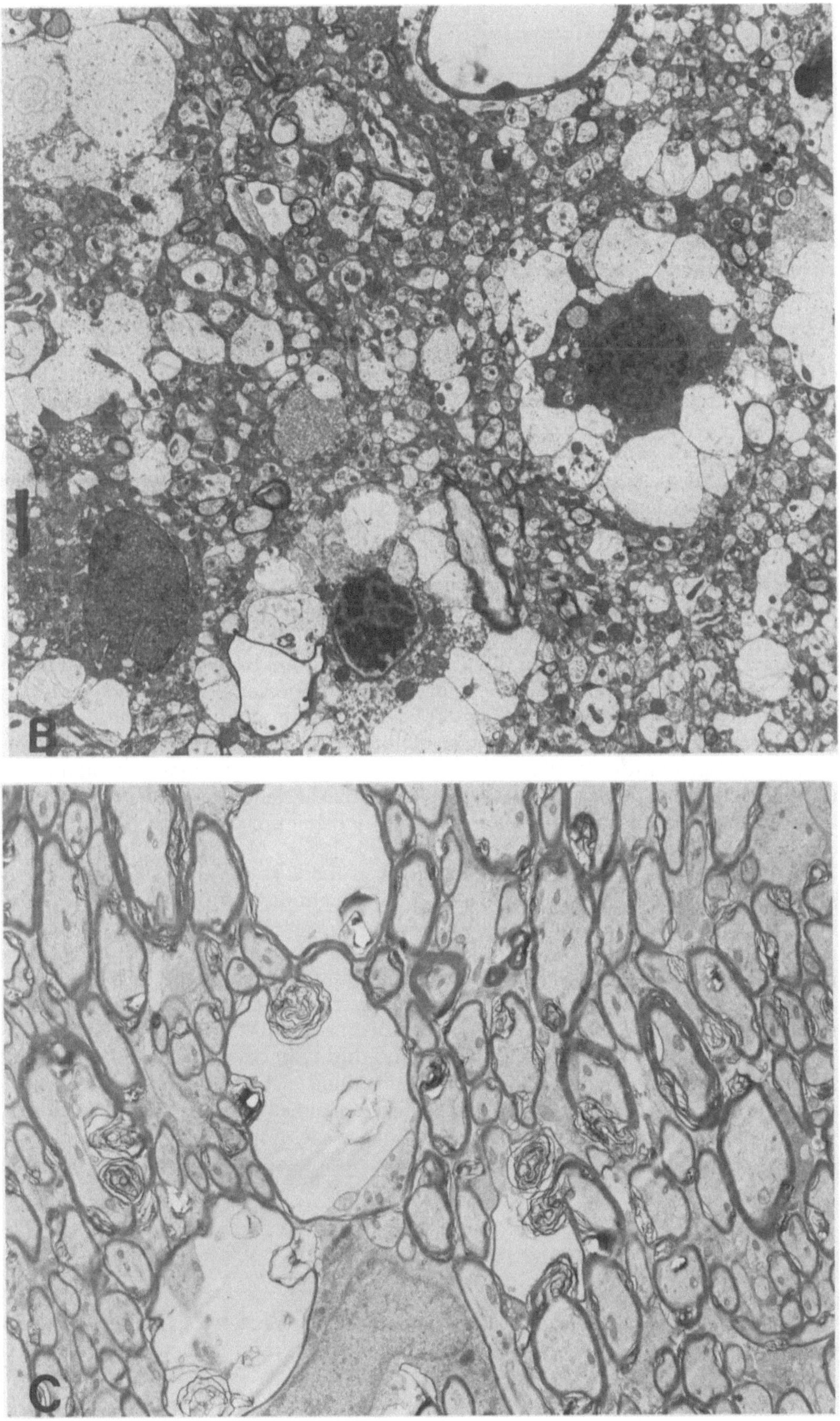

neurons can be interpreted as cytologic abnormalities of an acute nature that develop during or shortly after the time when the brain is biopsied.

Red neurons are cells with intensively eosinophilic cytoplasm having a pyknotic nucleus (Fig. 6-25). This cellular change has traditionally been regarded as an indicator of acute lethal injury, especially ischemic in origin. Red neurons are a reliable indicator of acute injury. When the structural/staining abnormalities involve almost exclusively neurons, in the absence of cellular inflammatory changes, it is safe to interpret this neuronal alteration as being of ischemic origin. Dark neurons are equally reliable indicators of preoperative injury provided these cellular changes coexist with other indicators of ischemia such as vacuolation of neuropil and astrocytic swelling. The environmental conditions necessary to induce the transformation of a normal neuron into a red one can be developed in vitro only when the medium's pH is maintained close to 7.0.[156] Postmorten ischemia is accompanied by marked acidosis attributed to lactate accumulation. Consequently, red neurons in human tissues are reliable indicators of in vivo lethal cell injury of a recent age. In experimental ischemic brain injuries, red neurons are seen mostly at sites of incomplete ischemia (i.e., interface between infarcted and normal tissues) of about 12–18 hours' duration.[45,49] Brierley[13] has suggested that in addition to ischemia, red neurons are indicators of acute neuronal injury by either hypoglycemia or hypoxemia.

During the early stages (15–60 minutes) of regional or incomplete brain ischemia, two sets of structural alterations are characteristic: heterogenous, multifocal changes of neuronal soma (Figs. 6-26 A–C); and sponginess of neuropil.[45,50] The low-magnification appearance given by this type of multivacuolated neuropil has been designated status spongiosus, an abnormality that does not develop in the complete absence of energy substrates, (e.g., postmortem).[83] Status spongiosus is an identifying feature of either incomplete ischemia (as is typical of incipient brain infarctions) or transmissible encephalopathy of "slow viruses"[47] (Fig. 6-27). In the United States, the most common of the transmissible spongiform encephalopathies is Creutzfeldt-Jakob disease (C-J). The differential diagnosis between this disease and an early ischemic process could pose difficulties, especially because all brain biopsies are partially ischemic. Nevertheless, the otherwise normal appearance of the vacuolated neurons in the C-J, the ultrastructural demonstration of curled membranes in either astrocytes or neurons, and the intense astrocytosis of C-J can help identify this condition in most cerebral or cerebellar biopsies.[88] Spongiform changes involving the very superficial or molecular layer of the cerebral cortex have been found also in patients with senile dementia of the Alzheimer type.[37] Some dementing processes are transmissible when tissues (e.g., cornea) from patients having status spongiosus are grafted onto normal recipients. Because the risk that such transmissibility poses to the laboratory personnel, special procedures aimed at inactivating the tissue infectivity have been recommended for the handling of biopsies from patients with dementia of unknown origin.[7] These procedures are aimed at protecting the laboratory personnel from potentially infectious tissues. Brain tissues from patients with spongiform encephalopathy lose their infectivity after being submerged for a short period in a weak hypochlorite solution.[7]

Inborn Errors of Metabolism

Reasonably good evidence exists that inborn enzymatic defects are the underlying cause of at least 150 metabolic disorders, many of which result in neurologic disorders

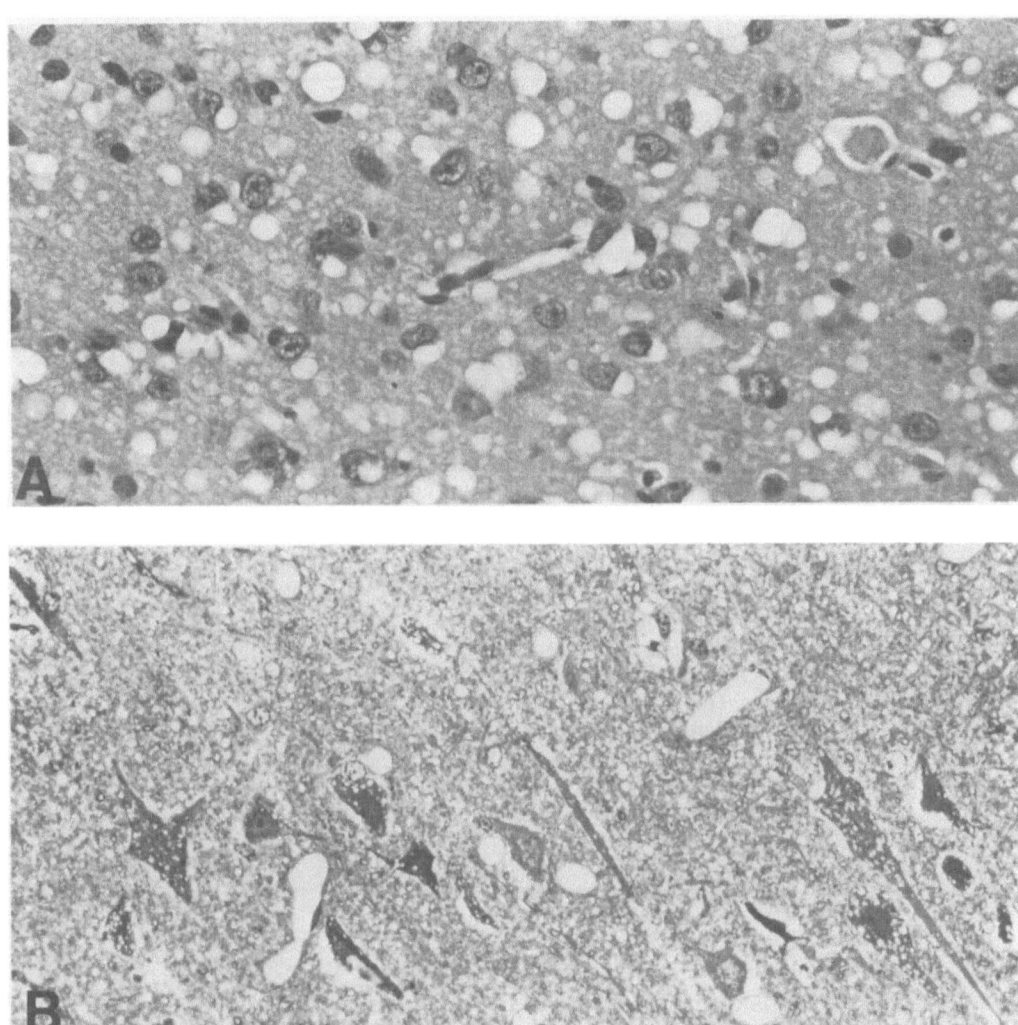

Fig. 6-27. (A) Status spongiosus from a case of spongiform encephalopathy. Multiple vacuoles of various sizes (some of them in the neuronal perikaryon) contribute to the spongy appearance of the cortex; preservation of nuclear features in the neurons and absence of leukocytic infiltrates are also apparent (×64); (B) Cerebral cortex from an area made ischemic by arterial ligation 60 min. before *in situ* fixation to demonstrate the nature of sponginess. Numerous vacuoles are visible in the neuronal perikarya. (Toluidine blue; ×100).

that usually become manifest during childhood.[12] Prominent members of this group are the lysosomal storage diseases (Table 6.1). In past years the diagnosis of these conditions was sometimes attempted by brain biopsy. Nowadays, and with few exceptions, the diagnosis of inherited metabolic disorders of the CNS can be achieved through: (1) assays of enzyme activity in serum, peripheral blood leukocytes, and cultured skin fibroblasts; (2) the microscopic evaluation of biopsies from the skin, conjunctiva, or peripheral nerve, and (3) ulstructural examination of circulating white blood cells, cultured fibroblasts, and amniotic cells.

Table 6-1.
Lysosomal Storage Diseases

1. Glycogenoses
   Type II (Pompe disease)
2. Sphingolipidoses
   GM 1 gangliosidosis
       Type 1 generalized; Type 2, juvenile
   GM 2 gangliosidosis
       Tay-Sachs disease; Sandhoff disease
   Sulfatidoses (metachromatic leukodystrophy)
       Type 1, infantile; Type 2, juvenile; Type 3, adult;
       Type 4, multiple sulfatase deficiency
   Krabbe disease (globoid cell leukodystrophy)
   Fabry disease (hereditary dystopic lipidosis)
   Gaucher disease (glucosylceramide lipidosis)
       a. chronic non neuronopathic; b. acute neurono-
       pathic, infantile; c. subacute neuronopathic, juve-
       nile
   Niemann Pick disease (sphingomyelinosis)
       a. acute neuronopathic; b. chronic non neurologic;
       c. chronic neuronopathic; d. Nova Scotia variant
   Farber disease (lipogranulomatosis)
3. Mucopolysaccharidoses (MPS)
   Hurler syndrome (MPS I-H)
   Hunter syndrome (MPS II)
   Sanfilippo disease (MPS III)
   Morquio disease (MPS IV)
   Maroteaux Lamy syndrome (MPS VI)
   Beta glucuronidase deficiency (MPS VII)
4. Oligosaccharidoses
5. Miscellaneous

Modified from Kolodny[85] and Becker, Yates.[8]

Three large groups of inborn errors of metabolism are recognized:[85]

1. Disorders of amino acid metabolism, (e.g., phenylketonuria).
2. Lysosomal storage diseases, (e.g., sphingolipidoses).
3. Inherited metabolic diseases without known enzyme deficiencies. Particularly prominent in this group are adrenoleukodystrophy and neuronal ceroid-lipofuscinoses.

Diagnostic approaches commonly used in presumptive cases of inborn metabolic errors include:[85]

1. CT scan or MRI of the head and evoked potential recordings (in cases of suspected leukodystrophy).
2. Ultrastructural evaluation of skin, conjunctiva, circulating leukocytes, peripheral nerve, cultured skin fibroblasts, and (for prenatal diagnosis) electron microscopy of cultured amniotic cells.
3. Thin layer chromatography of a few drops of urine is particularly useful for the identification of some gangliosidoses, mannosidosis, fucosidosis, and mucolipidoses.[75]

4. High-performance liquid chromatography (HPLC) has been applied to the study of urine, plasma, and tissues for the diagnosis of various diseases including GM-2 gangliosidosis and Fabry disease.[24]

Brain tissues biopsied for the purpose of establishing the diagnosis of a suspected metabolic disorder should be both fresh frozen and fixed in aldehydes for light and electron microscopic evaluation. Becker and Yates[8] recommend, as a minimum, applying the following special staining methods to both paraffin-embedded and fresh-frozen histologic sections: oil red 0, Sudan black B, and Luxol fast blue for lipids; periodic acid-Schiff with and without diastase for glycogen and other carbohydrate derived products; acid cresyl violet and toluidine for metachromatic substances; and mucicarmine and Alcian blue for mucopolysaccharides.

Most glycogenoses (eleven varieties have been described) involve tissues other than the brain with the exception of glycogenosis type II (Pompe disease). In the infantile form, neuronal perikarya distended with fine droplets of PAS positive material have been described in dorsal root ganglia, spinal anterior horns, and motor neurons of the brain stem. In the cerebral white matter glycogen deposits may be found in astrocytes and various other cells, including the smooth muscle cells of small arteries.[41] The tissue diagnosis of Pompe disease and most other glycogenosis may be readily established in a skeletal muscle biopsy, as discussed in Chapter 8.

Of the sphingolipidoses shown in Table 6.1, *GM-2 gangliosidosis* (Tay-Sachs disease) is the most common in a group of rare disorders. GM-2 gangliosidosis is characterized, in cerebral or cerebellar cortices, by swollen and deformed neuronal perikarya. The Nissl substance and nucleoplasm are eccentrically displaced; this change is accompanied by minimal cellular inflammation (Figs 6-28, 6-29). Swollen, deformed axons, called perikaryal torpedoes (or meganeurites) are found in the late stages of the disease. The ganglioside can be recognized by the ultrastructural appearance of the cytoplasmic inclusions (Fig. 6-30), which also can be detected in lymphocytes[109] and in neurons located outside the central nervous system such as those of the autonomic ganglia and myenteric plexus.[1] During the early stages of the disease, structural changes are limited to the neuromal soma, but later either magalencephaly or brain atrophy may be observed, and severe neuronal loss is accompanied by extensive gliosis.[158]

The structural abnormalities (light and electron microscopy) of brain biopsies from children with *GM-1 gangliosidosis* (or familial neuroviscerolipidosis) may overlap with those of GM-2 gangliosidosis;[62,143] however, the clinical features of the two diseases (GM-2 and GM-1 gangliosidosis) are significantly different from one another. Somatic deformities, similar to those found in Hurler syndrome (MPS-I), evidence of multisystem involvement at birth are common in GM-1 gangliosidosis, whereas these features are not seen in patients with GM-2 gangliosidosis.

Cerebral cortical neurons do not accumulate lipid in cases of glucosylceramide lipidosis (Gaucher's disease), even in the neuronopathic infantile form or type II.[39] Neuronal storage of the ganglioside has been observed in basal ganglia, thalamus, Purkinje cells, brain stem, and spinal motor neurons; neuronophagia is usually evident at the same sites.[8]

Sphingomyelinosis (Niemann Pick disease) may be indistinguishable by light microscopy from GM-2 gangliosidosis (Fig. 6-31), although some ultrastructural features (Fig. 6-32) partly differentiate the two conditions.[4] Systemically, abundant foamy cells may be found in most tissues derived from patients with sphingomyelinosis.

In Table 6.1, mucopolysaccharidosis type I (Hurler's syndrome; gargoylism) in brain

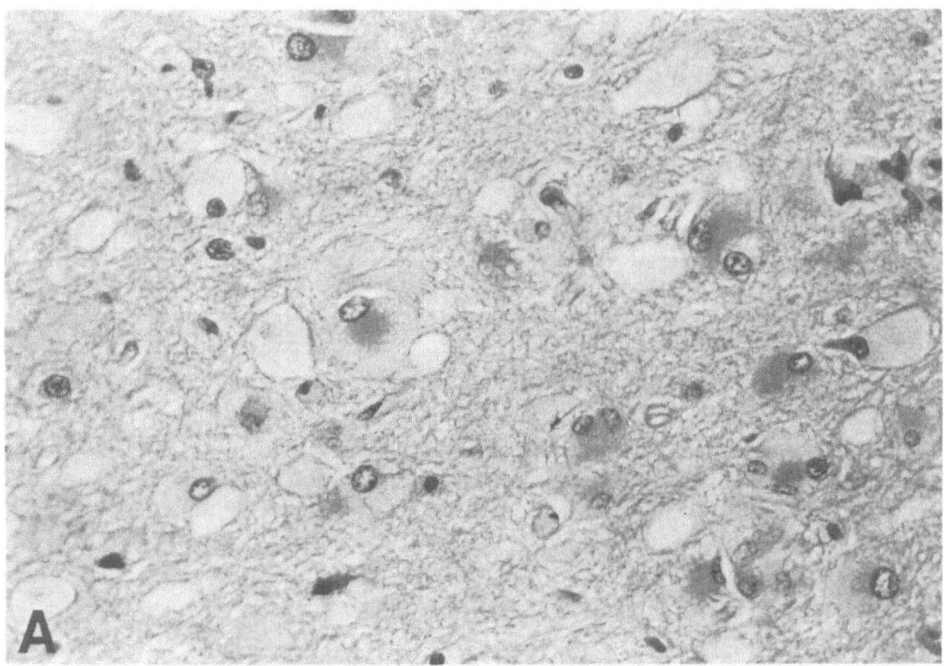

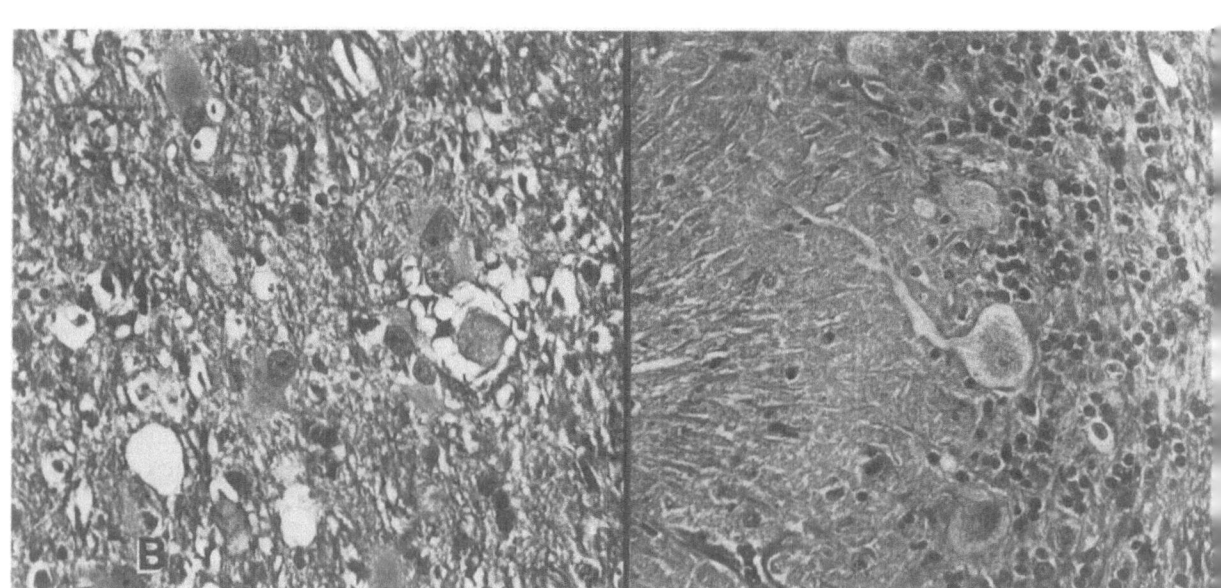

Fig. 6-28. Gangliosidosis GM-2. (A) Cerebral cortex: several large neurons are distended and globular; smaller cells are macrophages and astroglia (×16). (B) Cerebellar cortex (right) showing depletion of internal granular cells and swelling of Purkinje cells. White matter (left) showing rarefaction, gliosis, and spheroids.

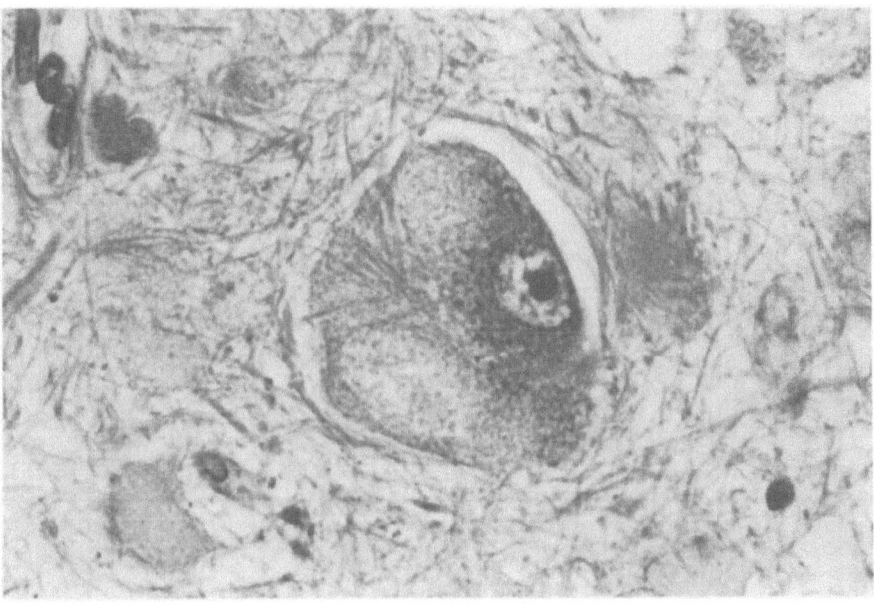

Fig. 6-29. Gangliosidosis GM-2. This is same case as in Fig. 6-28 and demonstrates the detail of abnormalities in neuronal perikaryon (×100).

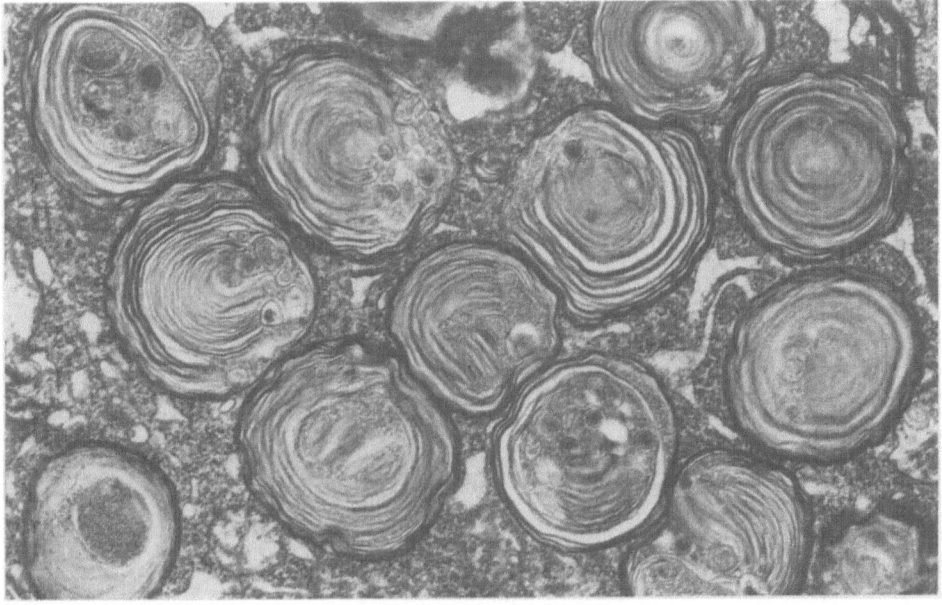

Fig. 6-30. Gangliosidosis GM-2. Characteristic ultrastructural features of the stored lipid (membranous concentric bodies) in the perikaryon of affected neurons (×25,000).

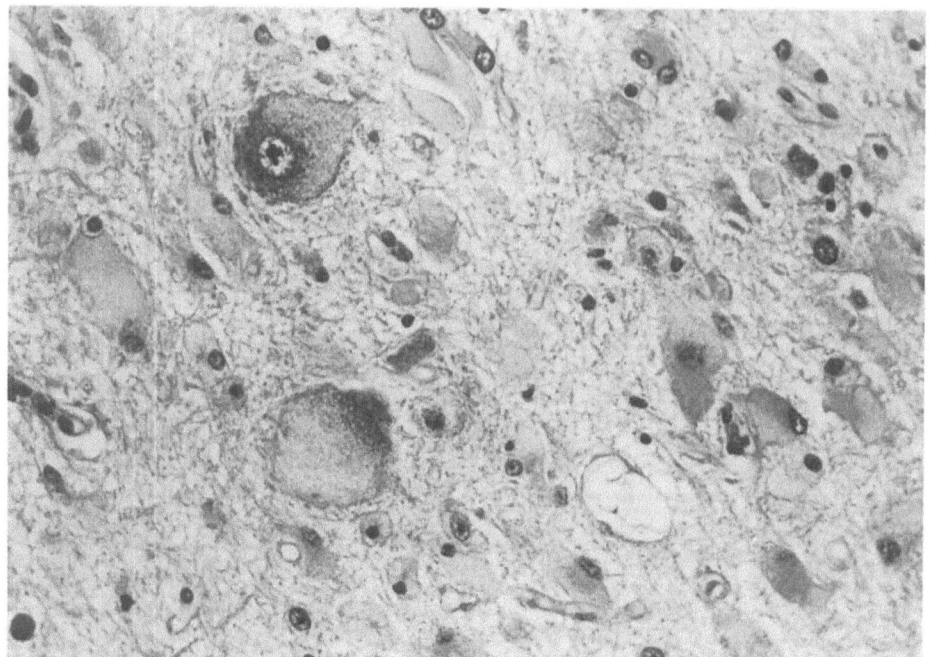

Fig. 6-31. Sphingomyelinosis (Niemann-Pick). Cerebral cortex showing enlarged neurons, filled with finely granular material, and reactive glial cells (×16).

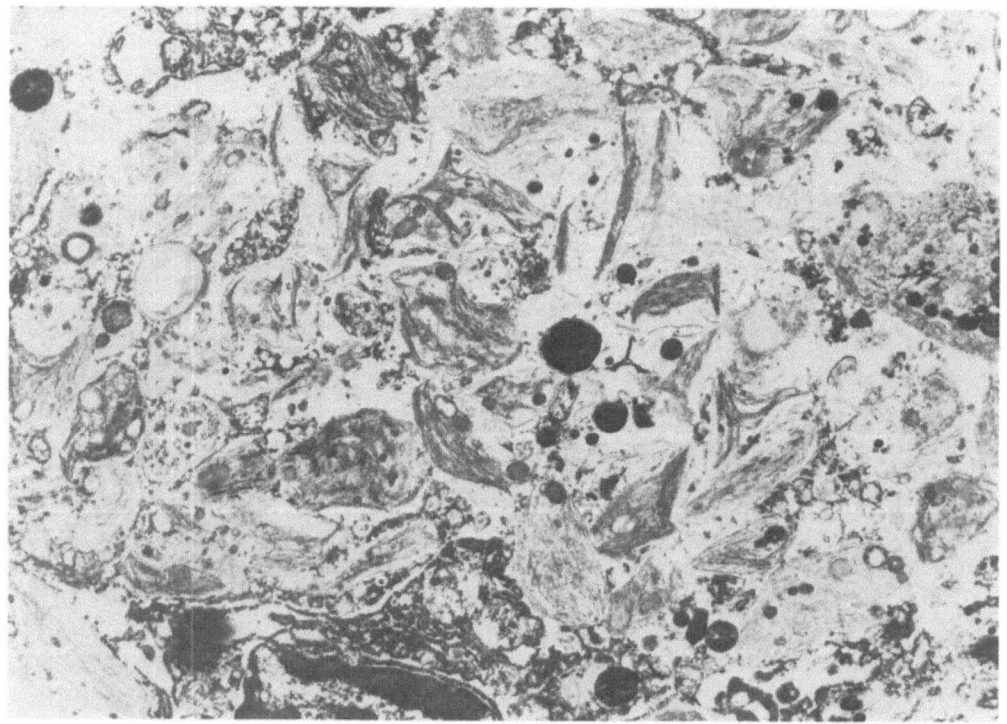

Fig. 6-32. Sphingomyelinosis (Niemann-Pick). In most instances, the lipid particles differ substantially from the membranous concentric bodies of gangliosidosis GM-2 shown in Fig. 6-30. (Original magnification ×15,000).

biopsies shares a few light-microscopic features with some of the previously described lipidoses; however, the ultrastructural appearance of most glycosaminoglycans (GAGs) is that of "zebra bodies," and these substances are strongly PAS-positive.[29] Additional differentiating features (at the ultrastructural level) include a large number of membrane-bound pleomorphic bodies that are easily seen in cerebral cortical neurons and in many extraneural tissues such as the liver, spleen and rectal mucosa.[8]

Mucopolysaccharidosis and oligosaccharidosis are best diagnosed by applying thin-layer chromatography to the examination of urine.[75] Neuronal ceroid lipofuscinosis, adrenal leukodystrophy, and Alexander's disease are conditions lacking a known metabolic defect. Their diagnostic features are described under the respective headings of: pigments in the neuronal perikaryon and meningeal cells, and leukodystrophies.

Neuronal Inclusion Bodies

Inclusion bodies are discrete, roughly round, or spherical structures appearing as extraneous, intracellular material[23] described in brain tissues as two types of *intranuclear* inclusions (A and B) visible with the light microscope. Of these, only type A is consistently found in association with viral infections. This inclusion body is usually single, eosino-philic, homogeneous, and displaces the nuclear chromatin in a symmetrical and centrifugal manner (Fig. 6-33). Although many types of inclusion bodies occur in neurons,[133] only a few types are discussed here because of their potential significance in the interpretation of cortical brain biopsies.

Negri bodies were originally described in 1903 in the brains of patients with rabies encephalitis. In H&E preparations, they appear as sharply defined, round, dark eosino-philic, intracytoplasmic structures measuring 5–10 µm (Fig. 6.34). More than one inclu-

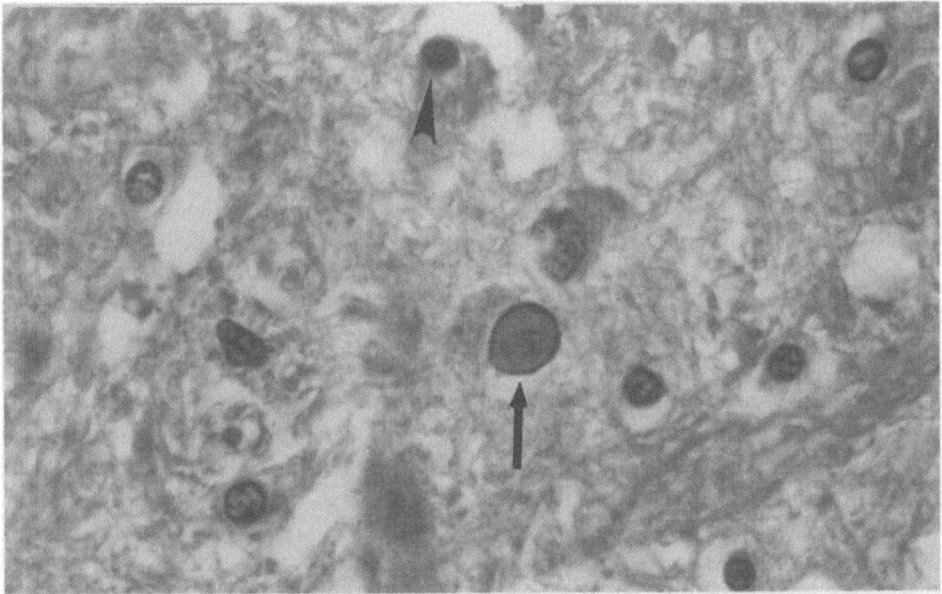

Fig. 6-33. Intranuclear inclusion body (Cowdry type A) in oligodendrocyte (arrow), to be contrasted with the appearance of normal oligodendrocyte (arrowhead) (×100).

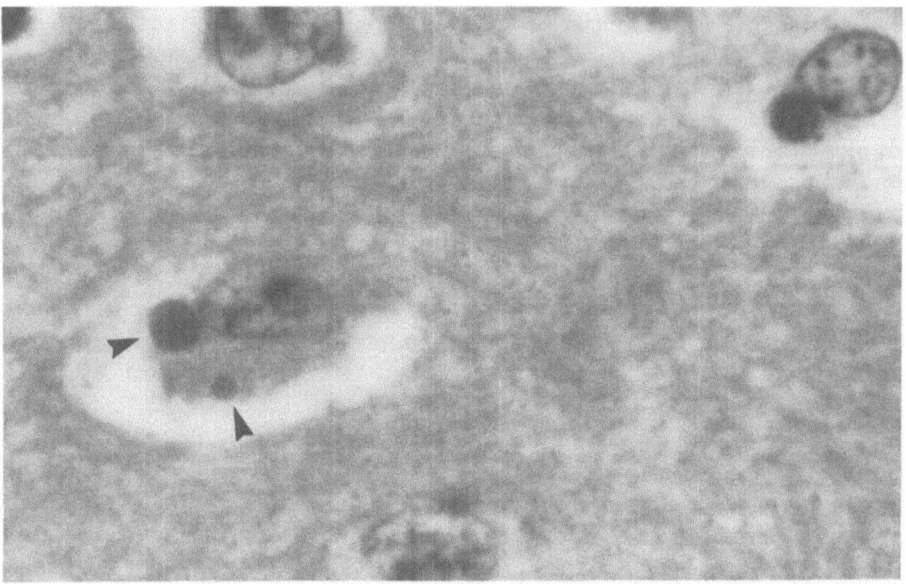

Fig. 6-34. Brain sample from a 40-year-old man with fever, stupor, and hydrophobia of 3 days' duration. Two intracytoplasmic inclusion bodies (arrowheads) are visible in this cortical neuron. A diagnosis of rabies encephalitis was confirmed serologically (×400).

sion may be visible in a single neuron. Inflammation is sparse in areas where Negri bodies are abundant.[30] In patients with confirmed rabies, Negri bodies are more abundant in the neurons of the hippocampus, cerebellar cortex, and brain stem. Some Negri bodies are aggregates of virions and cell membranes,[117] but neither they nor the lyssa (i.e., rabies) bodies[30] are reliable indicators of rabies encephalitis. This diagnosis of rabies requires identification of the antigen by immunohistochemical methods.[27]

Lafora bodies are the structural hallmark of Lafora disease. The inclusion bodies are usually found in the neuronal perikaryon, but can also exist in other parts of the neuron. They also occur outside the neuron and may be abundant in the cerebral cortex; they are round and have an average diameter of 4.5 μm (range: 3–15 μm) (Fig. 6-35). Some inclusion bodies are dense and solid, but others have a Y-shaped split in the center. Lafora bodies may be seen both in neurons and glial cells. In H&E stained preparations, these inclusions may be difficult to distinguish from corpora amylacea. Lafora bodies occur in many tissues outside the central nervous system, particularly in muscle fibers and the liver.[135] Some glycogenoses with involvement of liver and skeletal muscle may be associated with intracellular structures resembling Lafora bodies. Electron microscopically, Lafora bodies are not membrane-bound; they are made of filaments and amorphous material easily impregnated with silver proteinate. Lafora bodies may be aggregates of polyglucosan,[42] and they are the hallmark of Lafora disease, one of the familial forms of organic epilepsy.

Pick's disease (PD) is a form of adult dementia having clinical features similar or identical to those of Alzheimer's disease (AD). In the absence of characteristic clinical or laboratory features by which these diseases may be diagnosed with certainty, brain biopsy usually constitutes a last resort procedure. Histologically, the two diseases may share a widespread loss of cortical neurons, especially apparent in the temporal lobe.

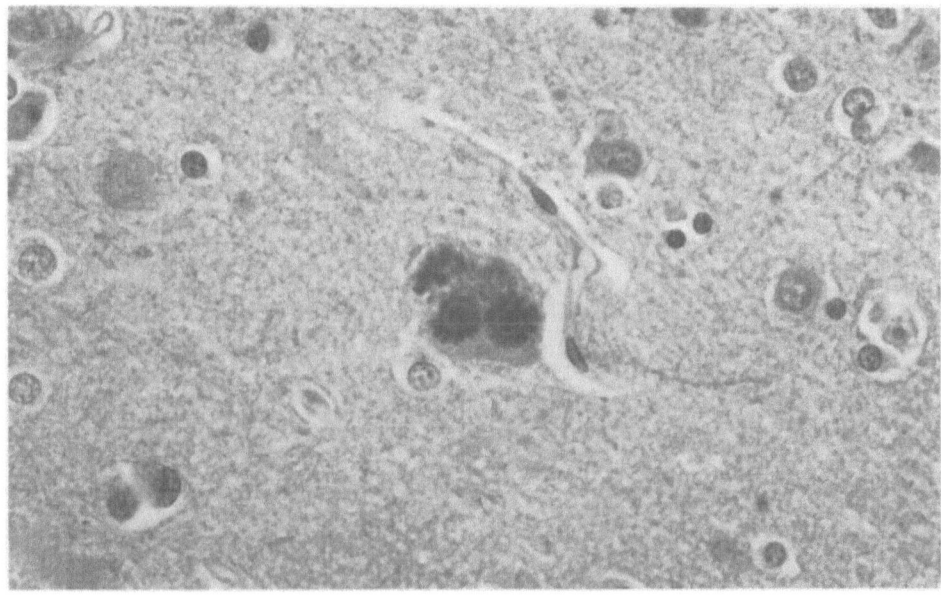

Fig. 6-35. Lafora body. Cerebral cortex: two types of intraneuronal inclusions (Lafora body) are shown in this presumably neuronal perikaryon (×250).

Two abnormalities are generally considered either characteristic of or compatible with a diagnosis of PD: (1) intracytoplasmic structures known as Pick inclusion bodies, and (2) profuse astroglial proliferation in the subcortical white matter.[165]

Pick inclusion bodies in hematoxylin-eosin preparations are often poorly defined cytoplasmic structures (Fig. 6-36) found in neurons having a ballooned appearance reminiscent of that seen in neurons after axonal transection (i.e., retrograde cell change or central chromatolysis).

Two types of inclusions have been described in the Ammon's horn and the temporal allocortex, respectively. In the latter location, "complete" Pick bodies are usually found in the superficially placed neurons.[15] The Pick body is better demonstrated by silver impregnation as a large (about 25 μm) paranuclear structure. Electron microscopically, a Pick body is composed primarily of neurofilaments.[165] The osmophilic inclusions contain many filaments (10 nm) and a few neural tubules (24 nm); the former are more argentophilic than the microtubules. The inclusion body also contains vesicles and complex lipid compounds and is not surrounded by a discernible membrane.[149] The pathogenesis of the cellular changes of Pick's disease is unknown.

Other forms of cytoplasmic inclusion bodies (such as the Lewy type) have been described in cortical neurons among patients afflicted with dementia of undetermined origin, which sometimes develops in the late stages of Parkinson's disease.[111] Inclusion bodies of the Lewy type are usually single, round eosinophilic structures surrounded by a clear halo; the core consists of a tangle of 7–8 nm filaments without surrounding, limiting membrane.[69] In rare occasions, Lewy inclusion bodies have been found in cortical neurons of demented patients.[170]

Dense microspheres and Hirano bodies, described previously in this chapter, may be included in the category of neuronal cytoplasmic inclusions of nonspecific significance.

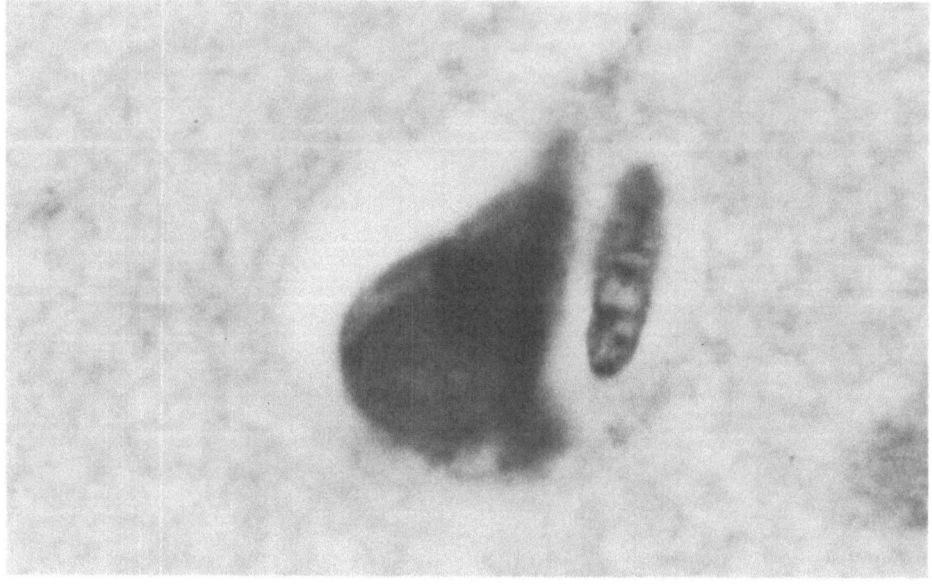

Fig. 6-36. Pick inclusion body: a large, round structure adjacent to the neuronal nucleus in most instances stains lightly with hematoxylin but is strongly argentophilic. (Courtesy R.D. Terry, M.D.) (×630).

Intranuclear inclusion of bodies accompanying viral infections are described under the heading of white matter alterations.

Pigments in the Neuronal Perikaryon and Meningeal Cells

A biologic pigment is an intrinsically colored substance that can be seen in the absence of staining. In standard histologic preparations of human samples, pigments do not bind either to hematoxylin or eosin.

Neuronal ceroid lipofuscinosis (NCL): The presence of light, golden-yellow pigment (ceroid or lipofuscin) in neuronal perikarya is normal (even in infancy) in locations such as the dorsal root, autonomic ganglia, cerebellar dentate nuclei, thalamic nuclei, and inferior olivary nucleus among others. Lipofuscin is a heterogeneous substance containing lipids, proteins, and carbohydrates. Because of the abundant hydrolytic enzymes at sites of lipofuscin accumulation, the inclusions are considered residual bodies in nondividing cells.[133] Lipofuscin pigment in the neuronal perikaryon of the neocortex may be abnormal, particularly if it fulfills certain histochemical and ultrastructural characteristics such as the expression of fingerprints and curvilinear bodies.[172]

Excessive amounts of lipofuscin in the neuronal perikaryon of the cerebral cortex are characteristic of a group of conditions called neuronal lipofuscinosis. Because differences in tinctorial or fluorescent properties between lipofuscin and ceroid are not apparent in light-microscopic preparations, the nature of a pigment should be verified by electron microscopy.[60] NCL includes a group of disorders characterized by accumulation of ceroid-lipofuscin pigment in the cytoplasm of neurons, glia, and many other cells. The biochemical nature of lipofuscin is undetermined, and although various elements or components have been described ultrastructurally at sites of pigment aggregation, only one type (curvilinear bodies) is commonly found in neurons and glia of patients with NCL who develop symptoms before 4 years of age.[31] Skeletal muscle, skin biopsies, or ultrastructural evaluation of lymphocytes may prove sufficient for the diagnosis of NCL.[21,35,96]

Pigment accumulation in renal tubules and other forms of visceral involvement have also been described in patients with NCL.[26] At present, curvilinear profiles are the most reliable morphologic indicator of NCL. Some forms of this group of diseases are accompanied by structural abnormalities in circulating leukocytes.[95,167] In addition to the neuronal accumulation of pigment, brain biopsies from patients with neuronal ceroid lipofuscinosis may reveal "loss" of nerve cells and gliosis. The pigment (lipofuscin) is autofluorescent, PAS-positive, and acid-fast. Senescence is accompanied by lipofuscin deposits in many cells; hence, the appraisal of neuronal lipofuscinosis in a brain biopsy must be weighed with this thought in mind.

A rare, inherited disorder with prominent neurological symptoms, common to human and several other species in which cytoplasmic, pigmented inclusion bodies or giant granules are visible in brain neurons is *Chediak-Higashi disease*. The structures seen in this disease may be differentiated from those of neuronal ceroid lipofuscinosis by the larger size and the ultrastructural features of the pigment, some of which are similar to those of hemosiderin.[70,142]

Other pigments encountered in human brain biopsies include: leptomeningeal melanin (Fig. 6-37), present in melanocytes. These cells are particularly abundant in the leptomeninges at the base of the brain, on the convexity of the cerebellum, and on the ventral surface of the brain stem. Melanin is bleached by hydrogen peroxide or potassium permanganate, does not contain iron, and is revealed in Fontana stains. Neuromelanin (Fig. 6-38) is a normal organelle of many adult dopaminergic neuronal perikarya, such as those of the substantia nigra. Neuromelanin is also visible in the locus ceruleus and dorsal motor nucleus of the vagus nerve; it is not found in normal cortical neurons. Formaldehyde pigment (Fig. 6-39) is a dark brown, crystalline substance that precipitates on the surface of erythrocytes. This pigment results from the reaction between formalin and hemoglobin. The pigment becomes particularly abundant when the pH of the fixative is less than 7.0.

Formaldehyde pigment should be differentiated from malarial pigment (Fig. 6-40), an intracellular substance that results from the interaction between hemoglobin and *Plasmodium falciparum*. Formalin pigment precipitates on the erythrocyte surface, is iron-negative (Perl's reaction), birefringent with polarized light, and can be bleached by carbonic, nitric, and formic acids.[90]

Cerebral Senile Changes

Aging in nondemented persons (i.e., senescence) is accompanied by a progressive decrease of brain weight,[73,74] which is attributed to the physiologic of loss of nerve cells and white matter fibers. The latter may be reflected in slight dilatation of the ventricular system. Other features of aged brains include the appearance of neuronal abnormalities known as: (1) senile or neuritic plaques, (2) neurofibrillary tangles, (3) granulovacuolar changes,[154] and (4) Hirano bodies.

All these microscopic features of brain aging are found in increased numbers among persons who are afflicted with senile dementia of the Alzheimer type (SDAT). This condition is the most frequent type of organic dementia among adults (over the age

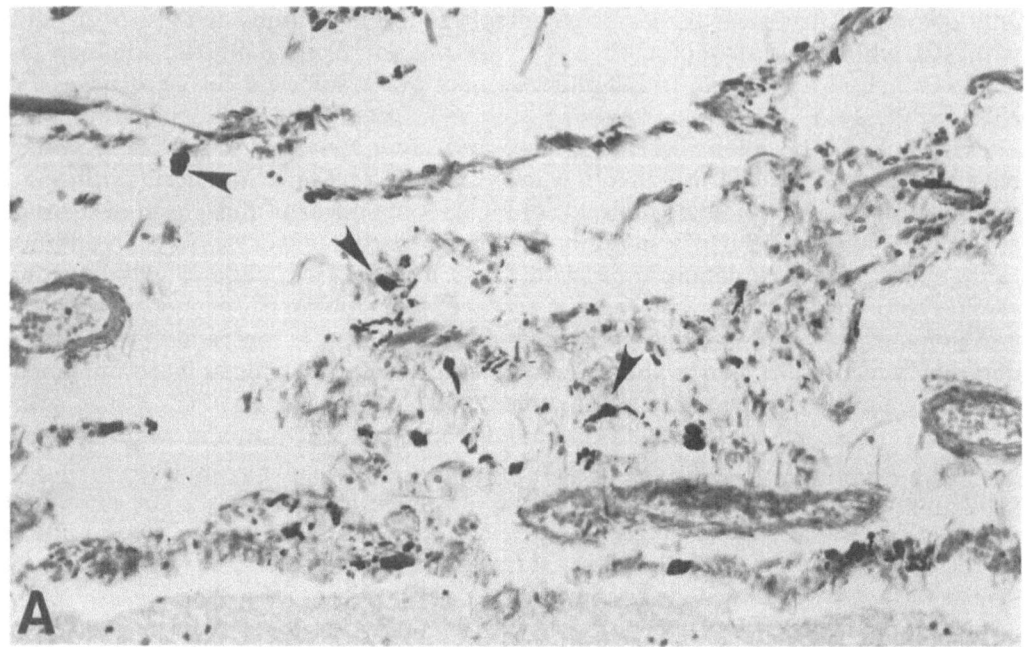

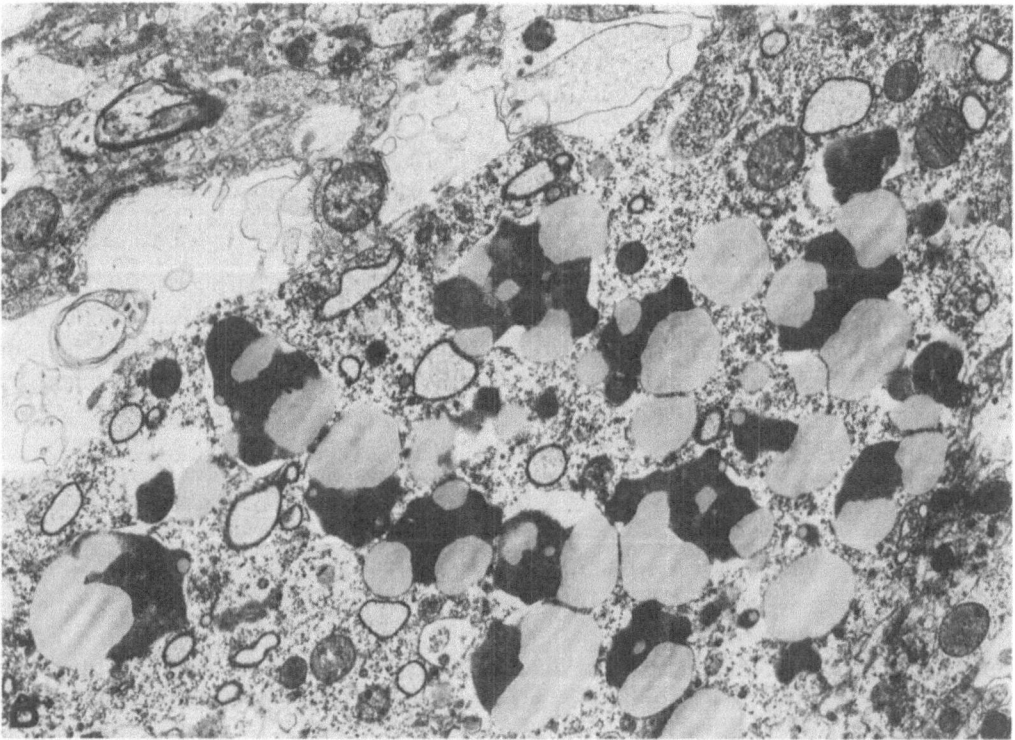

Fig. 6-37. (A) Cerebellar leptomeninges (normal); sample from a 27-year-old black person who died in an automobile accident. Melanin-containing cells are indicated by arrowheads (×40); (B) Detail of lipofuscin pigment in the neuronal perikaryon of an adult human (×35,000).

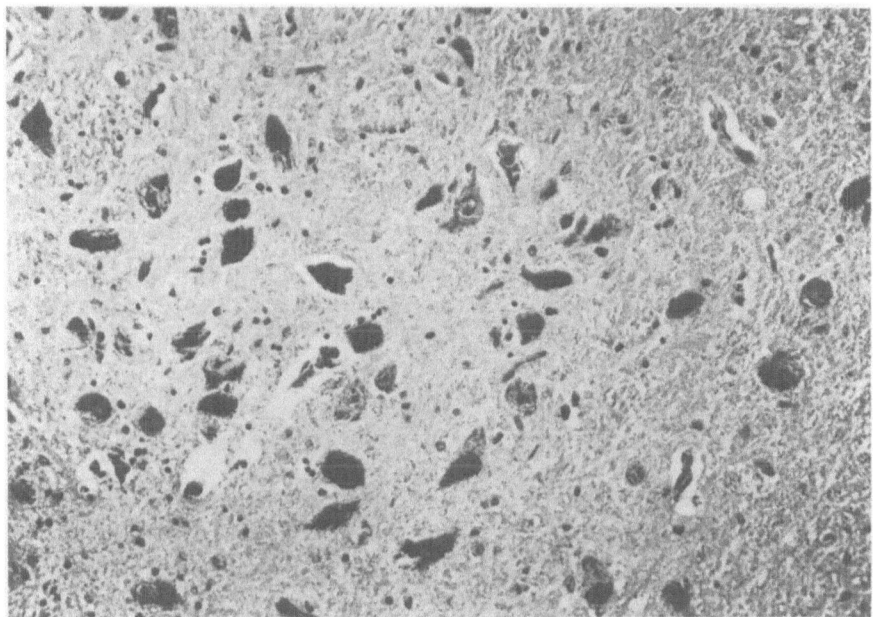

Fig. 6-38. Neurons of the substantia nigra from a 67-year-old patient. This pigment is normally not visible by naked-eye inspection in brains of persons younger than 18 years of age (×160).

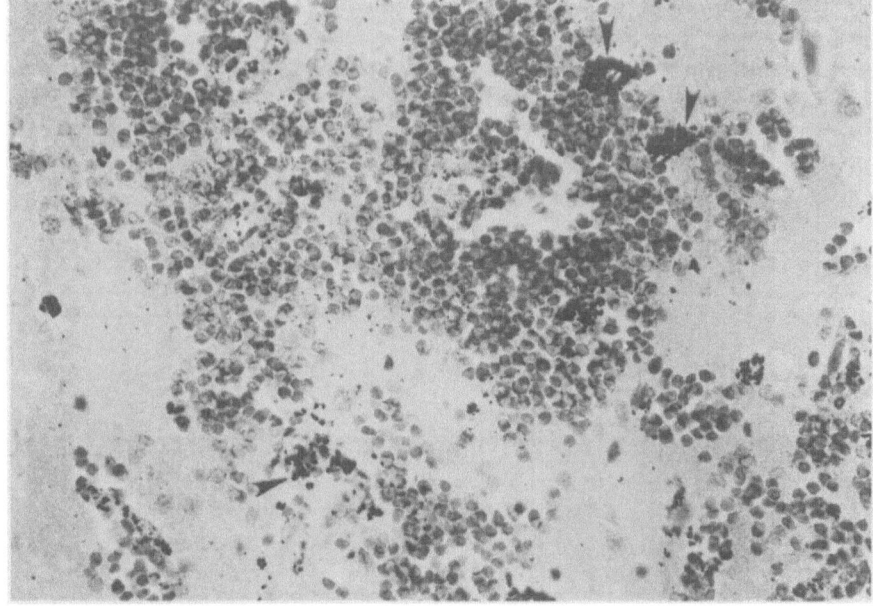

Fig. 6-39. Formalin pigment (arrows) at the site of a recent brain hemorrhage. Formation of this pigment can be considerably prevented by using appropriately buffered fixative solutions (×100).

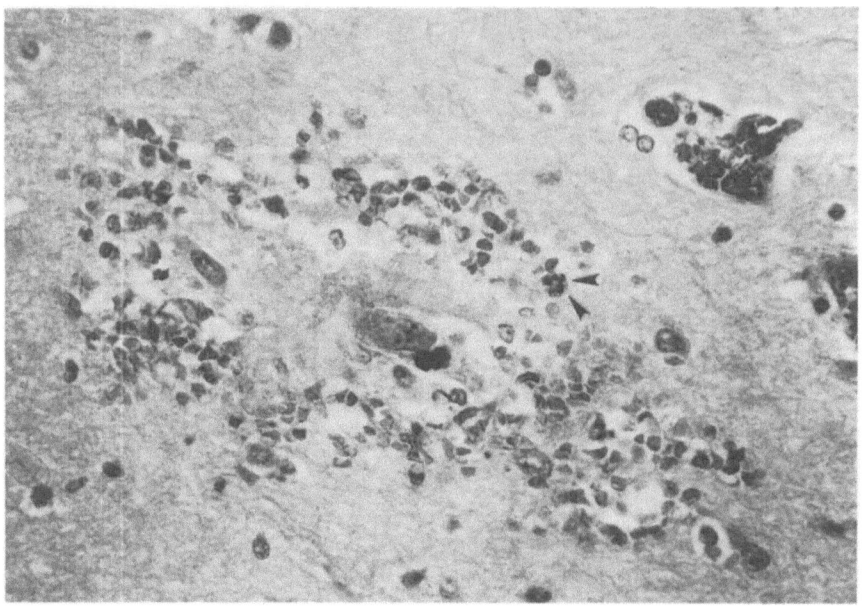

Fig. 6-40. Cerebral malaria. This "ring" or perivascular brain hemorrhage occurred at the site of vascular necrosis, secondary to the effects of infection by *Plasmodium falciparum.* The malarial pigment is indicated by the arrowheads (×100).

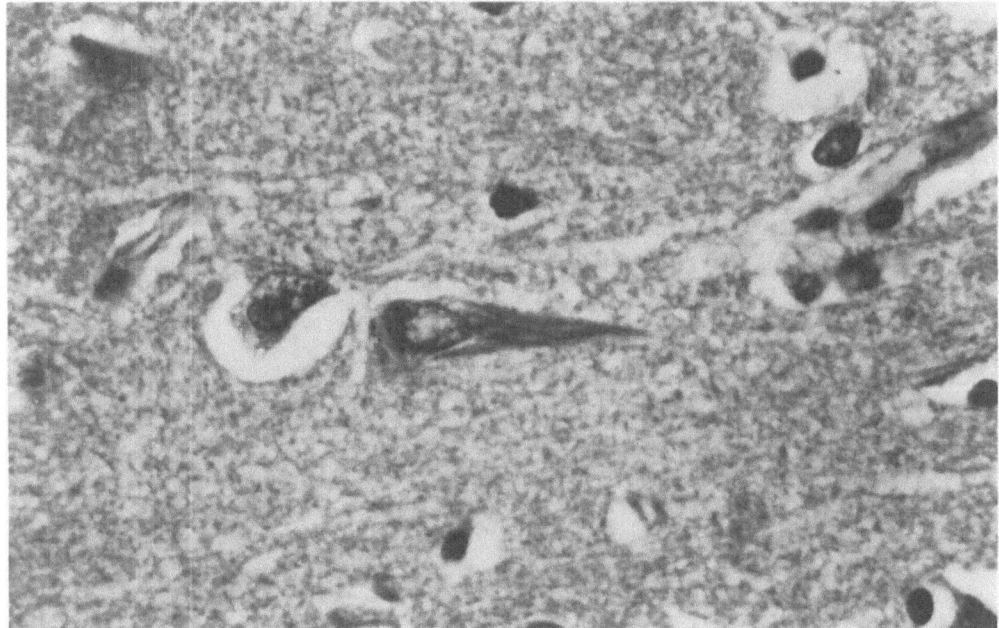

Fig. 6-41. Neurofibrillary tangles fill most of the perikaryon of this pyramidal neuron in the hippocampus (×250).

of 65) in the United States,[6,168] Great Britain,[154a] and probably in most industrialized societies.

Anatomically, Alzheimer's disease (presenile dementia) is synonymous with senile dementia. Both are characterized by two identical histologic abnormalities appearing in the cerebral neocortex: neurofibrillary tangles and abundant senile (neuritic) plaques. In the current literature, the two conditions are included under the designation of senile dementia of the Alzheimer type (SDAT) or simply, Alzheimer's disease.

Neurofibrillary tangle (NFT) (Fig. 6-41) is a neuronal abnormality made up of a cluster of paired helically wound 10 nm filaments with the twist occurring every 80 nm. These tangles are particularly abundant in the cerebral cortex of patients with AD, but NFT also can be found in other neurologic diseases (e.g., Parkinsonism, dementia pugilistica, and subacute sclerosing panencephalitis) and in nondemented, aged persons in whom the NFT's are generally confined to the entorhinal cortex and the hippocampus. Neurofibrillary tangles, although visible in H&E preparations, can be demonstrated better through impregnation with silver salts. Staining with thioflavin T is the preferred method for demonstrating NFT.[149,150]

Senile (neuritic) plaques (Fig. 6-42) range widely in diameter (15–250 μm) and may have amyloid (Congo red-positive protein) in the center (Fig. 6-43); the peripheral component of a senile plaque is a roughly circular aggregate of abnormal unmyelinated neuronal processes, mostly presynaptic boutons. For this reason, senile plaques may also be called neuritic plaques.[150] A circulating protein, amyloid, is thought by some to be deposited secondarily at the core of the senile plaque,[166a] but the nature of the amyloid in the plaque is not yet agreed upon.[150] Both neurofibrillary tangles and senile plaques can be seen to great advantage after staining with thioflavine T and examination with fluorescent illumination. Neurofibrillary tangles and senile plaques are found in elderly persons with normal mentation. However, the numbers of these structures, particularly

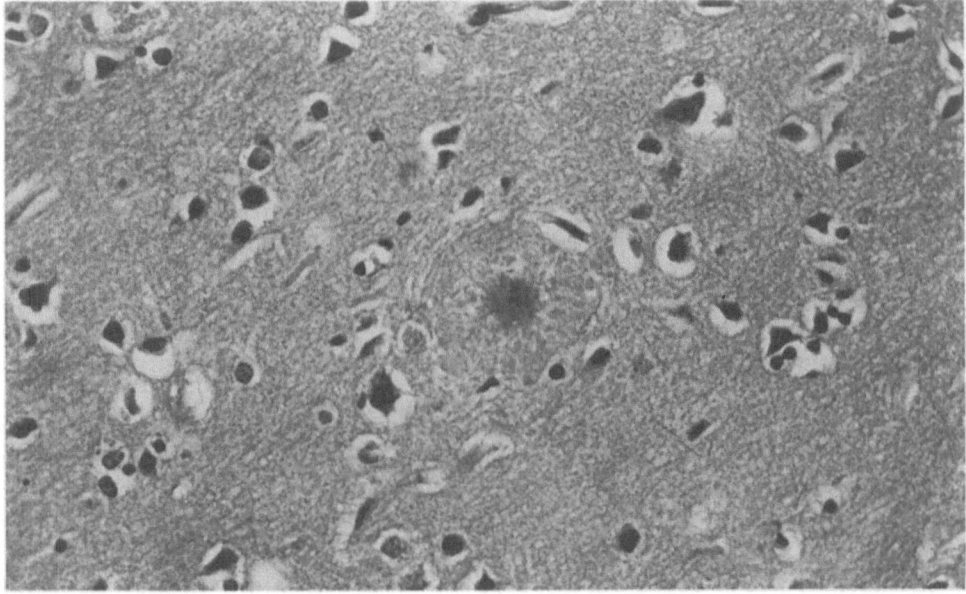

Fig. 6-42. Senile plaque in hippocampus. The amyloid core is surrounded by altered neurites and a few glial cells (×160).

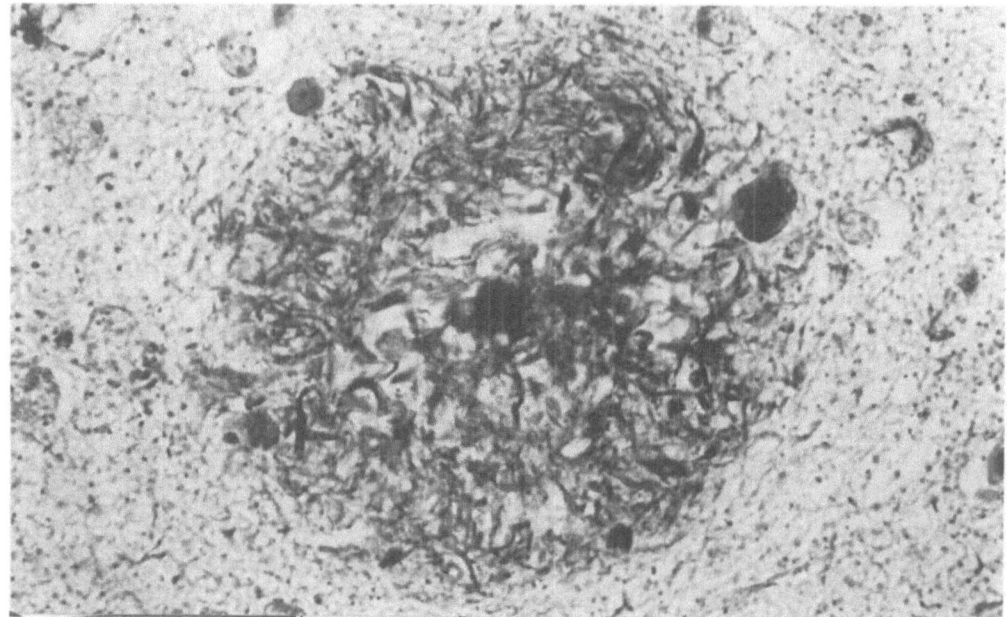

Fig. 6-43. Senile plaque showing argentophilia of the central and peripheral components of the plaque. (Silver carbonate ×400).

in the cerebral neocortex, are greater in individuals afflicted with SDAT, in some of whom diffuse symmetrical cerebral hemispheric atrophy is particularly evident in the limbic system.[76,154a] The clinical criteria for the diagnosis of Alzheimer's disease correlates best with the presence of NFT and neuritic plaques in the hippocampus, regardless of neocortical findings.[151] The appearance of histologic abnormalities typical of SDAT is virtually inevitable in persons with Down's syndrome who live past 40 years.[6] Granulo-vacuolar changes, another common feature of senile dementia (Fig. 6-44), occurs mainly (or exclusively) in the pyramidal cells of the hippocampus[55] and, therefore, is unlikely to be found in brain biopsies.

Although abnormally high neuronal loss is frequently mentioned as a feature of senility and other forms of dementia, a decrease of neuronal numbers is extremely difficult to ascertain in the usual brain biopsy,[6] among other reasons, because of lack of standardization of section thickness. A second type of organic dementia of adulthood (i.e., "senile") is characterized by an abnormality in the neuronal perikaryon that includes peripheral displacement of the nucleus and appearance in the cytoplasm of a round inclusion body (Pick bodies). These are illustrated in the section on inclusion body disease (Fig. 6-36). Inclusion bodies of the Pick type are preferentially abundant in the hippocampus and the entorhinal cortex. Some have suggested separation of two subgroups of patients with Pick disease: the classical one is characterized by predominantely cortical (lobar) atrophy and Pick bodies in the hippocampus and neocortex; the second group shows both subcortical and cortical atrophy but also had inclusion bodies, although in fewer numbers.[107]

Creutzfeldt-Jakob disease is another type of organic dementia, whose precise identification cannot be achieved, without microscopic evaluation of brain tissues. In H&E preparations of cerebral cortex, the changes characteristic of this condition have been

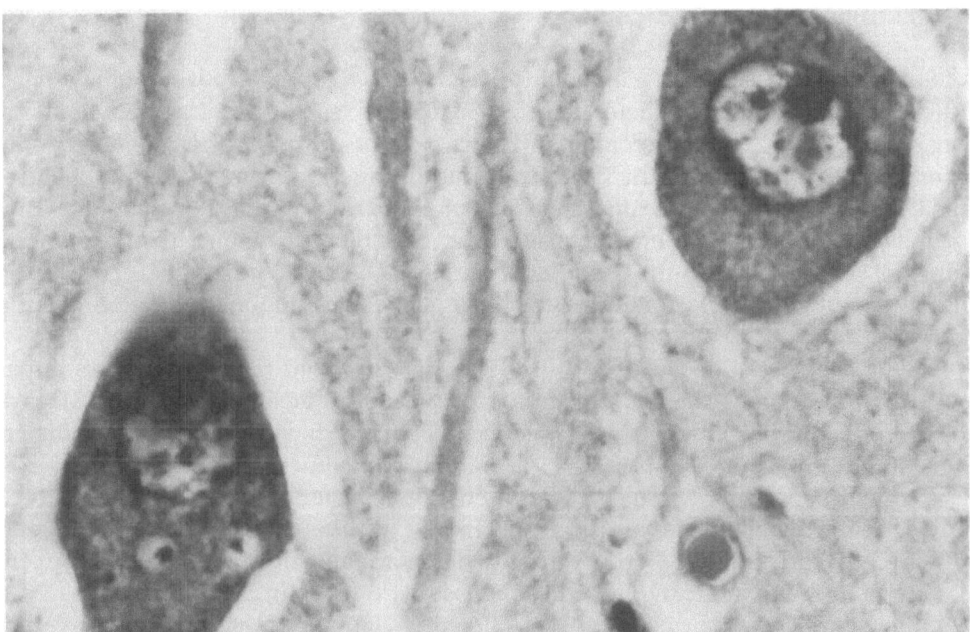

Fig. 6-44. Granulovacuolar changes in a pyramidal cell (hippocampus) from an elderly person; the neuronal perikaryon of the cell at left side shows at least two large "vacuoles" each containing a "granule." A normal cell is visible at right (×400).

described under the designation of status spongiosus to signify the multivacuolated appearance of the cerebral or cerebellar cortices (Fig. 6-27a). This vacuolation reflects, in part, the presence of numerous intracellular vacuoles in the dendrites and neuronal perikarya as well as in the astrocytic cytoplasm. The astroglia are usually markedly increased in numbers and size and cellular inflammatory infiltrates are not observed.[88] The absence of these changes in a brain biopsy does not rule out the diagnosis of Creutzfeldt-Jakob, as the disease can have selective localization in a few cortical sites or in CNS structures other than the cerebral cortex, including the spinal cord.

Huntington's disease (HD): Patients afflicted with dementia and chorea may suffer from an autosomal-dominant disease first described by Huntington.[78] In brain biopsies, the disease is said to be characterized by diffuse or circumscribed variable loss of neurons and the accumulation of large amounts of lipofuscin in neurons and glia; this pigment is well seen in frozen sections examined for autofluorescence and for acid phosphatase activity. Electron microscopically, abundant glial cells are present, some in close proximity to neuronal perikarya, as well as numerous lipofuscin-laden, large astrocytes.[147] Increased amounts of ceroid-lipofuscin pigment are a nonspecific histologic feature. Because of the nonspecific nature of the change described in the cerebral cortex of patients with HD, the diagnosis of this condition should not be attempted by means of cortical biopsy. A restriction enzyme marker has been found in patients with Huntington disease indicating that a specific gene for the disease is located in chromosome 4.[134] The earliest and most characteristic changes in Huntington disease are detectable in the medial paraventricular portion of the caudate nucleus where marked loss of medium-sized spiny neurons (up to 50% decrease initially, compared to matched controls) occurs simultaneously with increased numbers of reactive astrocytes.[159]

Axonal Changes

Spheroids (or "schollen") are cylindrical, ovoid, or circular eosinophilic structures measuring 5–40 μm in diameter (Fig. 6-45) that correspond to fragmented, beaded, swollen axis cylinders. Spheroids can be part of the features of ischemic, traumatic, or inflammatory injuries to the CNS. In these conditions, the axonal abnormalities are called reactive spheroids. Axonal swelling of a diffuse multifocal nature, particularly when it is visible in the cerebral/cerebellar cortices and in the absence of other significant structural abnormalities, is the hallmark of a group of hereditary disorders called neuroaxonal dystrophy (NAD); axonal abnormalities in these conditions are called dystrophic spheroids.[81]

Infantile NAD is an autosomal-recessive disorder that usually becomes apparent at about 6 months of age in the form of progressive motor, mental, and sensory disorders. The chief histologic features of NAD are axonal spheroids visible throughout the entire brain and the peripheral nerves. In decreasing frequency, the following CNS sites have shown spheroids: tegmentum of brain stem, posterior spinal funiculi, cerebellar cortex, basal ganglia/thalamus, spinal gray matter, and cerebral cortex.[81] Brain biopsies, examined by conventional light microscopy, sometimes fail to show axonal spheroids that are readily apparent by electron microscopy.[18] In brain biopsies of patients with NAD, most spheroids correspond to swollen axis cylinders containing either vesicular, tubular, or filamentous material. Apparently, only those spheroids filled with filaments are readily visible by light microscopy[130] (Fig. 6-46). In experimental animals and in some humans, vitamin E deficiency has been correlated with the presence of dystrophic axons, particularly in the medulla and the spinal cord.

Biopsies of mentally retarded persons, who are otherwise normal and whose karyo-

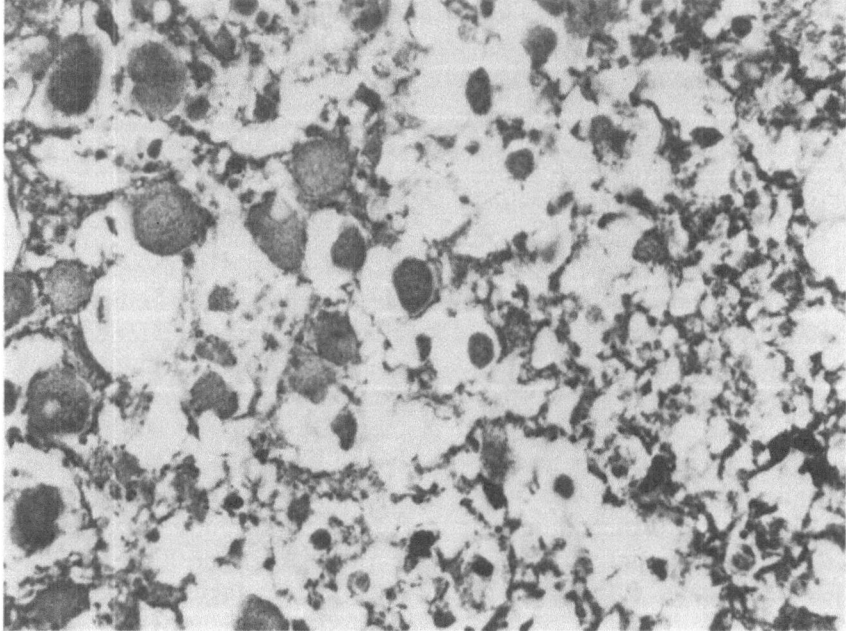

Fig. 6-45. Reactive spheroids are cross-sections of axis cylinders that in this case are severely swollen as a result of closed head trauma (×400).

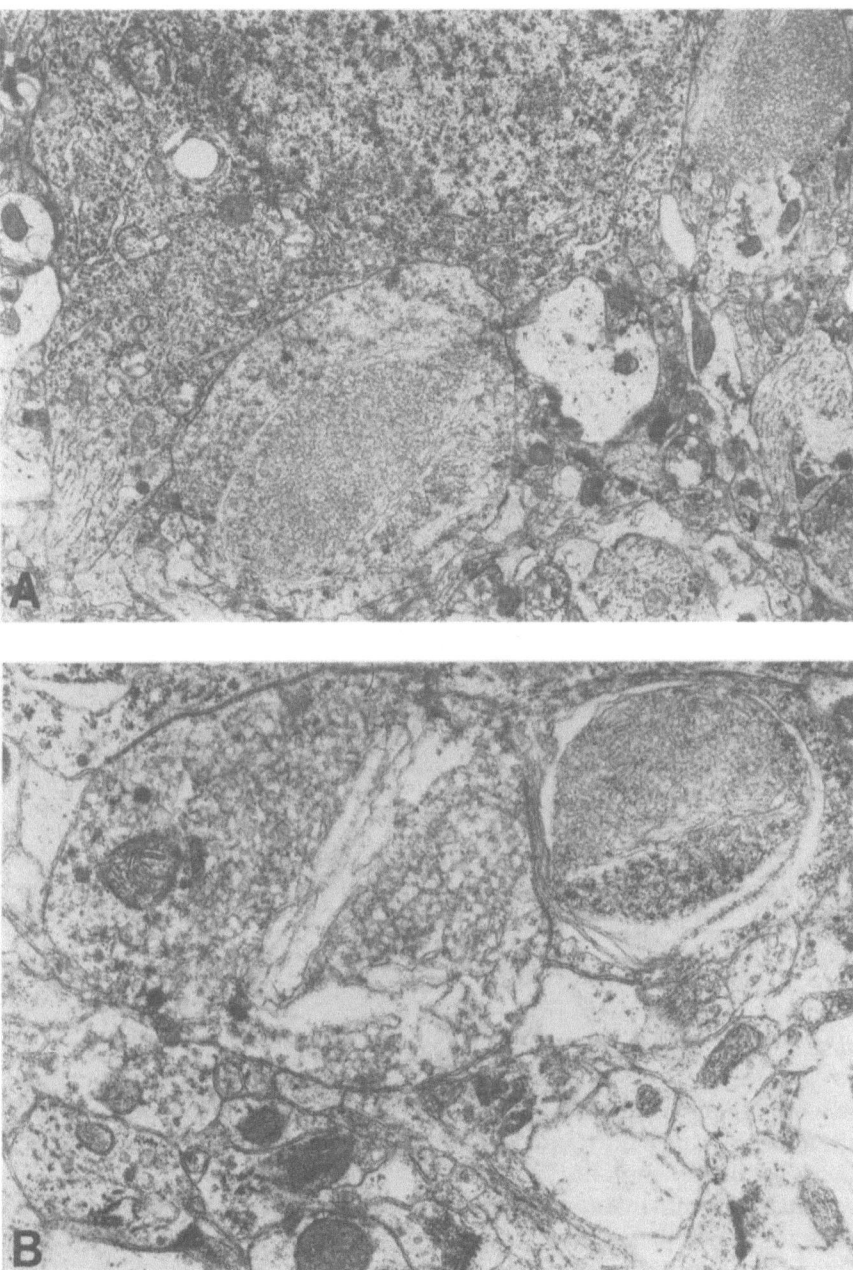

Fig. 6-46. (A&B) Neuroaxonal dystrophy. Dystrophic spheroids filled with vesicular and tubular materials. Spheroids are not visible by light microscopy of the brain biopsy (×15,000).

type is also normal, may disclose abnormalities in dendritic spines that can be detected only by the Golgi method[94] (Fig. 6-47). These structural changes consist of abnormally long, thin spines with absence of short, thick spines in the dendrites of cortical neurons.[120] These findings apply to a heterogeneous group of mentally retarded individuals and are not seen in brain biopsies of persons with normal intelligence. Additional axonal-

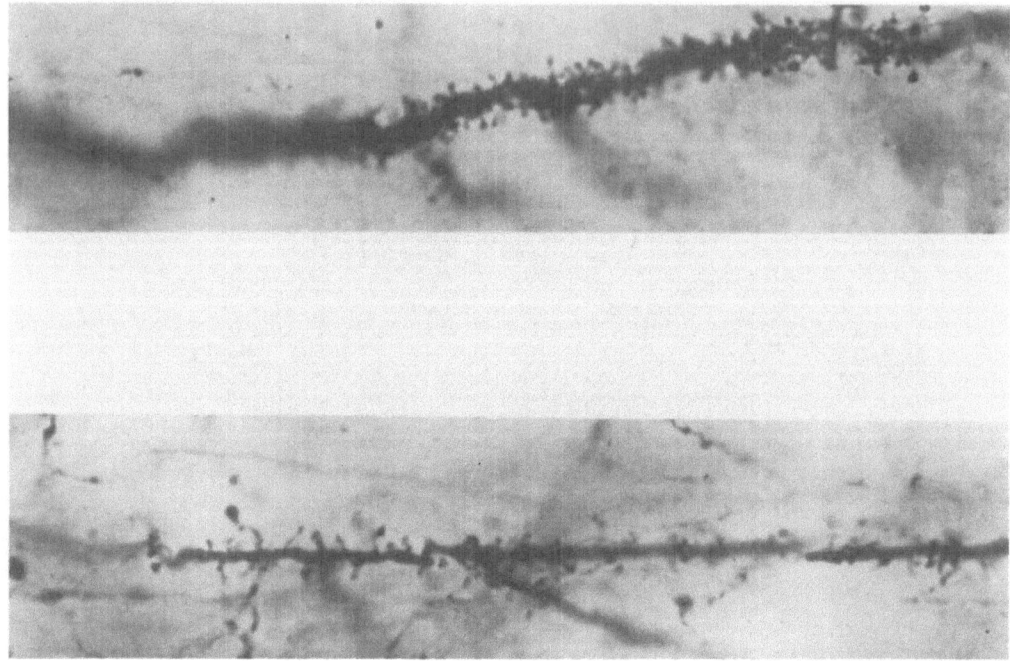

Fig. 6-47. Normal arborization of dendrites (top) is shown in the cerebral cortex of a child with normal intelligence. Marked decrease in the number of short, thick dendritic spines and presence of long, abnormally thin spines are apparent in the biopsy from a mentally retarded child (bottom) (Golgi-Cox ×640). (Courtesy D. Kristt, M.D.)

synaptic abnormalities in brain biopsies from patients with various forms of psychomotor retardation have detected three types of ultrastructural abnormalities: proliferation of tubulovesicular structures, abnormal mitochondria, and increased numbers of 8–10 nm filaments.[63] Some of these patients may belong in the late category of infantile NAD.

Encephalomalacia

This word literally means brain softening, a condition that is most commonly associated with either ischemic or traumatic injury to the brain. Tissue softening is a reflection of the increased water content typical of these conditions.

Focal areas of contusive (or traumatic) encephalomalacia may be surgically excised in patients in whom the progressive post-traumatic brain swelling leads to increases in intracranial pressure that are incompatible with long-time survival. The traumatic origin of a brain injury cannot be readily established by microscopic examination; this is because the microscopic features of brain lesions produced by physical force are similar to those of an ischemic injury. Nevertheless, contusive encephalomalacia tends to be much more hemorrhagic and edematous than brain infarctions caused by either vascular occlusion or hypotensive crises.

Localized areas of brain ischemia (visualized by CT scan of the head) may mimic the clinical expression of either a brain tumor or a viral encephalitis, herpetic or otherwise.[162] For this reason, the diagnosis of brain infarction may occasionally appear in brain biopsy reports.

Brain infarction is a designation usually reserved for necrotizing lesions resulting from the occlusion of either arterial or venous vessels. At the microscopic level and especially during the acute stage (i.e., the first few hours after the vascular occlusion), such lesions cannot be distinguished from focal brain injuries caused by hypotensive crises. Therefore, the designation of brain infarction is broadened to include ischemic lesions of either origin: vascular occlusion or hypotension.

The very early or acute stages of ischemic brain injuries have been studied prospectively in experimental animals.[46] Three types of abnormalities are characteristic of this lesion: (1) heterogeneous and multifocal alterations in volume and stainability of neuronal perikarya, including dark shrunken neurons and scalloped neurons, both of which are invariably present in the same microscopic field; (2) heterogeneous sponginess or vacuolation of the neuropil; and (3) in contrast to the neuronal shrinkage and hyperchromasia, marked swelling and hypochromasia of astrocytic nuclei (Figs. 6-22a, 6-23a-c).

The subacute or intermediate stage of brain ischemic lesions is characterized by the presence of inflammatory cells, such as neutrophils (in the 24–48 hour period) followed by monocytes and lipid-laden macrophages (usually abundant by days 7– 10). Blood vessel regeneration is usually expressed in the form of large, hyperplastic endothelial cells that become especially prominent in the lumen of venules and capillaries. During this period, swollen axons (spheroids) and reactive plump astrocytes may also be visible at the periphery of a brain infarction.[49] Brain infarctions secondary to either arterial embolism or venous occlusion contain perivascular leukocytic infiltrates that are much more abundant than they are in infarctions secondary to an arterial thrombus. The healing or chronic stage of a brain infarction is identifiable by the abundance of lipid-laden macrophages, the absence of axonal or vascular abnormalities, and the persistence of reactive astrogliosis at the interface between the infarction and the normal brain parenchyma. Vacuolation of the white matter at the periphery of old infarcts is a constant feature of the lesion that seemingly reflects the long-lasting effects of fluid accumulation.

Intracerebral Hemorrhage

The designation of brain or intracerebral hemorrhage (ICH) applies to bleeding in the brain *parenchyma* (cerebrum, cerebellum, and brain stem) and does not include epidural, subdural, and subarachnoid hemorrhages.[48]

Spontaneous brain hemorrhage can develop in the cerebral hemispheres (basal ganglia/thalamus and white matter), the cerebellum, or the pons. A significant number of cerebral and cerebellar hemorrhages are surgically removed, during the acute stage, in an attempt to reduce intracranial pressure and as a life-saving measure.

Brain fragments attached to large intracerebral hemorrhages of nontraumatic origin have revealed the following features under microscopic examination: neoplastic cells (either primary or metastatic tumors), angiomatous malformations, and at least two types of angiopathies involving small or medium caliber blood vessels: arteriolarsclerosis, and cerebral amyloid angiopathy.[68]

In addition to the cause of the brain hemorrhage, the microscopic examination of blood clots and adjacent brain helps determine the approximate age of a hemorrhage as indicated by deformities of the erythrocytes (for example in sickle cell disease), lysis of erythrocytes, and presence/absence of leukocytic infiltrates at the periphery of the hemorrhage.[166] Both brain hemorrhages and brain ischemic lesions heal in the same manner, (i.e., a fluid-filled cavity, devoid of capsule, is formed at the site of the original lesion). Causes of brain hemorrhage are numerous; among the most prominent are: arterial hypertension, trauma to the head, blood dyscrasias, angiopathies (congenital or acquired), and brain neoplasms.[48]

White Matter

The normal components of the cerebral white matter in adult human tissues include: abundant myelinated axons, oligodendrocytes, astrocytes, blood vessels (Fig. 6-48), and probably, occasional microglial elements. The interpretation of brain biopsies obtained from young children (under the age of 5 years) must take into account that myelination of the human brain, in general, proceeds in a caudal-rostral direction over a period of 2 decades; the peripheral nerves, spinal cord, and most of the brain stem are almost fully myelinated in the full-term infant. In contrast, myelinated fibers, in the cerebrum and at 41 weeks gestation, are mostly confined to the subcortical nuclei and the association fiber tracts.[127] After the rapid pace of the perinatal period, myelination of the cerebral hemispheres continues at a progressively slower rate to the age of 16–20 years. The progression of the myelination pattern is indicated by a numerical scale that corresponds to the regional designation of the brain devised by Flechsig,[38] and used by Brodman in his cytoarchitectural studies of the cerebral cortex.

Few myelin abnormalities noted in brain biopsies are sufficiently characteristic to permit the diagnosis of a specific disease. Instead, most structural changes in myelin suggest one of the following groups of disorders: (1) demyelination, (2) leukodystrophy, (3) inflammation/neoplasia, (4) vascular-circulatory changes, (5) inflammatory conditions with abundant intranuclear inclusion bodies, and (6) miscellaneous leukoencephalopathies.

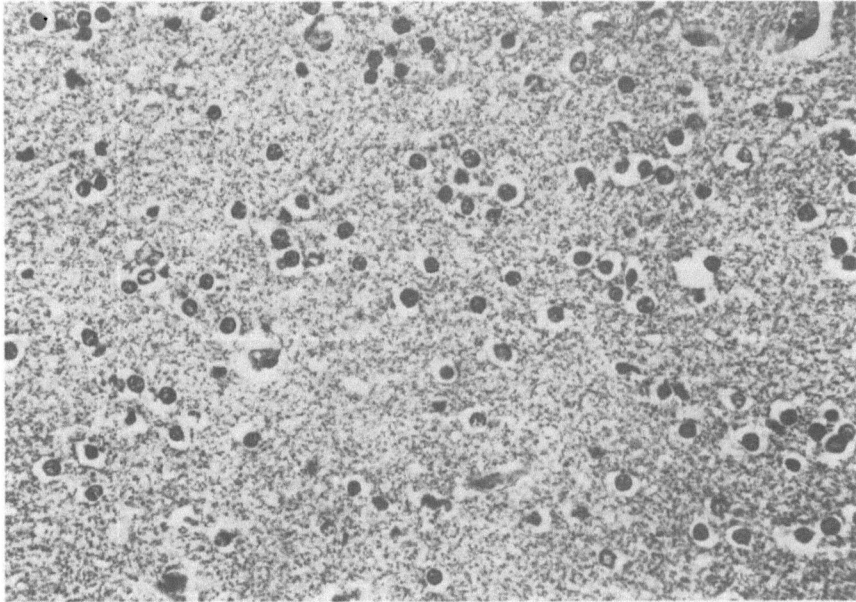

Fig. 6-48. Normal white matter (frontal lobe) of adult human who died without neurologic deficits (×100).

Demyelinating Disease

Primary demyelinating or myelinoclastic diseases, of which multiple sclerosis (MS) is the prototype, are conditions in which myelin sheaths are focally and selectively destroyed (Figs. 6-49A and B). Three premises are implied in the concept of MS: (1)

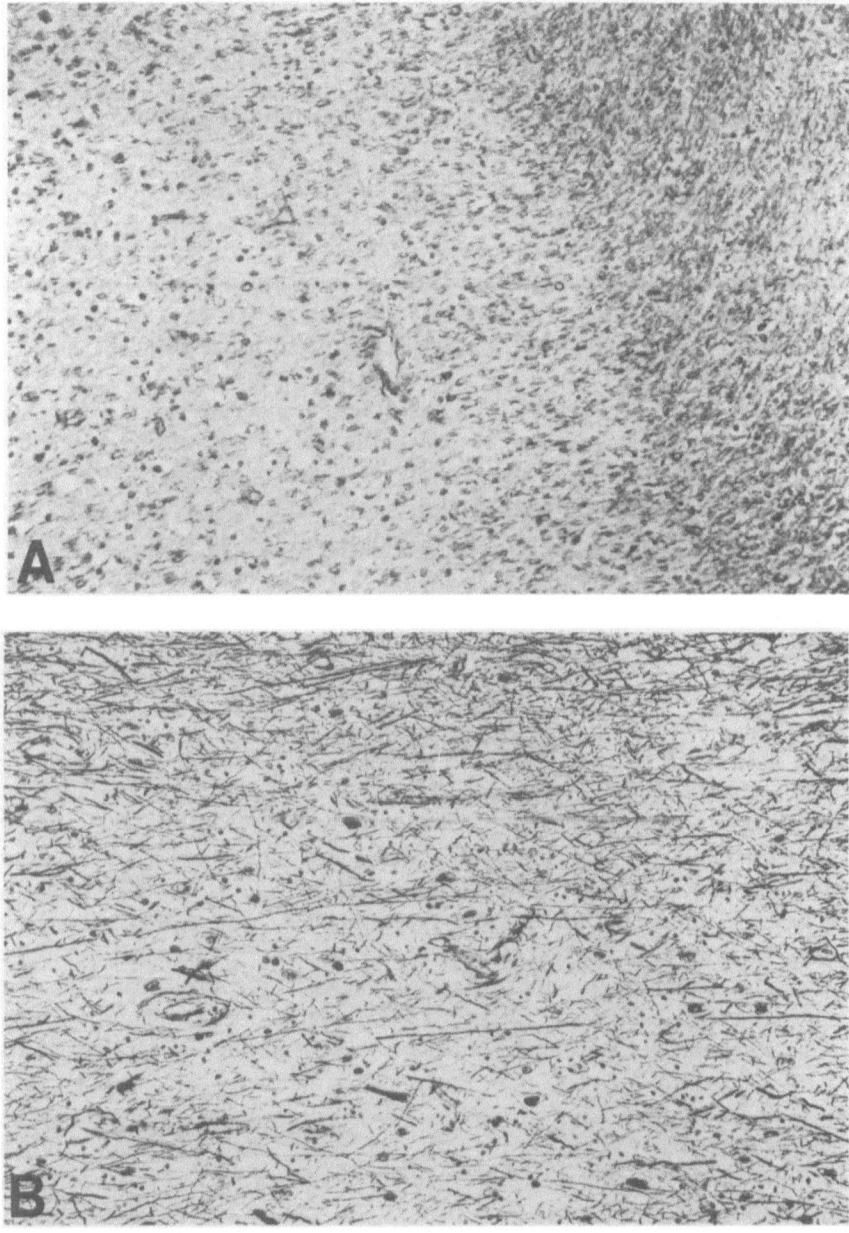

Fig. 6-49. (A) Plaque of myelin loss in the cerebral white matter of a patient with multiple sclerosis of long duration. Normal-staining myelin is visible at right (Luxol-fast blue ×250); (B) Same lesion as in Fig. 6-49A. Axis cylinders in the center of the plaque are better preserved than the myelin sheaths (Bodian technique ×250).

myelination of the CNS has normally progressed and is reflected in the normal development of neurologic functions; (2) the localized, circumscribed lesions of MS (called *plaques*) appear either successively or simultaneously at multiple sites in the CNS as sharply demarcated, focal, irregularly shaped lesions; and (3) the initial lesion involves selective destruction of myelin sheaths, with preservation of all other white matter components; these changes are accompanied, in most instances by minimal cellular inflammation.[119] Although the plaques can develop anywhere in the neuraxis, when they involve the cerebral hemispheres they are most common around the lateral ventricles and in the subcortical white matter. Biopsies of these plaques have been obtained in the course of doing a thalamotomy for the treatment of tremor.[142a] The histologic abnormalities found in these specimens are not specific for this group of diseases. In addition to patchy loss of myelin with preservation of axis cylinders, the following changes may be seen in biopsies of MS plaques: mononuclear infiltrates (sometimes in a perivascular location), astrocytic proliferation, cavitation associated with lipid-laden macrophages, and rarely diffuse as opposed to focal demyelination.[145] In plaques of recent origin, ultrastructural observations have been interpreted as indicating that macrophages are responsible for the ingestion of structurally normal myelin sheaths.[119] Large plaques of MS have been mistaken clinically and radiologically (including CT scan) as being compatible with the expression of a brain tumor,[129] a misconception that has resulted in the biopsy of the lesion. In a chronic MS plaque, this error could be compounded at the time of histologic evaluation because the intense gliosis of a "burnt-out" MS plaque may be misinterpreted as representing a well-differentiated "astrocytoma."

Equivalent demyelinating disorders with selective involvement of peripheral myelin are described under the heading of "Nerve Biopsies."

Leukodystrophies

The concept of leukodystrophy differs from that of demyelination in several ways. Leukodystrophies are a heterogeneous, usually progressive group of diseases having in common, abnormalities of cerebral white matter in which myelin sheaths as well as other white matter components (e.g., axons) are involved by the initial injury. Leukodystrophies tend to involve the cerebrum in a diffuse, poorly defined and relatively symmetrical fashion that contrasts with the rather focal, well-circumscribed, and haphazardly scattered lesions of MS. These respective morphologic features of MS and leukodystrophies can be best appreciated by magnetic resonance imaging (MRI) of the head. Many leukodystrophies are associated with inherited metabolic defects; for this reason, they tend to be more common in childhood and may involve the central and peripheral nervous systems simultaneously. In contrast, MS is a disease of young adults in which the myelin disappearance is selective in two ways: it initially spares the axons and is confined to the central myelin. For this reason, the diagnosis of MS could not be achieved by nerve biopsy.

Adrenoleukodystrophy (ALD) is an X-linked disorder associated with progressive destruction of the cerebral white matter (Fig. 6-50), atrophy of the adrenal cortex (reflected in adrenal insufficiency in about one-third of the cases) and accumulation (in brain and adrenal tissues) of substances rich in long-chain fatty acids.[105,106] The name reflects the fact that ultrastructurally identical deposits found in macrophages of the white matter are also detectable in the zona fasciculata-reticularis of the adrenal cortex. Demonstrable adrenal insufficiency is rare, despite the almost constant involvement of

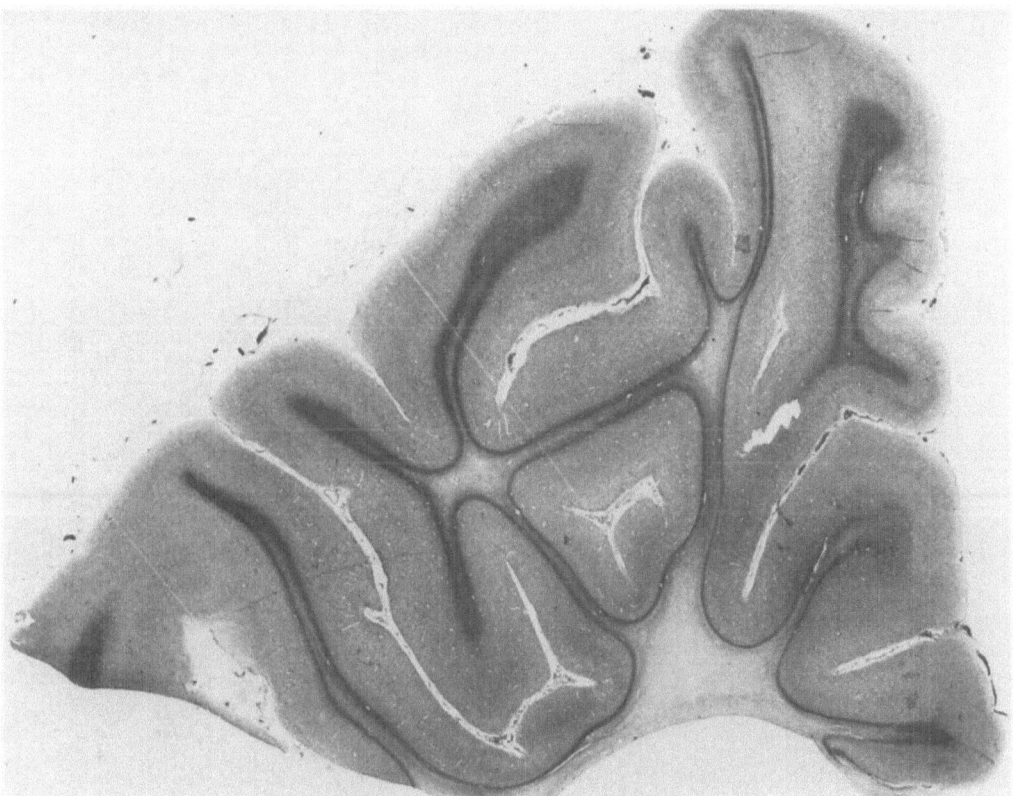

Fig. 6-50. Metachromatic leukodystrophy: parietal lobe. The subcortical myelinated fibers stain normally; there is no stainability of the deeper white matter sheaths (Loyez method ×4).

the adrenal gland. By light microscopy, incomplete destruction of cerebral white matter is associated with the presence of PAS-positive, orthochromatic and sudanophilic cells, identified as macrophages. Residual myelin sheaths and many denuded axons are common in areas of intense mononuclear (lymphocytes and plasma cells) perivascular infiltrates, dense gliosis, and occasional areas of cavitation. Electron microscopically, axoplasmic filaments undergo granular disintegration and numerous macrophages contain membrane-bound, electron-dense leaflets enclosing a cleft or clear space (Fig. 6-51). These characteristic leaflets can be seen also in biopsies of adrenal cortex, testes, peripheral nerve, skin, and conjunctiva.[96] Although most ALD patients have predominant cerebral involvement of the parietal and occipital lobes, this localization cannot be predicted by clinical tests.[131] In the adrenal cortex cells of the zona fasciculata and reticularis initially show, birefringent striations composed of lamellar profiles that contain both cholesterol esters and long chain fatty acids.[118a] Variants of classic ALD involving primarily spinal cord or becoming manifest at birth have been described.[8]

Globoid cell leukodystrophy (GLD) or Krabbe's disease, is a progressive neurologic disorder characterized by an inherited deficiency of galactocerebroside β-galactosidase, which is demonstrable in circulating leukocytes. In brain biopsies, the histologic diagnosis of GLD is based on the identification of globoid cells that are usually located in the white matter near the vascular adventitia (Fig. 6-52). Individual cells range in diameter

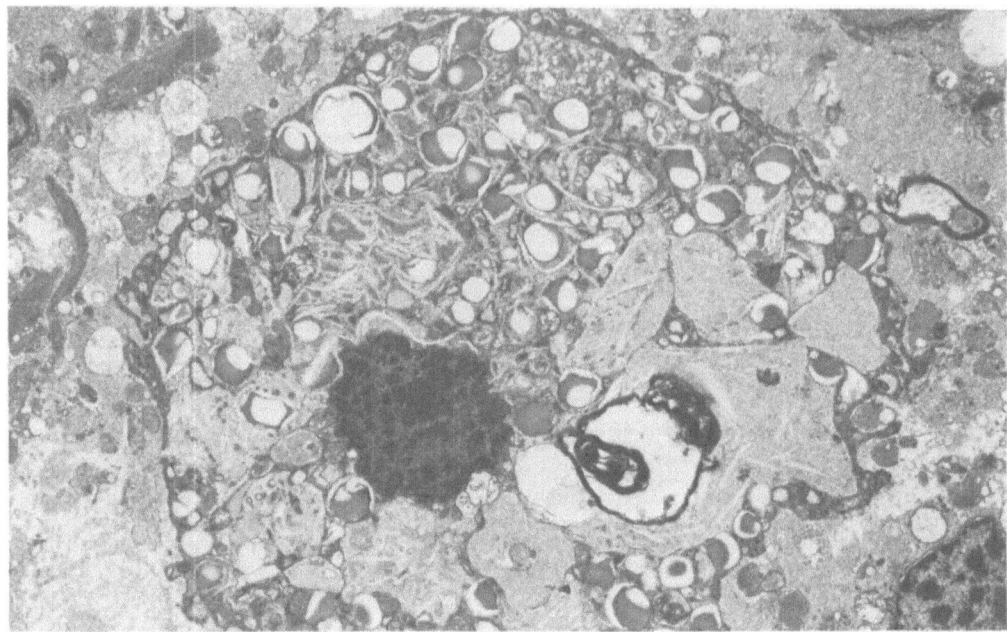

Fig. 6-51. Adrenoleukodystrophy. The perikaryon of this phagocyte is filled with abundant lipid droplets and spicules (×3,000) (Courtesy H. Schaumburg, M.D.).

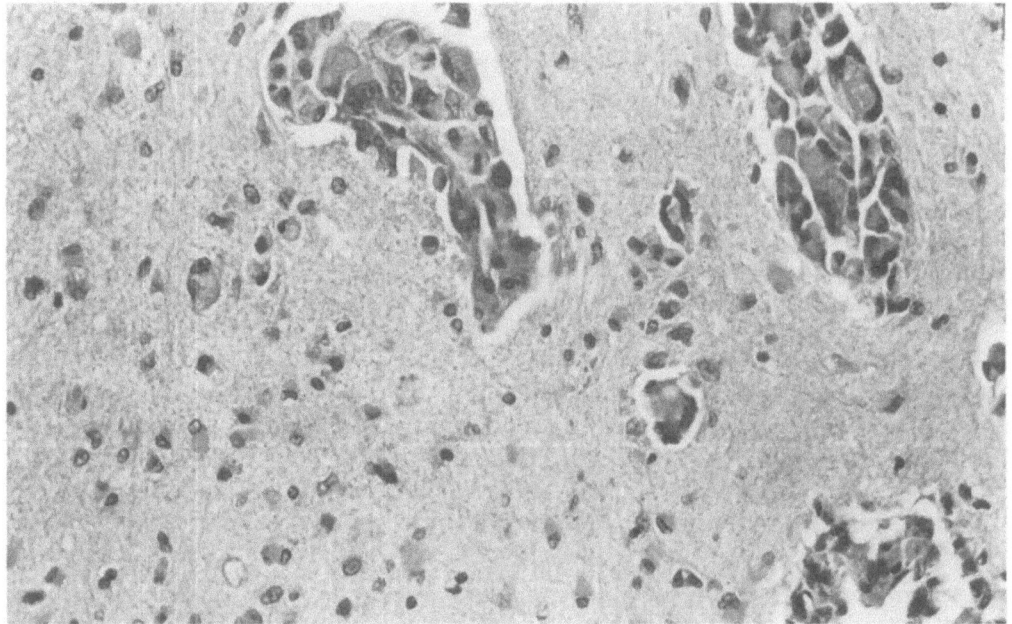

Fig. 6-52. Krabbe disease. A 4-year-old child with progressive neurologic deterioration since age 3 months. Sample of white matter from the parietal lobe showing nests of globoid and epitheloid cells, myelin pallor, and astroglial proliferation (×165) (Courtesy E.J. Yunis, M.D.).

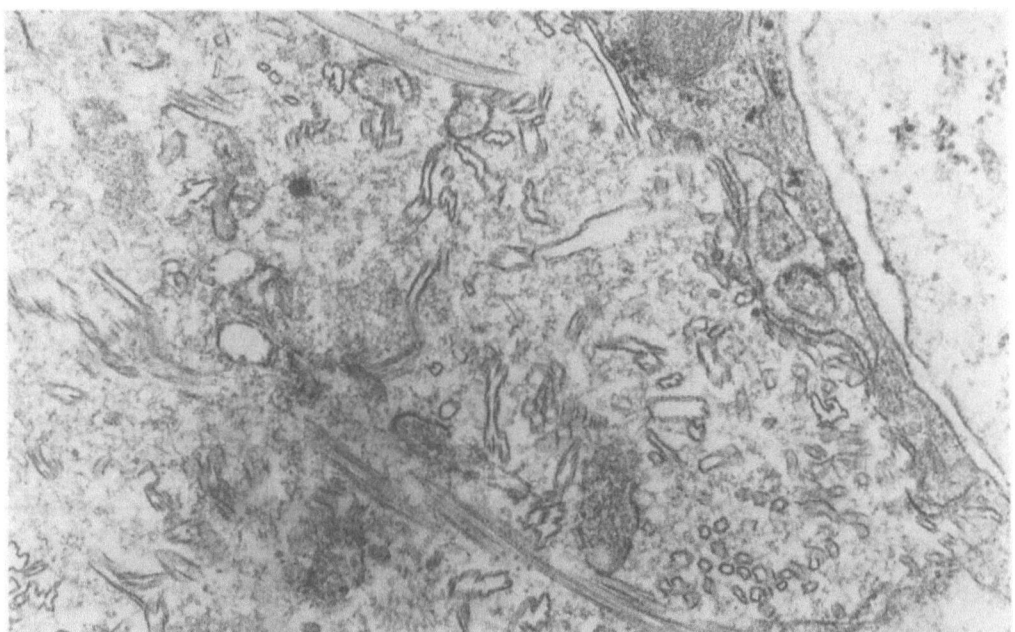

Fig. 6-53. Globoid cell leukodystrophy. The characteristic material (galactocerebroside) is visualized as tubules either straight or twisted (not shown here) in the globoid cell cytoplasm (×16,000) (Courtesy E.J. Yunis, M.D.).

from 20 to 50 μm and may have as many as 15 peripherally placed nuclei; some globoid cells are mononuclear measure 2–10 μm in diameter and are sometimes called epithelioid. The cytoplasmic content is PAS-positive and also stains faintly with sudan black and sudan IV: acid phosphatase activity is strong. Except for the subcortical areas, loss of myelinated fibers is extensive and is accompanied by dense astroglial proliferation. The cerebral cortex is essentially normal. The electron-microscopic features of the stored cerebroside include straight and periodically twisted tubules (Fig. 6-53) that are considered characteristic for both the human and the canine forms of GLD, a condition that can also be diagnosed by nerve biopsy.[171] These inclusions usually are up to 5 μm long and 200 nm wide. In addition to the globoid cells, the inclusions can also be found in endothelial and perithelial cells.[144]

Metachromatic leukodystrophy (MLS) is a progressive neurologic disorder chiefly affecting cerebral white matter and peripheral nerve and featuring a marked deficiency of cerebroside sulfate (sulfatide) sulfhydrolase (arylsulfatase A) in all tissues. Inheritance is autosomal recessive and at least three clinical forms (infantile, juvenile, and adult) are recognized, according to the age at onset of symptoms.[34] Diagnosis can be achieved by assaying arylsulfatase A in urine and leukocytes, as well as by sural nerve biopsy. Abnormalities in leukocytes are useful in the identification of the homozygous individual. Brain biopsy has revealed, in addition to the white matter abnormalities and the typical sulfatide deposits that stain metachromatically with crystal violet (Fig. 6-54), various intraneuronal deposits whose recognition may require ultrastructural evaluation of the sample[58a] (Fig. 6-55).

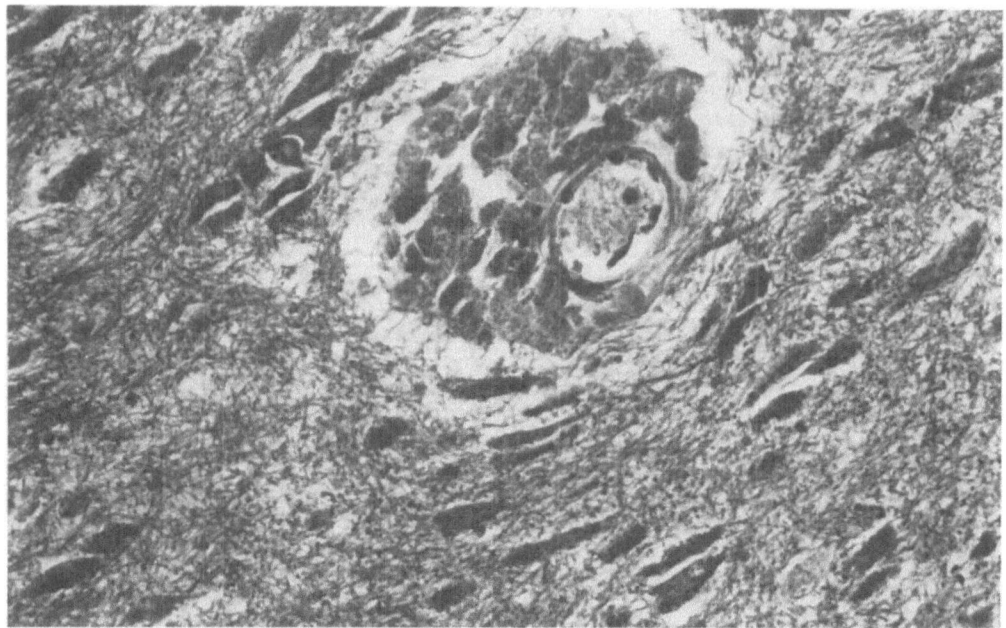

Fig. 6-54. Metachromatic leukodystrophy. A 7-year-old girl with progressive mental impairment, motor difficulties, and rigidity. Sample from parietal white matter showing collection of macrophages containing granular, metachromatic substances (×165).

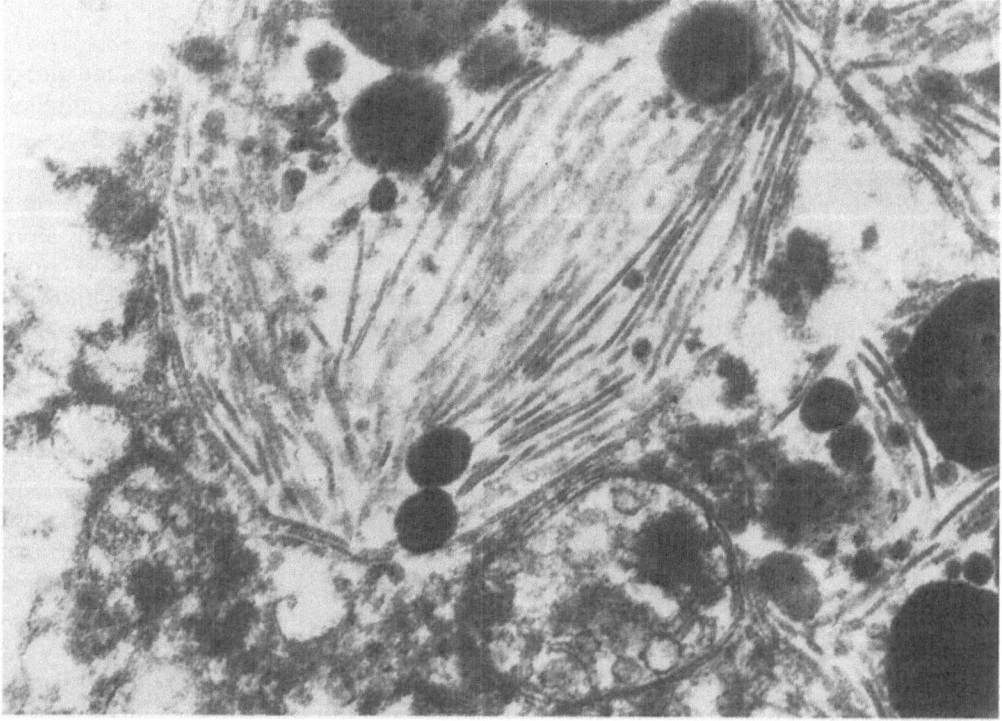

Fig. 6-55. Residual lipid molecules (dense granules and spicules) from a case of metachromatic leukodystrophy. (Original magnification ×35,000).

Inflammation/Neoplasia

In the early stages of the development of a brain abscess, microscopy reveals partly necrotic brain tissue in which protein-rich exudates in the form of pale eosinophilic amorphous materials, and perivascular clusters of neutrophils are easily observed. Bacteria (or fungi) may be demonstrable at this stage with the appropriate staining methods. At the interface between the inflamed and the normal brain tissues, edema, macrophages, reactive astrocytes, and microglia are accompanied by fibrin deposits in the walls of small veins. The designation of cerebritis is sometimes applied to diffuse inflammatory changes of this type that precede the development of a cavity filled with pus. During the stage of liquefaction necrosis protein-rich exudate, disintegrating neutrophils, and other cellular debris fill the center of the lesions, while the periphery is walled off by granulation tissue (within approximately 2 weeks). Soon this is replaced by a two-layered capsule: the inner layer is made up of degenerating neutrophils and fibrin; the outer layer is made of collagen fibers that are encircled by lymphocytes, plasma cells, and reactive astrocytes in the midst of an edematous brain.[157] Approximately 25% of brain abscesses are sterile; Gram-positive (*Staphylococcus aureus*, aerobic *Streptococcus*) and Gram-negative bacteriae (*Proteus*) are recovered from most brain abscesses.[169]

Among the less suppurative causative agents of both cerebritis and brain abscesses are the fungi, in particular aspergillus, cryptococcus, blastomyces, and histoplasm.[36] Brain infections by these organisms are more common among immunocompromised patients, such as the recipients of organ transplants. A large number of localized fungal infections of the brain do not show the discrete pus-filled cavity typical of bacterial abscesses. Rather, fungal lesions may at first appear as either an "infected infarction" or an "infected brain hemorrhage." A more exotic type of fungal infection of the CNS not associated with immune deficiencies and seemingly more common in temperate than in tropical climates has been called "chromoblastomycosis" because of the pigmented nature of the etiologic agent. The fungus, *Cladosporium trichoides*, is different from those producing cutaneous infections of which the most common one is *Cladosporium carrionii*. The presence of *C. trichoides* induces in the CNS a combination of parenchymal (abscess), ventricular, and leptomeningeal inflammatory lesions with abundant scarring.[114]

Localized areas of tissue necrosis and inflammation caused by tuberculous infection of the CNS may occur either on the brain surface (e.g., cerebellopontine angle) or in the brain parenchyma. These localized tuberculous lesions may mimic brain abscesses or tumors and are called tuberculomas. In children, tuberculomas are more frequent in the infratentorial compartment (cerebellum and pons) than in the cerebral hemispheres. In adults, the parietal-occipital lobes seem to be more frequently involved by tuberculomas than the rest of the brain.[25]

Tuberculomas are well-circumscribed and usually, well-encapsulated, relatively avascular lesions whose center is occupied by typically cheesy, white, homogeneous material, (i.e., caseation necrosis). The histologic diagnosis is predicated on the recognition of abundant granulomata at the periphery of the site of necrosis and the identification of the organism. These tuberculous granulomata are usually typical and easy to recognize because they contain abundant multinucleated cells, epithelioid cells, and lymphocytes/monocytes. In most instances, the acid-fast bacilli are easily demonstrable with the appropriate staining methods unless the patient has received many doses of antituberculous drugs immediately before the biopsy was obtained.

A less common type of localized infection of the CNS is called gumma, because of its somewhat rubbery consistency. Gummas are produced by a localized parenchymal type of neurosyphilis. The necrosis in the central part of the lesion differs from that in tuberculomas in that many of the stroma fibers, i.e., reticulin are preserved in the syphilitic lesions.

Small-cell infiltrates in the white matter may indicate a neoplastic condition or an infectious process; a diagnosis of encephalomyelitis should be considered when the small cell infiltrates are accompanied by additional cellular responses such as increased numbers of plump astrocytes, rod cells, and intranuclear inclusion bodies (Fig. 6-56). As discussed below, white matter lesions, where lipid-laden macrophages, plump astrocytes and intranuclear inclusion bodies are abundant, strongly suggest a diagnosis of progressive multifocal leukoencephalopathy (PML). Isolated increases in the number of small cell nuclei (Fig. 6-57) may indicate either proximity to a large collection of neoplastic glial cells or a diffuse growth by cells of a mesenchymal derivation, (e.g., malignant lymphoma).[108] Under such circumstances, a diagnosis of neoplasia is strongly supported by the demonstration of atypical mitotic figures, nuclear pleomorphism, angiocentricity on the part of the presumed neoplastic cells, and endothelial hyperplasia.

White Matter Necrosis

Brain edema is defined as an increase in the volume of brain secondary to the accumulation or retention of fluid, either protein-free or protein-rich. During the acute stage, post ischemic edema is almost exclusively intracellular and primarily astrocytic;[13] chronic brain edema, the type that accumulates at the periphery of intracerebral tumors

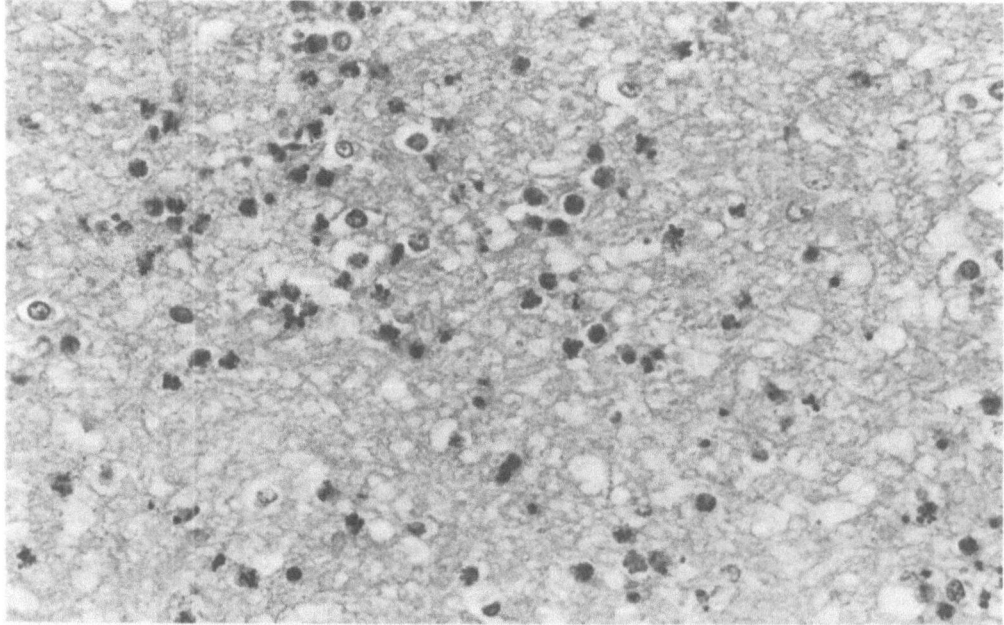

Fig. 6-56. Acute disseminated encephalomyelitis (human). Frontal white matter showing vacuoles, swollen astrocytes, and many neutrophils (×250).

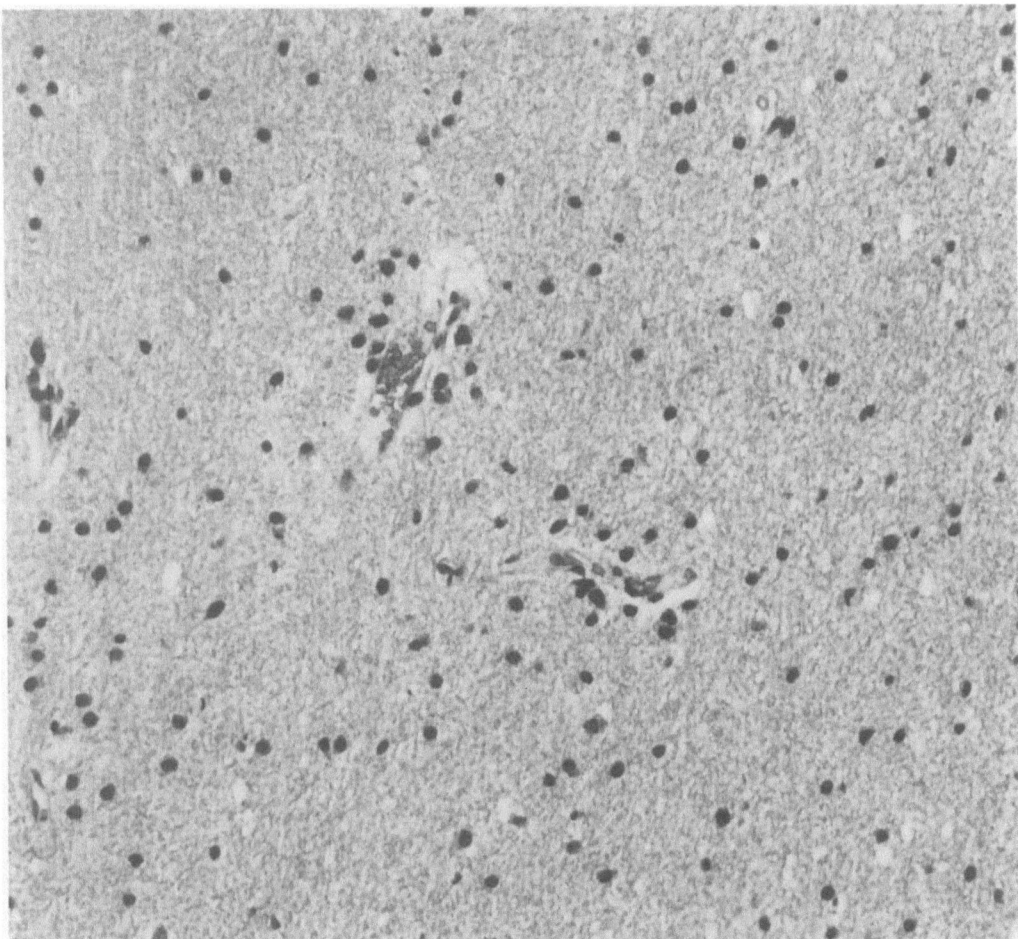

Fig. 6-57. Increased number of mononuclear cells, particularly abundant around blood vessels, in this white matter sample from a patient with a primary brain lymphoma (×400).

(primary or metastatic), is characterized by widening of the extracellular space and myelin splitting.[92] The evidence of brain edema, as measured by the wet weight/dry weight method for example, is easier to demonstrate during the acute stage. Histologically, the sequelae of excessive fluid accumulation remain evident several weeks after the acute episode. Structural abnormalities compatible with a diagnosis of brain edema include persistence of circular, lucent spaces, and the presence of plump, reactive astrocytes.[45,45a] Acute edema in an area of ischemia secondary to an arterial occlusion, is characterized by pallor of myelin, vacuolation, swelling of astrocytic nucleus and cytoplasm, preservation of the stainability of oligodendrocytic nuclei, and occasional spheroids (Fig. 6-58). Disintegration of myelin sheaths and some astrocytes during the subacute stage of edema is accompanied by mononuclear leukocytic infiltrates and by the appearance of abundant lipid-laden macrophages (Fig. 6-59). In chronic edema, the stainability of myelin is probably restored through remyelination.[16] There may be occasional spheroids, abundant plump astrocytes, and large (up to 100 µm in diameter)

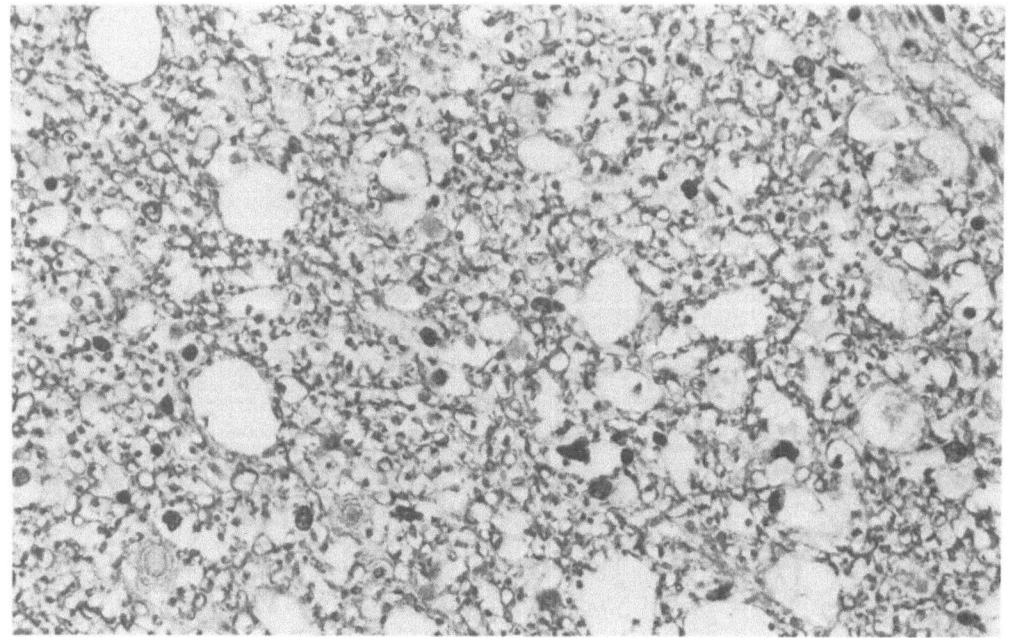

Fig. 6-58. Acute brain edema characterized by large vacuoles, myelin pallor, and normal nuclear stainability (×400).

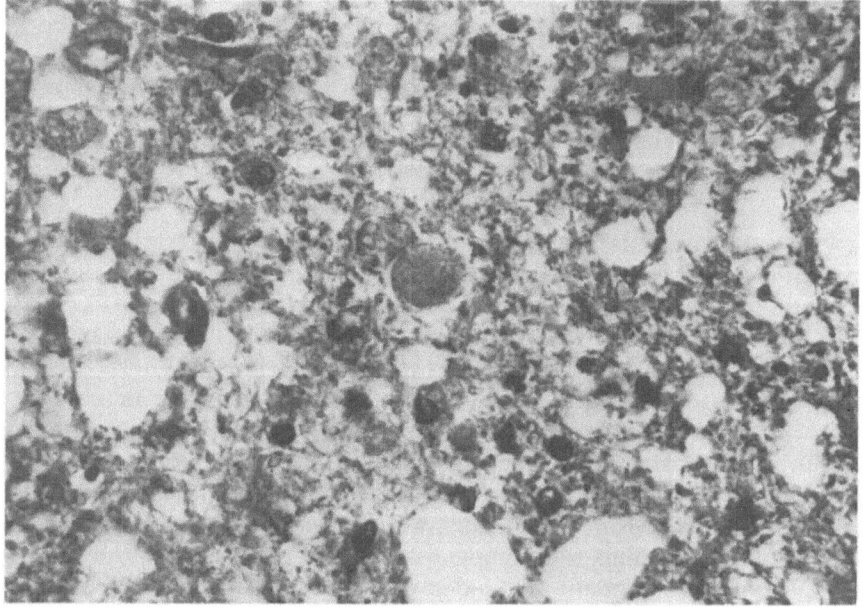

Fig. 6-59. White matter from an area made ischemic by arterial occlusion about one week before death to show vacuolation, at least a spheroid, macrophages, and reactive astrocytes (×640).

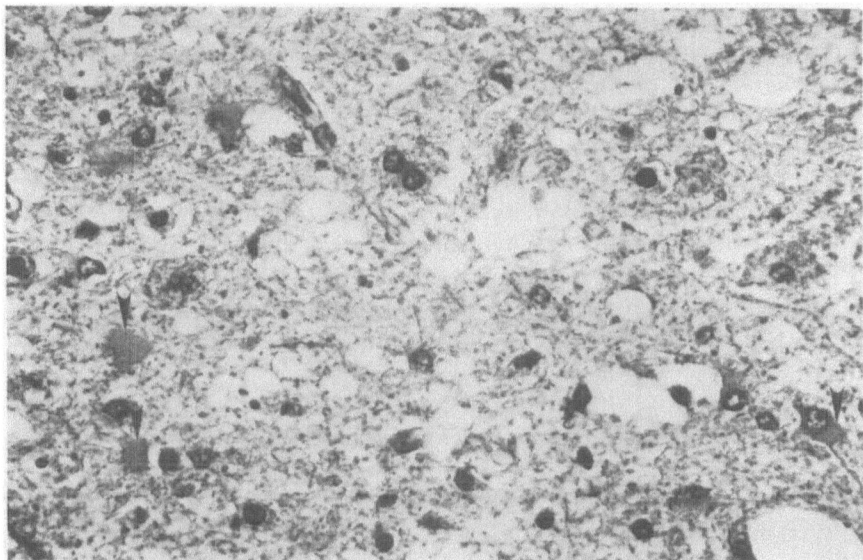

Fig. 6-60. Swollen white matter surrounding a metastic carcinoma; mostly circular enlarged spaces and plump astrocytes are apparent (arrowheads) (×640).

vacuoles, which are probably the remnants of spaces where massively swollen axis cylinders have eventually disintegrated (Fig. 6-60).

Subcortical arteriosclerotic encephalopathy is the designation adopted for a diffuse and slowly progressive disease of the cerebral white matter that develops in association with structural abnormalities involving the penetrating small arteries and arterioles of the brain. These vessels characteristically show thickening of the tunica media with replacement of the smooth muscle fibers by collagen (i.e., hyalinization) (Figs. 6-61,

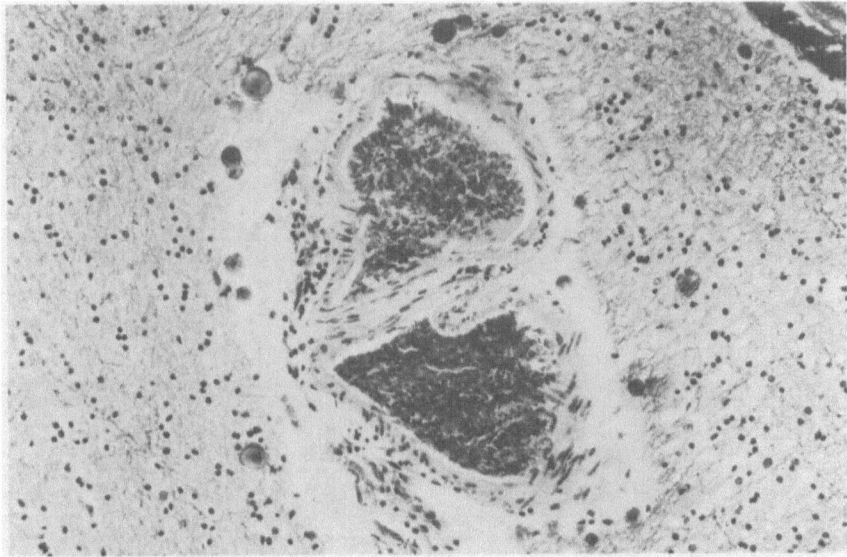

Fig. 6-61. Cross-section of normal arterioles in a 67-year-old patient; a few, perivascular mononuclear cells and occasional corpora amylacea are visible (×400).

and 6-62). In some of the larger vessels such as the lenticulostriate branches of the MCA, lipid-laden macrophages may be visible. The white matter is intact in the subcortical areas, whereas the deeper, periventricular portions show considerable rarefaction or loosening of the myelinated fibers accompanied by astrogliosis. This appears to be a result of two phenomena: enlargement of extracellular space caused by retention of protein-free fluid and destruction of axons and myelin sheaths; and oligodendrocytic nuclei retain their normal stainability. Some of the prominent symptoms observed in these patients include: various focal neurologic deficits usually appearing in progressive episodes that may end in a dementing syndrome.[20] Considerable controversy exists over the relationship that may exist between subcortical white matter lucency (as demonstrated by MRI) and the syndrome of multi-infarction dementia.[32]

Non-Suppurative Inflammatory Lesions: Viral Encephalitis

A large number of patients admitted to the hospital with a presumptive diagnosis of acute viral encephalitis (not otherwise specified) have been evaluated prospectively in a nationwide collaborative study. The analysis of these 182 patients, all of whom had a lobe of their brain biopsied, revealed that a significant percent of such patients had in fact noninfectious brain diseases, such as an infarction and brain tumor, or were afflicted with cerebral infections other than herpetic encephalitis.[162] This and subsequent analyses of similar studies have led to the conclusion that brain biopsy is necessary for the diagnosis of acute viral encephalitis, of which the three major causative agents are: herpes simplex virus, toga virus, and St. Louis encephalitis virus.[161] The light-microscopic features of these conditions are not significantly different from one another;

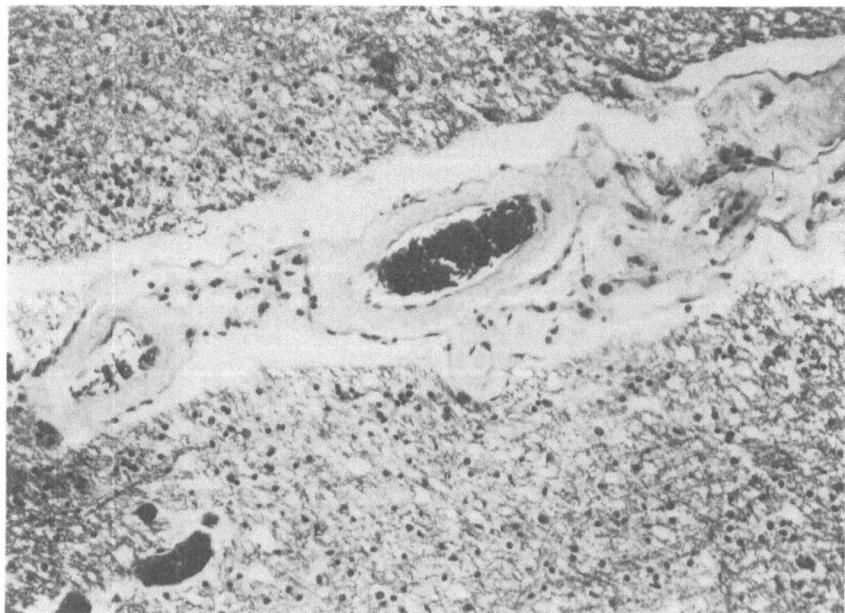

Fig. 6-62. The smooth muscle cell in these arterioles appear thickened, hyalinized, and homogeneous in this white matter biopsy obtained from a person with chronic arterial hypertension (×400).

however, when intranuclear inclusion bodies can be found and immunohistochemical identification of the antigen can be achieved, microscopy may allow a conclusive diagnosis of (for example) herpes encephalitis. The potential benefits derived from the early start of the antiviral therapy require in most instances brain biopsy to confirm the diagnosis.

The demonstration of mononuclear infiltrates either in the subarachnoid space or the brain parenchyma (Fig. 6-63), usually permit an intraoperative diagnosis "compatible with viral encephalitis," which may be sufficient to start the administration of the antiviral agent.

A more definitive diagnosis of herpetic infection may be advanced within a few hours through the application of immunohistochemical methods, (i.e., light-microscopic demonstration of the herpes antigen by the peroxidase-antiperoxidase method).[46] In addition to the typical Cowdry type A inclusion body, brain biopsies from patients with herpes simplex may show a variety of other nuclear abnormalities that may not necessarily qualify as typical inclusion bodies.[46] Moreover, even in biopsies where the intranuclear inclusion bodies are not seen, the ultrastructural evaluation may reveal viral particles suggestive of a specific diagnosis, (e.g., herpes simplex and togavirus encephalitis).[46] (Figs. 6-64 and 6-65). Other conditions characterized by the presence of intranuclear inclusion bodies either in gray or white matter structures are described below.

Subacute sclerosing panencephalitis (SSPE) is a slowly progressive neurologic disorder of childhood that may be identified in brain biopsies by inflammation consisting of slight mononuclear infiltrates in leptomeninges, presence of lymphocytes, plasma

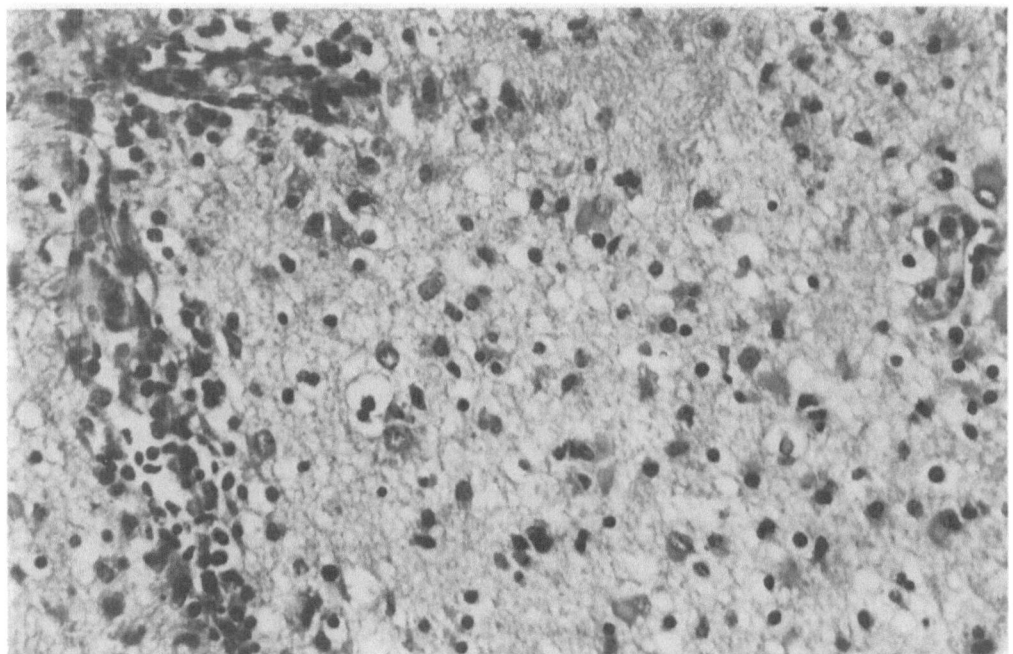

Fig. 6-63. Eight-year-old boy with myoclonic jerks and personality changes. Lymphocytic infiltrates, myelin breakdown, astrogliosis, and intranuclear inclusion bodies (not shown) made this biopsy compatible with a diagnosis of SSPE (×250).

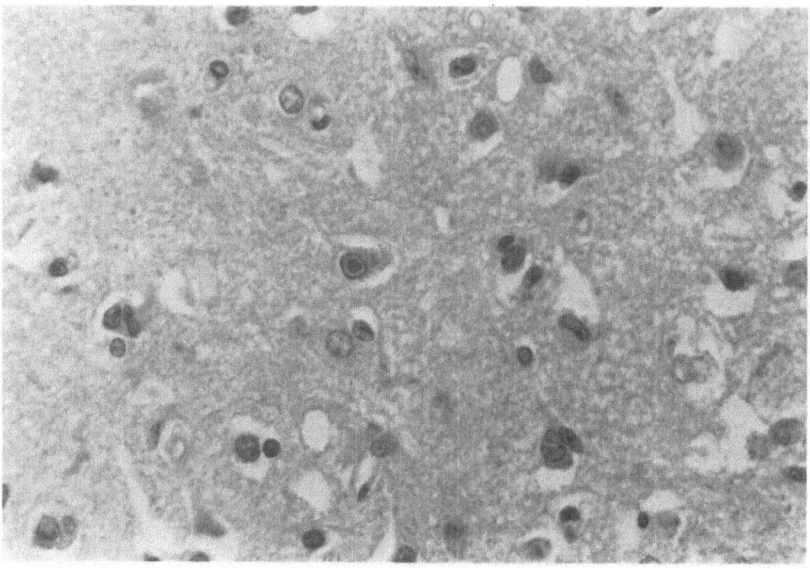

Fig. 6-64. Two-and-one-half-month-old boy with a 3-week history of sleepiness, vomiting, fever, and generalized seizures. Sample from temporal lobe showing an intranuclear inclusion body (×630).

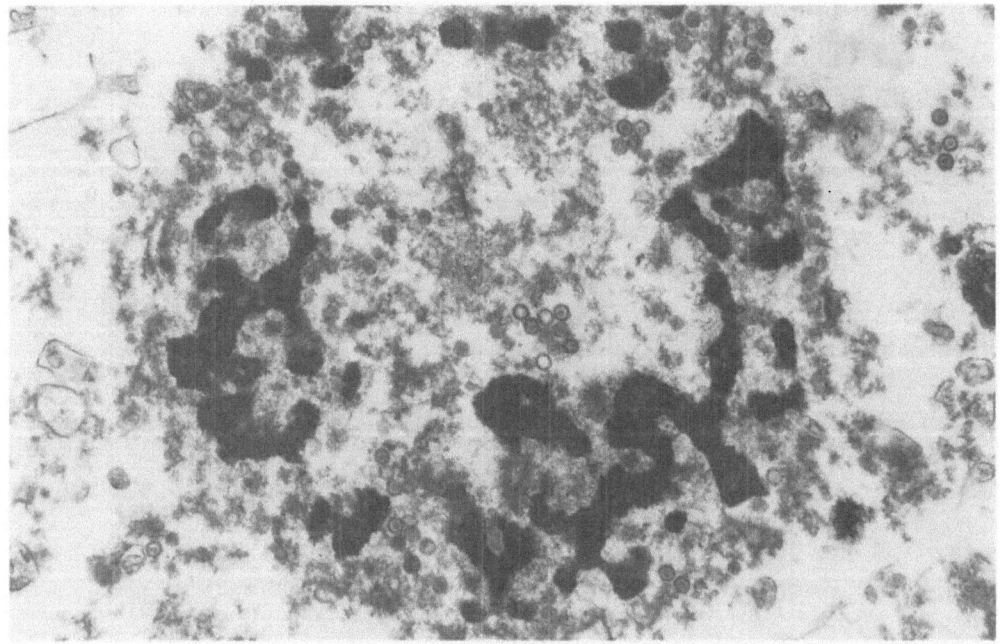

Fig. 6-65 Herpes simplex encephalitis. The hexagonal viral particles (each measuring about 200 μm in diameter) are shown here in the nucleus and cytoplasm. Tissues were kept in fixative for several months before being processed for electron microscopy (×28,000) (Courtesy E.J. Yunis, M.D.)

cells, and macrophages in the cortex, but particularly in the white matter where the mononuclear infiltration may be either diffuse or nodular. Abundant plump astrocytes may be visible, and occasional intranuclear inclusion bodies (Fig. 6-66) can also be found; myelin stains poorly or not at all. By electron microscopy, one can confirm that both myelin and axons disintegrate. The intranuclear inclusion bodies are particularly abundant in astrocytes, but they can also be found in neurons, oligodendrocytes, phagocytes, and other cells. Ultrastructurally, the typical inclusion bodies (Cowdry type A) are confined to astroglia and are composed of tubular myxovirus-like structures measuring 17–23 nm in diameter. Many other nonspecific intranuclear inclusions have been described in biopsies from patients with SSPE.[148,97] In some cases, the cerebral cortex is almost exclusively involved, but more often there is diffuse inflammation and astrogliosis of the white matter. In addition to the characteristic clinical features, the diagnosis of SSPE can be strongly inferred from the well known abnormalities of the EEG and the CSF.[80]

A second condition characterized histologically by multiple zones of myelin loss, inflammatory infiltrates, alterations in glial nuclei, and intranuclear inclusion bodies is progressive multifocal leukoencephalophthy (PML). The usual circumstances in which the disease occurs involve an immunocompromised patient (i.e., patients afflicted with lymphoma, leukemia, tuberculosis, sarcoidosis, organ transplant recipients, and HIV positive patients) who develops multifocal neurologic abnormalities usually confined to the white matter as demonstrated by CT scan of the head. In most patients, there are widespread lesions of the entire CNS, but in about 10% of the cases, the initial symptoms suggest primarily unifocal disease of either the brain stem or cerebellum.[102] The primary abnormality consists of focal destruction to myelin sheaths accompanied

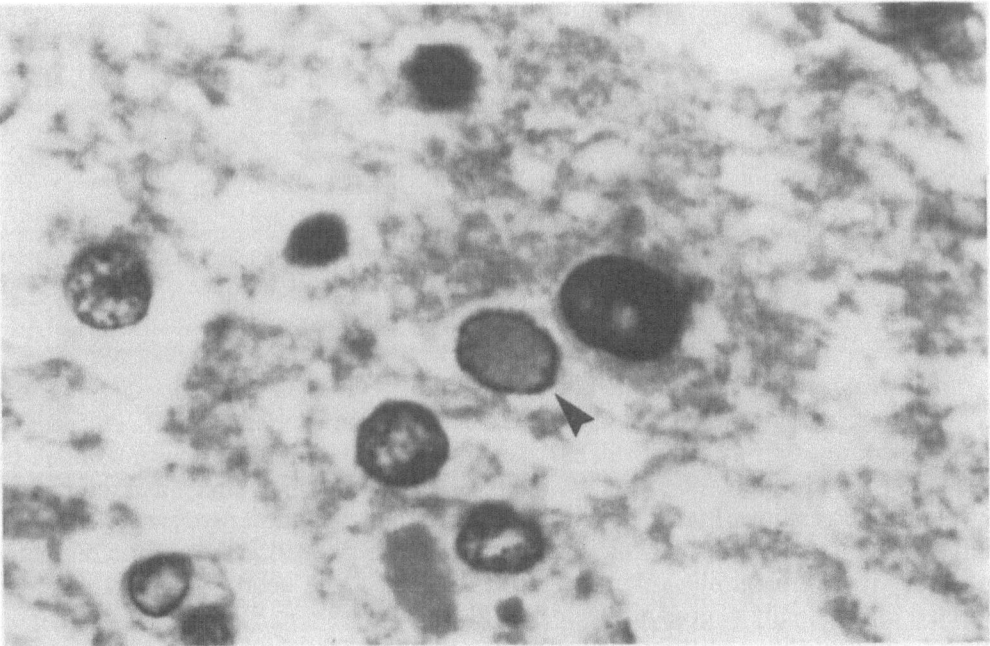

Fig. 6-66. SSPE. The chromatin of the cell in the center (arrowhead) is displaced eccentrically by a collection of virions that collectively correspond to the "inclusion body" (×630) (Courtesy of E.J. Yunis, M.D.).

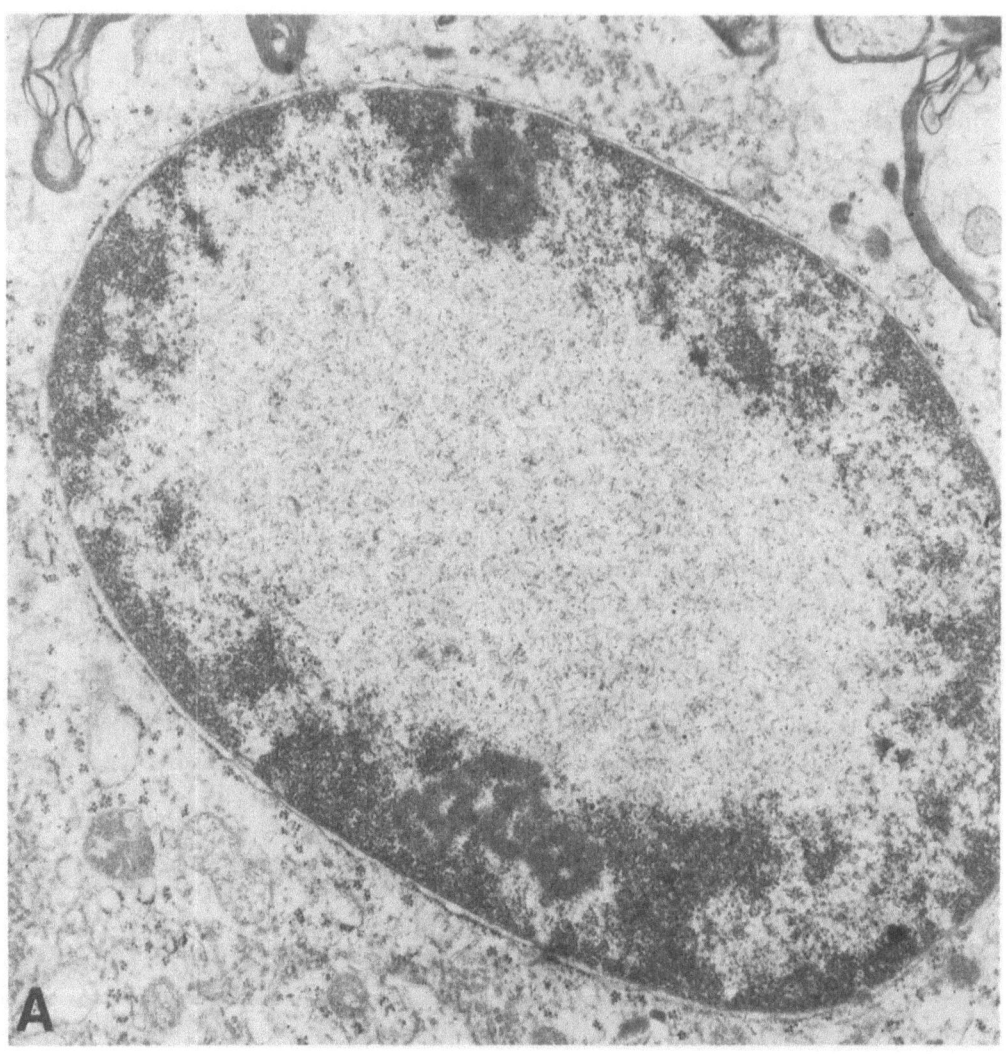

Fig. 6-67. (A and B) Progressive multifocal leukoencephalopathy. Numerous uncoated viral particles (papova viruses), each measuring about 35 nm in cross-diameter, partially fill the nucleus (×10,000 and ×50,000).

by inflammatory changes that include a few lymphocytes, plasma cells, and abundant lipid-laden phagocytes. Two microscopic features are characteristic of PML: enlargement of oligodendrocytic nuclei with dense basophilia and clumping of chromatin. A less frequently found cellular abnormality involves astrocytes that exhibit a marked increase in volume with changes in nuclear chromatin pattern that suggest neoplastic transformation (Alzheimer's type I).[125] By electron microscopy (Fig. 6-67) and immunofluorescent methods, two serologically different papova viruses have been demonstrated in the infected cells (usually oligodendrocytes) of PML: JC virus and SV-40 virus.[160] Serologic studies indicate that about 50% of adults worldwide have had at least one infection with JC virus;[102] therefore, it is presumed that the development of PML reflects the recrudescence of a latent infection.

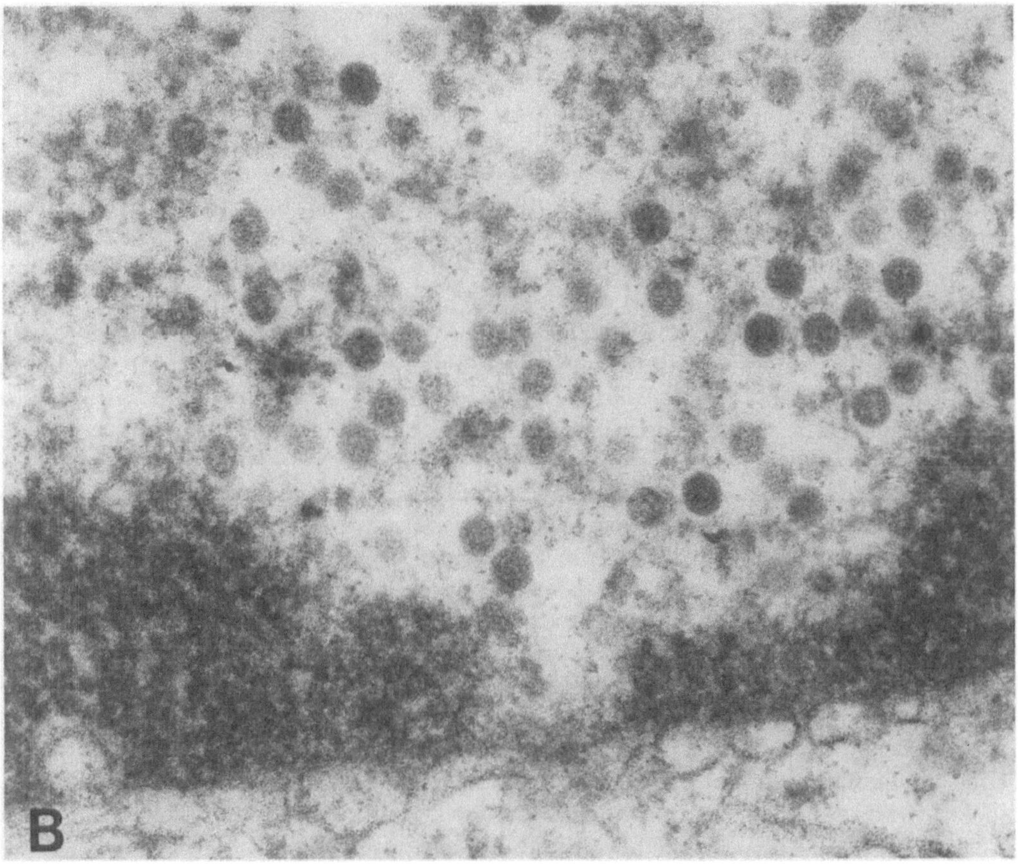

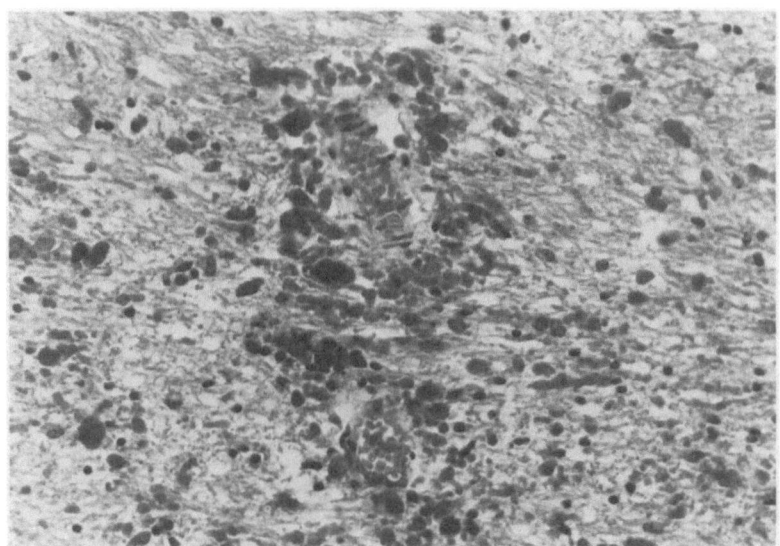

Fig. 6-68. Alexander disease. Abundant Rosenthal fibers around blood vessels in this white matter biopsy obtained from a child whose main symptoms included dementia and megalencephaly (×250).

Miscellaneous White Matter Disorders

Alexander's disease is a rare disorder of infancy, characterized clinically by progressive spasticity, mental retardation, and megalencephaly. In light-microscopic preparations, Alexander's disease can be recognized by the almost total absence of myelin sheaths and oligodendrocytes, the severe decrease in number of axis cylinders, and the luxuriant irregular astrogliosis with numerous Rosenthal fibers (RF).[51] These fibers are homogeneous, eosinophilic masses forming elongate, tapered rods (measuring up to 30 μm in length and 2–20 μm in diameter) that are diffusely scattered throughout the cortex and white matter, and are specially numerous in subpial, perivascular, and subependymal locations (Fig. 6-68). RF are conspicuously absent from the cerebellar cortex, while large numbers are usually present in a periaqueductal location. Rosenthal fibers are not specific for Alexander's disease. They also can be found in cases of syringomyelia, in areas of gliosis, in the vicinity of cerebral, spinal, and cerebellar astrocytomas (including optic nerve gliomas), and in demyelinating processes such as multiple sclerosis.[66] Rosenthal fibers are intracytoplasmic, electron-dense, amorphous materials almost always seen in astrocytic processes and areas of marked astrogliosis. Despite their intracellular presence in astrocytes, RF are antigenically different from glial filaments. The existence of localized type of Rosenthal fiber accumulation has been interpreted as being a variant of the diffuse, typical Alexander's disease.[59]

Cerebral radiation necrosis is the designation given to histologic changes that appear in the brain of some patients subjected to radiotherapy directed to the head. Several months or years may elapse between the radiotherapy and the beginning of symptoms. The white matter is more commonly involved than the cortex and involvement of the cerebrum is more frequent than that of the infratentorial tissues. The histologic appearance of the acute lesions in the white matter resembles that of multiple sclerosis plaques (Fig. 6-69). In the delayed variety of radiation disease, telangiectasis, fibrinoid vascular changes, and astroglial alteration (Fig. 6-70) have been observed.[79] Radiation induced changes may mimic (in the imaging studies) the histologic features of an astrocytoma or even those of a fibrosarcoma. A usually reliable sign of radiation effect can be appreciated in the form of fibrinoid changes in medium caliber arterioles.

Cerebral spongy degeneration of infancy, sometimes called Canavan disease, is a fatal autosomal-recessive disorder of unknown cause. Prominent clinical features include: megalencephaly, blindness, spasticity, and progressive psychomotor deterioration. Brain biopsy shows striking vacuolation in both cortex and subjacent white matter. Vacuolation in the former is caused by marked astrocytic swelling. In the white matter, vacuoles correspond to intramyelinic and extracellular fluid accumulation.[2] In the cerebellum, vacuoles are most prominent at the interface between cortex and white matter; abnormalities in astrocytic nuclei (commonly known as Alzeheimer's type II) are prominent in the absence of any evidence of hepatic disease. Ultrastructural and histochemical studies suggest a metabolic abnormality of astroglial mitochondria as a cause of the structural abnormalities.[8]

Additional spongy abnormalities of the white matter, or cerebral sponginess, may be seen in subcortical areas of either the cerebellum or cerebrum of young children or infants in association with hexachlorophene intoxication, disorders of gangliosides metabolism, and several other causes such as administration of triethyltin sulfate, cuprizone, and isonicotinic acid hydrazide.[146] Disorders of amino acid metabolism, such as phenylketonuria, may coexist with defects in myelination, astrogliosis, and vacuolation of white

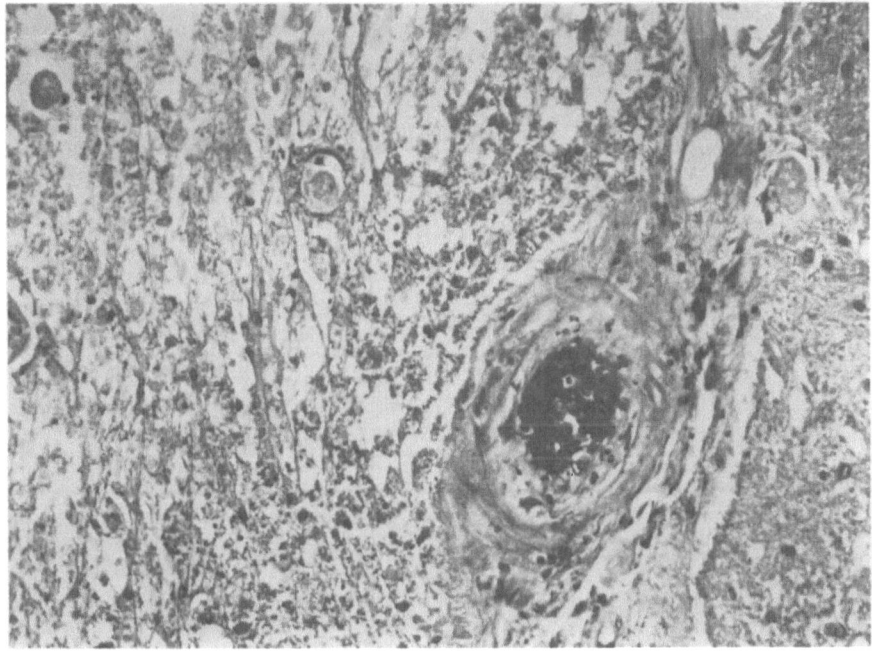

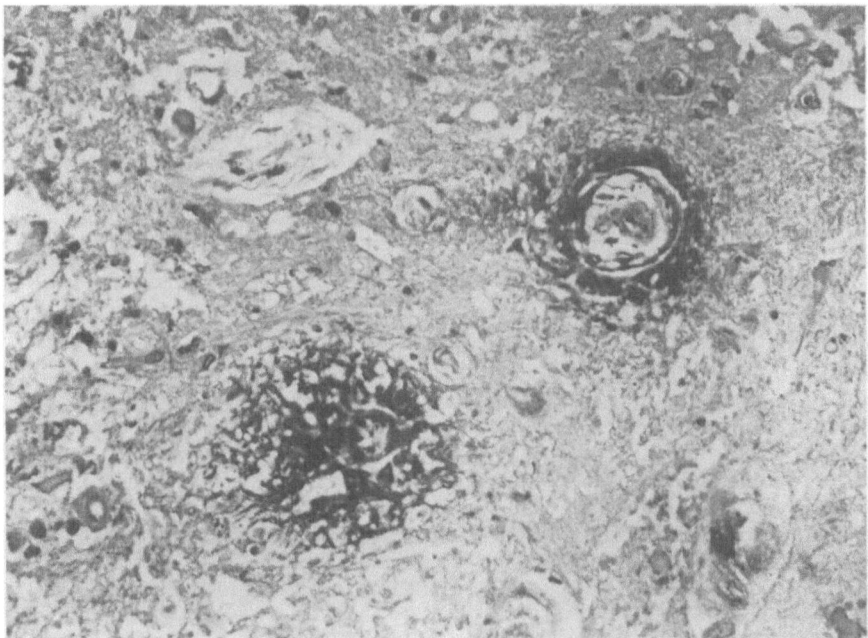

Fig. 6-69, 6-70. Fragment of spinal white matter from a 61-year-old man (with carcinoma of the lung) who received 8,500 rads 8 weeks before death. Destruction of myelin and axons, and angiitis can be observed at the top. The bottom figure shows fibrinoid changes in the vessel walls (×640).

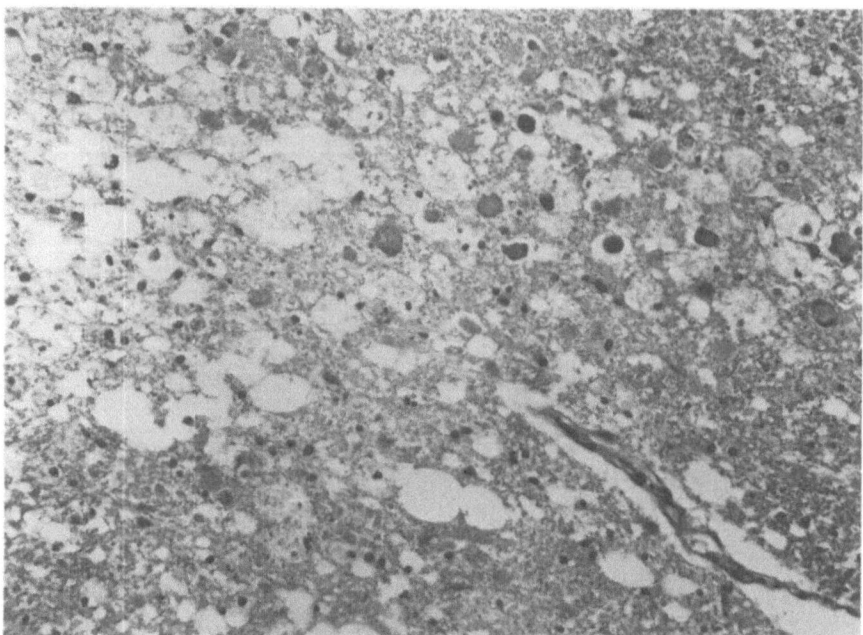

Fig. 6-71. Focal vacuolation, myelin pallor, spheroids, and lipid laden macrophages from the spinal white matter of a leukemic patient who became paraplegic 8 weeks before death (×640).

matter, that are especially prominent in the cerebral hemispheres. These changes are associated with a decrease in lipids and proteolipids.[137]

Multifocal areas of white matter vacuolation, collections of macrophages, spheroids, and astroglia (Fig. 6-71) in the brains of leukemic patients have been attributed by some authors to the combined effects of drugs used in the treatment of these patients (such as methotrexate) and radiotherapy directed to the brain or spinal cord.[97a,128]

References

1. Adachi M, Volk BW, Schneck L, et al: Fine structure of myenteric plexus in various lipidoses. *Arch Pathol* 87:228–236, 1969
2. Adornato BT, O'Brien JS, Lampert PW, et al: Cerebral spongy degeneration of infancy. A biochemical and ultrastructural study of affected twins. *Neurology* 22:202–210, 1972
3. Alexander CB, Burger PC, Gore JA: Dissecting aneurysms of the basilar artery in two patients. *Stroke* 10:294–299, 1979
4. Anzil AP, Blinzinger K, Mehraein P, et al: Niemann-Pick disease type C: A case report with ultrastructural findings. *Neuropediatrie* 4:207–225, 1973
5. Averback P: Dense microspheres in normal human brain. *Acta Neuropathol (Berl)* 61:148–152, 1983
6. Ball MJ: Alzheimer's disease. A challenging enigma. *Arch Pathol Lab Med* 106:157–162, 1982
7. Baringer JR, Gajdusek DC, Gibbs CJ, et al: Transmissible dementias: Current problems in tissue handling. *Neurology* 30:302–303, 1980
8. Becker LE, Yates A: Inherited Metabolic disease. In: *Textbook of Neuropathology* (eds) RL Davis and DM Robertson. Baltimore, Williams and Wilkins, 1985, 284–371
9. Bentz MS, Towfighi J, Greenwood S, et al: Sturge-Weber syndrome. A case with thyroid and choroid plexus hemangiomas and leptomeningeal melanosis. *Arch Pathol Lab Med* 106:75–78, 1982
10. Berger MS, Wilson CB: Epidermoid cysts of the posterior fossa. *J Neurosurg* 62:214–219, 1985

11. Bostrom K, Liliequist B: Primary dissecting aneurysm of the extracranial part of the internal carotid and vertebral arteries. *Neurology* 17:179–186, 1967
12. Brady RO: Biochemical genetics in neurology. *Arch Neurol* 33:145–151, 1976
13. Brierley JB: Pathology of cerebral ischemia, in McDowell FH, Brennan RH (eds): *Cerebral Vascular Diseases, Eighth Princeton Conference.* New York, Grune & Stratton, 1973, 59–66
14. Brightman MW, Broadwell RD: The morphological approach to the study of the normal and abnormal brain permeability. *Adv Exp Med Biol* 69:41–54, 1976
15. Brion S, Mikol J, Psimaras A: Recent findings in Pick's disease, in HM Zimmerman (ed): *Progress in Neuropathology, Vol 2,* New York, Grune & Stratton, 1973, 421–452
16. Bunge RP: Glial cells and the central myelin sheath. *Physiol Rev* 48:197–251, 1968
17. Burger P, Burch JG, Kunze U: Subcortical arteriosclerotic encephalopathy (Binswanger's disease) A vascular etiology of dementia. *Stroke* 7:626–631, 1976
18. Butzler JF, Schochet SS, Bell WE: Infantile neuroaxonal dystrophy. *Acta Neuropathol (Berl)* 31:35–43, 1975
19. Cammermeyer J: Is the solitary dark neuron a manifestation of postmortem trauma to the brain inadequately fixed by perfusion? *Histochem* 56:97–115, 1978
20. Caplan LR, Schoene WC: Clinical features of subcortical arteriosclerotic encephalopathy (Binswanger disease). *Neurology* 29:1206–1215, 1978
21. Carpenter S, Karpati G, Wolfe LS: A type of juvenile cerebromacular degeneration characterized by granular osmiophilic deposits. *J Neurol Sci* 18:67–87, 1973
22. Cohen EB, Pappas GD: Dark Profiles in apparently normal central nervous system: A problem in the electron microscopic identification of early anterograde axonal degeneration. *J Comp Neurol* 1136:375–395, 1969
23. Cowdry EV: The problem of intranuclear inclusions in virus diseases. *Arch Pathol* 18:527–542, 1934
24. Daniel PF, DeFeudis DF, Lott IT, et al: Quantitative microanalysis of oligosaccharides by high performance liquid chromatography. *Carbohydrate Res* 97:161–180, 1981
25. Dastur DK, Lalitha VS: The many facets of neurotuberculosis: An epitome of neuropathology, in Zimmerman HM (ed): *Progress in Neuropathology, Vol 2,* New York, Grune & Stratton, 1973, 351–408
26. DeBaecque CM, Pollack MA, Suzuki K: Late infantile neuronal storage disease with curvilinear bodies. Systemic pathologic features. *Arch Pathol Lab Med* 100:139–144, 1976
27. Deraksham I, Bahmanyar M, Noorsalehi S, et al: Light-microscopic diagnosis of rabies. A reappraisal. *Lancet* 1:302–303, 1978
28. Dolman CL: Diagnosis of neurometabolic disorders by examination of skin biopsies and lymphocytes. *Semi Diagn Pathol* 1:82–97, 1984
29. Dorfman, Matalon R: The mucopolysaccharidoses, in Stanbury JB, Wyngaarden, JB, Frederickson, DS, et al (eds): *The Metabolic Basis of Inherited Disease,* New York, McGraw-Hill, 1972, 1218–1272
30. DuPont JR, Earle KM: Human rabies encephalitis. A study of forty-nine fatal cases with a review of the literature. *Neurology* 15:1023–1034, 1965
31. Elfenbein IB Cantor HE: Late infantile amaurotic idiocy with multilamellar cytosomes: An ultrastructural study. *J Pediatr* 75:353–364, 1969
32. Erkinjuntti T, Haltia M, Palo J, et al: Accuracy of the clinical diagnosis of vascular dementia: A prospective clinical and post mortem neuropathological diagnosis. *J Neurol Neurosurg Psych* 51:1037–1044, 1988
33. Escobar E: The pathology of neurocysticercosis, in Palacios E, Rodriguezcarbajal J, Taveras JM (eds): *Cysticercosis of the Central Nervous System,* Springfield, Illinois, Charles C. Thomas, 1983
34. Farrell DF, MacMartin MP, Clark AF: Multiple molecular forms of arylsulfatase A in different forms of metachromatic leukodystrophy. *Neurology* 29:16–20, 1979
35. Farrell DF, Sumi SM: Skin punch biopsy in the diagnosis of juvenile neuronal ceroid-lipofuscinosis. A comparison with leukocyte peroxidase assay. *Arch Neurol* 34:39–44, 1977
36. Fetter BF, Klintworth GK, Hendry WF: *Mycoses of the Central Nervous System.* Baltimore, Williams & Wilkins, 1967
37. Flament-Durand J, Rouck AM: Spongiform alterations in brain biopsies of presenile dementia. *Acta Neuropathol (Berlin)* 46:159–162, 1979
38. Flechsig P: *Anatomie des Menschlichen Gehirns und Rueckenmarks auf Myelogenetischer Grundlage, Band 1,* Leipzig, 1920
39. Fredrickson DS, Sloan HR: Sphingomyelin lipidoses: Niemann-Pick disease, in Stanbury JB, et al (eds): *The Metabolic Basis of Inherited Disease,* New York, McGraw-Hill, 1972, 783–799
40. French BN, Rewcastle, NB: Sequential morphological changes at the site of carotid endarterectomy. *J Neurosurg* 4:745–754, 1974

41. Gambetti P, DiMauro S, Baker SL: Nervous system in Pompe disease: Ultrastructure and biochemistry. *J Neuropathol Exp Neurol* 30:412–430, 1971
42. Gambetti P, DiMauro S, Hirt L, et al: Myoclonic epilepsy with Lafora bodies. Some ultrastructural, histochemical, and biochemical aspects. *Arch Neurol* 25:483–493, 1971
43. Garcia JH, Mitchem HL, Briggs L, et al: Transient focal ischemia in subhuman primates: Neuronal injury as a function of local cerebral blood flow. *J Neuropathol Exp Neurol* 42:44–60, 1983
44. Garcia JH, Kamijyo Y, Kalimo H, et al: "Dark" neurons and red neurons: Ultrastructural evaluation. *J Neuropathol Exp Neurol* 37:84, 1975
45. Garcia JH, Lossinsky AS, Kauffman FC, et al: Neuronal ischemic injury: Light microscopy, ultrastructure and biochemistry. *Acta Neuropathol (Berl)* 43:85–95, 1978
45a. Garcia JH: Experimental ischemic stroke: A review. *Stroke* 15:5–14, 1984
46. Garcia JH, Colon LE, Whitley RJ, Wilmes FJ: Diagnosis of viral encephalitis by brain biopsy, in Santa Cruz DJ (ed): *Seminars in Diagnostic Pathology*, San Diego, Grune & Stratton, 1984, 78–81
47. Garcia JH: The neuropathology of stroke. *Hum Pathol* 6:583–598, 1975
48. Garcia JH: Circulatory disorders of the brain, in Davis RL, Robertson D (eds): *Textbook of Neuropathology*, Baltimore, Williams & Wilkins, 1985, 548–631
49. Garcia JH, Kamijyo Y: Cerebral infarction. Evolution of histopathological changes after occlusion of a middle cerebral artery in primates. *J Neuropathol Exp Neurol* 33:409–421, 1974
50. Garcia JH, Kamijyo Y, Kalimo H, et al: Cerebral ischemia. The early structural changes and correlations of these with known metabolic and dynamic abnormalities, in Whisant JP, Sandok B (eds): *Cerebral Vascular Disease Ninth Conference*, JP Whisnant, B Sandok (eds), New York, Grune & Stratton, 1975, 313–323
51. Garret R, Ames RP: Alexander disease. Case report with electron microscopical studies and review of the literature. *Arch Pathol* 98:379–385, 1974
52. Geer JC, McGill HC, Strong JP: The fine structure of human atherosclerotic lesions. *Am J Pathol* 38:263–271, 1961
53. Geer JC, Garcia JH: Atherosclerosis, in Wilkins RH, SS Rengachary (eds): *Neurosurgery*. New York, McGraw-Hill, 1985, 1189–1192
54. Ghatak NR, Mushrush GJ: Supratentorial intra-arachnoid cyst. Case report. *J Neurosurg* 35:477–482, 1971
55. Gibson PH, Stones M, Tomlinson BE: Senile changes in the human neocortex and hippocampus compared by the use of the electron and light microscopes. *J Neurol Sci* 27:289–406, 1976
56. Gil DR, Ratto GD: Contribution to the study of the origin of the leptomeninges in the human embryo. *Acta Anat (Basel)* 85:620–623, 1973
57. Glenner GG: Amyloid deposits and amyloidosis. The β-fibrilloses. *N Engl J Med* 302:1283–1344, 1980
58. Go KG, Houthoff HJ, Blaaw EH, et al: Arachnoid cysts of the sylvian tissue. Evidence of fluid secretion. *J Neurosurg* 60:803–810, 1984
58a. Goebel HH, Argyrakis A, Shimokawa K, et al: Adult metachromatic leukodystrophy. IV. Ultrastructural studies on the central and peripheral nervous system. *Eur Neurol* 19:294–307, 1980
59. Goebel HH, Bode G, Caesar R, et al: Bulbar palsy with Rosenthal fibers formation in the medulla of a 15-year-old girl. Localized form of Alexander's disease? *Neuropediatrics* 12:382–391, 1981
60. Goebel HH, Schulz F: The ultrastructural variability of nonspecific lipopigments. *Acta Neuropathol (Berl)* 48:227–230, 1979
61. Gold AP, Ransohoff J, Carter S: Vein of Galen malformation. *Acta Neurol Scan (Suppl 11)* 40:5–31, 1964
62. Gonatas NK, Gonatas J: Ultrastructural and biochemical observations on a case of systemic late infantile lipidosis its relationship to Tay-Sachs disease and gargoylism. *J Neuropathol Exp Neurol* 24:318–340, 1965
63. Gonatas NK, Moss A: Pathologic axons and synapses in human neuropsychiatric disorders. Hum Pathol 6:571–582, 1975
64. Hannieh A, Simpson DA, North JB: Arachnoid cysts: A critical review of 41 cases. *Child's Nerv Syst* 4:92–96, 1988
65. Harsh GR, Edwards MSB, Wilson CB: Intracranial arachnoid cysts in children. *J Neurosurg* 64:834–842, 1986
66. Herndon RM, Rubinstein LJ, Freeman JM, et al: Light and electron microscopic observations on Rosenthal fibers in Alexander's disease and in multiple sclerosis. *J Neuropathol Exp Neurol* 29:524–551, 1970
67. Herring AB, Urich H: Sarcoidosis of the central nervous system. *J Neurol Sci* 9:405–522, 1969
68. Hinton DR, Dolan E, Sima AAF: The value of histopathologic examination of surgically removed blood clots in determining the etiology of spontaneous intracerebral hemorrhage. *Stroke* 15:517–520, 1984
69. Hirano A: Neurons, Astrocytes and Ependyma, in Davis RL, Robertson DM eds: *Textbook of Neuropathology* Baltimore, Williams and Wilkins, 1985, 30–32

70. Hirano A, Zimmerman HM, Levine S, et al: Cytoplasmic inclusions in Chediak-Higashi and wobbler mink. An electron microscopic study of the nervous system. *J Neuropathol Exp Neurol* 30:470–487, 1971

71. Hirano A, Terry RD: Aneurysm of the vein of Galen. *J Neuropathol Exp Neurol* 17:424–429, 1958

72. Hirano A, Ghatak NR: The fine structure of colloid cysts of the third ventricle. *J Neuropathol Exp Neurol* 33:333–341, 1974

73. Ho K-C, Roessmann U, Straumford JV, et al: Analysis of brain weight. II. Adult brain weight in relation to body height, weight and surface area. *Arch Pathol Lab Med* 104:640–645, 1980

74. Ho K-C, Roessmann U, Straumford JV, et al: Analysis of brain weight. I. Adult brain weight in relation to sex, race, and age. *Arch Pathol Lab Med* 104:635–639, 1980

75. Holmes EW, O'Brien JS: Separation of glycoprotein-derived oligosaccharides by thin layer chromatography. *Anal Biochem* 93:167–170, 1979

76. Hooper MW, Vogel FS: The limbic system in Alzheimer's disease. A neuropathologic investigation. *Am J Pathol* 85:1–20, 1976

77. Hudgins RW, Garcia JH: The effect of electrocautery, atmospheric exposure and surgical retraction on the permeability of the blood brain barrier. *Stroke* 1:375–380, 1970

78. Huntington G: On chorea. *Med Surg Rep, (Phila)* 26:317–321, 1872

79. Husain MM, Garcia JH: Cerebral "radiation necrosis": vascular and glial features. *Acta Neuropathol (Berl)* 36:381–385, 1976

80. Jabbour JT, Garcia JH, Lemmi H, et al: Subacute sclerosing panencephalitis—a multidisciplinary study of eight cases. *JAMA* 207:2248–54, 1969

81. Jellinger K: Neuroaxonal dystrophy: Its natural history and related disorders, in Zimmerman HM (ed): *Progress in Neuropathology, Vol 2*, New York, Grune & Stratton, 1973, 129–180

82. Jenkins LW, Povlishock JT, Becker DP, et al: Complete cerebral ischemia: An ultrastructural study. *Acta Neuropathol (Berl)* 48:113–125, 1979

83. Kalimo H, Garcia JH, Kamijyo Y, et al: The ultrastructure of "brain death": II. Electron microscopy of feline cortex after complete ischemia. *Virchows Arch B Cell Pathol* 25:207–220, 1977

84. Kistler JP, Ropper AH, Heros RC: Therapy of ischemic cerebral vascular disease due to atherothrombosis (first of two parts) *N Engl J Med* 311:100–105, 1984

85. Kolodny EH, Cable WJL: Inborn errors of metabolism. *Ann Neurol* 11:221–232, 1982

86. Krawchenko J, Collins GH: Pathology of an arachnoid cyst. Case report. *J Neurosurg* 50:224–228, 1979

87. Kumpe DA, Rao CVG, Garcia JH, et al: Intracranial neurosarcoidosis. *J Comput Assist Tomogr* 3:324–330, 1979

88. Lampert PW, Gajdusek DC, Gibbs CJ: Subacute spongiform virus encephalopathies Scrapie, Kuru and Creutzfeldt-Jakob disease: A review. *Am J Pathol* 68:626–652, 1972

89. Leech RW, Olafson R: Epithelial cysts of the neuroaxis: Presentation of three cases and a review of the origins and classification. *Arch Pathol Lab Med* 101:196–202, 1977

90. Lillie RD: *Histopathologic Technic and Practical Histochemistry*. New York, Blakiston Company, 1954, 239–240

91. Little JR, Gomez MR, MacCarty CS: Infratentorial arachnoid cysts. *J Neurosurg* 39:380–386, 1973

92. Long DM, Hartmann JF, French LA: The ultrastructure of human cerebral edema. *J Neuropathol Exp Neurol* 25:373–385, 1966

93. MacGregor DL, Humphrey RP, Armstrong DL, et al: Brain biopsy for neurodegenerative disease in children. *J Pediatrics* 92:903–905, 1978

94. Marin-Padilla M: Structural abnormalities of the cerebral cortex in human chromosome aberrations. A Golgi study. *Brain Res* 44:625–630, 1972

95. Markesbery WR, Shield LK, Engel RT, et al: Late-infantile neuronal ceroid-lipofuscinosis. An ultrastructural study of lymphocyte inclusions. *Arch Neurol* 33:630–635, 1976

96. Martin JJ, Jacobs K: Skin biopsy as a contribution to diagnosis in late infantile amaurotic idiocy with curvilinear bodies. *Eur Neurol* 10:281–291, 1973

97. Martinez AJ, Ohya T, Jabbour JT, et al: Subacute sclerosing panencephalitis (SSPE) reappraisal of nuclear, cytoplasmic and axonal inclusions. Ultrastructural study of eight cases. *Acta Neuropathol (Berlin)* 28:1–13, 1974

97a. Mena H, Garcia JH, Velandia F: Central and peripheral myelinopathy associated with systemic neoplasia and chemotherapy. *Cancer* 48:1724–1737, 1981

98. McCormick GF, Zee C-S, Heiden J: Cysticercosis cerebri. Review of 127 cases. *Arch Neurol* 39:534–539, 1982

99. McCormick WF: The pathology of vascular (arteriovenous) malformations. *J Neurosurg* 24:807–816, 1966

100. McCormick WF: Vascular disorders of nervous tissue: Anomalies, malformations, and aneurysms, in

Bourne GH (ed): *Structure and Function of the Nervous System*, (Vol 3) New York, Academic Press, 1969, 537–596

101. Merei FT, Gallyas R, Horvath Z: Elastic elements in the media and adventitia of human intracranial extracerebral arteries. *Stroke* 11:329–337, 1980

102. Miller JR, Barrett RE, Britton CB, et al: Progressive multifocal leukoencephalopathy in a male homosexual with T-cell immune deficiency. *N Engl J Med* 307:1436–1437, 1982

103. Moossy J: Diagnostic cerebral biopsy, in Toole JF (ed): *Special Techniques for Neurologic Diagnosis*. Philadelphia, F. A. Davis Company, 1969, 183–191.

104. Morawetz RB, Whitley RJ, Murphy DM: Experience with brain biopsy for suspected herpes encephalitis: A review of forty consecutive cases. *Neurosurg* 12:654–657, 1983

105. Moser HW, Moser AB, Kawamura M, et al: Adrenoleukodystrophy: Elevated C-26 fatty acid in cultured skin fibroblasts. *Ann Neurol* 7:542–549, 1980

106. Moser HW, Moser AE, Singh I, et al: Adrenoleukodystrophy: survey of 303 cases: biochemistry, diagnosis, and therapy. *Ann Neurol* 16:628–641, 1984

107. Munoz-Garcia D, Ludwin SK: Classic and generalized variants of Pick's disease: A clinicopathological, ultrastructural, and immunocytochemical study. *Ann Neurol* 16:467–480, 1984

108. Neuwelt EA, Garcia JH, Kolar O, et al: Elevated CSF gamma globulins with cerebral "glioma." *Surg Neurol* 9:107–109, 1977

109. Noonan SM, Weiss L, Riddle JM: Ultrastructural observations of cytoplasmic inclusion in Tay-Sachs lymphocytes. *Arch Pathol* 100:595–600, 1976

110. Nystrom SHM: Development of intracranial aneurysms as revealed by electron microscopy. *J Neurosurg* 20:329–335, 1963

111. Okazaki H, Lipkin LE, Aronson SM: Diffuse intracytoplasmic ganglionic inclusions (Lewy type) associated with progressive dementia and quadriparesis in flexion. *J Neuropathol Exp Neurol* 20:237–244, 1961

112. Paillas JE, Berard M, Sedan R: The relative importance of atheroma in the clinical course of arteriovenous angioma of the brain. *Prog Brain Res* 30:419, 1968

113. Paljärvi L, Garcia JH, Kalimo H: The efficiency of aldehyde fixation for electron microscopy: Stabilization of rat brain tissues to withstand osmotic stress. *Histochem J* 11:267–276, 1979

114. Parker JC, Dyer ML: Neurologic infections due to bacteria, fungi, and parasites, in Davis RL, Robertson DM eds: *Textbook of Neuropathology*. Baltimore, Williams and Wilkins, 1986, 673–675.

115. Parker F, Healey LA, Wilske KR, et al: Light and electron microscopic studies on human temporal arteries with special reference to alterations related to senescence, atherosclerosis, and giant cell arteritis. *Am J Pathol* 79:57–80, 1975

116. Pascual-Castroviejo I: The association of extracranial and intracranial vascular malformations in children. *Can J Neurol Sci* 12:139–148, 1985

117. Perl DP: The pathology of rabies in the central nervous system, in Baer GM (ed): *The Natural History of Rabies, Vol 1*, New York, Academic Press, 1975, 235–269

118. Peters A, Palay SL, Webster HF: *The Fine Structure of the Nervous System: The Neurons and Supporting Cells*. Philadelphia, W.B. Sanders Co., 1976

118a. Powers JM, Schaumburg HH: Adrenoleukodystrophy (sex-linked Schilder's disease). *Am J Pathol* 76:481–500, 1974

119. Prineas J: Pathology of the early lesion in multiple sclerosis. *Hum Pathol* 6:531–554, 1975

120. Purpura DP: Dendritic spine "dysgenesis" and mental retardation. *Science* 186:1126–1128, 1974

121. Raimondi AJ, Shimojo T, Gutierrez FA: Suprasellar cysts: Surgical treatment and results. *Child Brain* 7:57–72, 1980

122. Ramsey HJ: Ultrastructure of corpora amylacea. *J Neuropathol Exp Neurol* 24:24–39, 1965

123. Regli F, Vonsattel J-P, Perentes E, Assal G: L'angiopathie amyloid cerebrale, Une maladie cerebro-vasculaire peu connue. Etude d'une observation anatomo-clinique. *Rev Neurol (Paris)* 137:181–194, 1981

124. Resch JA, Baker AB: Etiologic mechanisms in cerebral atherosclerosis. Preliminary study of 3,839 cases. *Arch Neurol* 10:617–628, 1964

125. Richardson EP: Progressive multifocal leukoencephalopathy. *N Engl J Med* 265:815–823, 1961

126. Roggendorf W, Cervós-Navarro J: Ultrastructure of arterioles in the cat brain. *Cell Tiss Res* 178:495–515, 1977

127. Rorke LB, Riggs HE: *Myelination of the Brain in the Newborn*. Philadelphia, JB Lippincot Company, 1969

128. Rubinstein LJ, Herman MM, Long TF, et al: Disseminated necrotizing leukoencephalopathy: A complication of treated central nervous system leukemia and lymphoma. *Cancer* 3:291–300, 1975

129. Sagar JH, Warlow CP, Sheldon PWE, et al: Multiple sclerosis with clinical and radiologic features of brain tumor. *JNNS Psychol* 45:802–808, 1982

130. Sandbank U, Lerman P, Gelfan M: Infantile neuroaxonal dystrophy. Cortical axonic and presynaptic changes. *Acta Neuropathol (Berlin)* 16:342–352, 1970

131. Schaumburg, H, Powers, JM, Raine CB, et al: Adrenoleukodystrophy: A clinical and pathological study of 17 cases. *Arch Neurol* 32:577–591, 1975

132. Schochet SS, Jr, McCormick WF; Ultrastructure of Hirano bodies. *Acta Neuropathol (Berl)* 21:50–60, 1972

133. Schochet SS: Neuronal inclusions, in Bourne GH (ed): *Structure and Function of Nervous Tissue*, Vol 4, New York, Academic Press, 1965, 129–177

134. Schoene WC: Degenerative Disease of the Nervous System, in Davis RL, Robertson, DM (eds): *Textbook of Neuropathology* Baltimore, Williams and Wilkins, 1985, 788–823

135. Schwartz GA, Yanoff M: Lafora's disease. Distinct clinicopathological form of Unverricht's syndrome. *Arch Neurol* 12:172–188, 1965

136. Shuangshoti J, Netsky MG, Nashold BS: Epithelial cysts related to sella turcica: Proposed origin from neuroepithelium. *Arch Pathol* 90:444–450, 1970

137. Stanbury JB, Wyngaarden JB, Frederickson DS, et al: *The Metabolic Basis of Inherited Disease*. Part 3. Disorders of amino acid metabolism, 5th Edition, New York, McGraw-Hill, 1983, 231–250

138. Starkman SP, Brown TC, Linell EA: Cerebral arachnoid cysts. *J Neuropathol Exp Neurol* 17:484–500, 1958

139. Stehbens WE: *Pathology of the Cerebral Blood Vessels*. St. Louis, C.V. Mosby, 1972, 351–456

140. Stehbens WE: Histopathology of cerebral aneurysms. *Arch Neurol* 8:272–276, 1963

141. Stein BM, Wolpert SM: Arteriovernous malformations of the brain: I. Current concepts and treatment. *Arch Neurol* 37:1–5, 1980

142. Sung JH, Okada K: Neuropathological changes in mink with Chediak-Higashi disease. A light and electron microscopic study. *J Neuropathol Exp Neurol* 30:33–62, 1971

142a. Suzuki K: Ultrastructural studies of multiple sclerosis. *Lab Invest* 20:444–450, 1969

143. Suzuki K, Suzuki Y, Chen GC: GM-1 gangliosidosis (generalized gangliosidosis) morphology and chemical pathology. *Pathol Eur* 3:389–408, 1968

144. Suzuki K, Suzuki Y: Galactosylceramide lipidosis: Globoid cell leukodystrophy, in Stanbury JB, Wyngaarden JB, Frederickson DS, et al. (eds): *The Metabolic Basis of Inherited Disease*. New York, McGraw HIll, 1983, 857–874

145. Tanaka J, Garcia JH, Khurana R, et al: Unusual demyelinating disease. A form of diffuse-disseminated sclerosis. *Neurology* 25:588–593, 1975

146. Tanaka J, Garcia JH, Max SR, et al: Cerebral sponginess and GM-3 gangliosidosis: Ultrastructure and probable pathogenesis. *J Neuropathol Exp Neurol* 34:249–62, 1975

147. Tellez-Nagel I, Johnson AB, Terry RD: Studies on brain biopsies of patients with Huntington's chorea. *J Neuropathol Exp Neurol* 33:308–332, 1974

148. Tellez-Nagel I, Harter DH: Subacute sclerosing leukoencephalitis. I. Clinico Pathological, electron microscopic and virological observations. *J Neuropathol Exp Neurol* 25:560–581, 1966

149. Terry RD: Dementia. A brief and selective review. *Arch Neurol* 33:1–4, 1976

150. Terry RD: Alzheimer's disease. in. Davis RL. Robertson DM eds: *Texthook of Neuropathology*. Baltimore, Williams and Wilkins, 1985, 824–841

151. Tierney MC, Fisher RH, Lewis AJ, et al: The NINCDS-ADRDA Work Group criteria for the clinical diagnosis of probable Alzheimer's disease: A clinicopathologic study of 57 cases. *Neurology* 38:359–364, 1988

152. Tomlinson BE, Blessed G, Roth M: Observations on the brains of nondemented old people. *J Neurol Sci* 11:205–242, 1970

153. Tomlinson BE: The pathology of dementia, in Wells CE (ed): *Dementia* (2nd ed), Philadelphia, F.A. Davis Company, 1977, 113–153

154. Tomlinson BE, Blessed G, Roth M: Observations on the brains of non-demented old people. *J Neurol Sci* 7:331–356, 1968

154a. Tomlinson BE: The pathology of dementia, in Wells CE (ed): *Dementia* (2nd ed), Philadelphia, F.A. Davis Company, 1977, pp. 113–153

155. Trump BF, Arstila AU; Cellular reaction to injury, in LaVia M, Hill R, (eds): *Principles of Pathobiology* (2nd ed) New York, Oxford University Press, 1975, 9–96

156. Vanderhaeghen JJ, Logan WJ: The effect of the pH on the *in vitro* development of Spielmeyer's ischemic neuronal changes. *J Neuropathol Exp Neurol* 30:99–104, 1971

157. Victor M, Banker BQ: Brain abscesses. *Med Clin North Am* 47:1355–1370, 1963

158. Volk BW, Adachi M, Schneck L: The gangliosidoses. *Hum Pathol* 6:555–569, 1975

159. Vonsattel JP, Myers RH, Stevens TJ, et al: Neuropathological Classification of Huntington's disease. *J Neuropathol Exp Neurol* 44:559–577, 1985

160. Weiner LP, Narayan O, Penney JB, et al: Papovavirus of JC type in progressive multifocal leukoencephalopathy. *Arch Neurol* 29:1–3, 1973
161. Whitley RJ, Song SF, Linneman E: Herpes simplex encephalitis: Clinical assessment. *JAMA* 247:317–320, 1982
162. Whitley R: Diagnosis and treatment of herpes simplex encephalitis. *Am Rev Med* 32:335–340, 1981
163. Wiener J, Spiro D, Lattes RG: The cellular pathology of experimental hypertension. II. Arteriolar hyalinosis and fibrinoid change. *Am J Pathol* 47:457–485, 1965
164. Wilkinson MS, Russell RWR: Arteries of the head and neck in giant cell arteritis. *Arch Neurol* 27:278–391, 1972
165. Wisniewski HM, Coblentz JM, Terry RD: Pick's disease. A clinical and ultrastructural study. *Arch Neurol* 26:97–108, 1972
166. Wisniewski H: The pathogenesis of some cases of cerebral hemorrhage (a morphological study of the margins of hemorrhagic foci and areas of the brain distant from the hemorrhage). *Acta Med Polona* 2:379, 1961
166a. Wisniewski HM, Ghetti B, Terry RD: Neuritic (senile) plaques and filamentous changes in aged Rhesus monkeys. *J Neuropathol Exp Neurol* 32:566–584, 1973
167. Witzleben CL, Smith K, Nelson JS, et al: Ultrastructural studies in late-onset amaurotic idiocy: Lymphocyte inclusions as a diagnostic marker. *J Pediatr* 79:285–293, 1971
168. Woodard JS: Alzheimer's disease in late adult life. *Am J Pathol* 49:1157–1169, 1966
169. Yang SY: Brain abscess: A review of 400 cases. *J Neurosurg* 55:794–799, 1981
170. Yamamoto T, Imai T: A case of diffuse Lewy body and Alzheimer's diseases with periodic synchronous discharges. *J Neuropathol Exp Neurol* 47:536–548, 1988
171. Yunis EH, Lee RE: Further observations on the fine structure of globoid leukodystrophy. Peripheral neuropathy and optic nerve involvement. *Hum Pathol* 3:371–388, 1972
172. Zeman W: Studies in the neuronal ceroid-lipofuscinosis. *J Neuropathol Exp Neurol* 33:1–12, 1974

7

Nerve Biopsy

Thomas W. Bouldin

Introduction

The biopsy of peripheral nerve has become an integral part of the diagnostic study of patients with disease of the peripheral nervous system (PNS). Nerve biopsy is a more sensitive indicator of peripheral neuropathy than electrodiagnostic studies, especially if the histologic assessment includes nerve-fiber teasing and morphometric analysis as well as light and electron microscopy.[15]

The sural nerve, a cutaneous sensory nerve, is the peripheral nerve most frequently biopsied. Muscular nerves are rarely biopsied.

Handling the Sural Nerve Specimen

The sural nerve is usually biopsied 4–6 cm proximal to the lateral malleolus. A biopsy of the soleus muscle may be obtained through the same incision when indicated. The segment of nerve should be at least 2 cm long so that sufficient material is available for light microscopy, electron microscopy, and nerve fiber teasing. Should additional material be needed for special tests, such as immunofluorescence, in vitro electrophysiologic studies, tissue culture, or biochemical measurements, an additional 1–2 cm of nerve must be taken.[233] Either a few fascicles or the whole nerve trunk may be biopsied; the latter is preferable for morphometric studies and for detecting amyloid deposits or vasculitis.[17,185]

Immediately upon receiving the specimen from the surgeon, the pathologist should place the nerve on a dry index card and gently stretch the specimen until it is straight and fully extended. After about 30 seconds, the unfixed nerve firmly adheres to the index card and then can be immersed in chilled fixative for 24 hours of primary fixation at room temperature. A 4% solution of glutaraldehyde, buffered with 0.05M sodium cacodylate, is an excellent primary fixative. One portion of the nerve is then cut into 1 mm thick, transverse and longitudinal sections, osmicated for two hours and then processed in the standard manner for plastic-embedding and electron microscopy. A second portion of the nerve, 5–10 mm long, is osmicated for 12–14 hours in buffered 1% osmium tetroxide, rapidly dehydrated in graded alcohols, and infiltrated with cedarwood oil for nerve fiber teasing. The remaining portion of the glutaraldehyde-fixed nerve is processed for standard paraffin embedding and light microscopy. A detailed description of the methods for handling and processing nerve specimens is given by Asbury and Johnson.[9]

Transverse, 1-μm-thick sections of the plastic-embedded nerve, stained with either toluidine blue or paraphenylenediamine, are excellent for both light microscopy of the nerve and for morphometric analysis of the myelinated fibers. Transverse and longitudinal, paraffin-embedded sections of the nerve are routinely stained with hema-

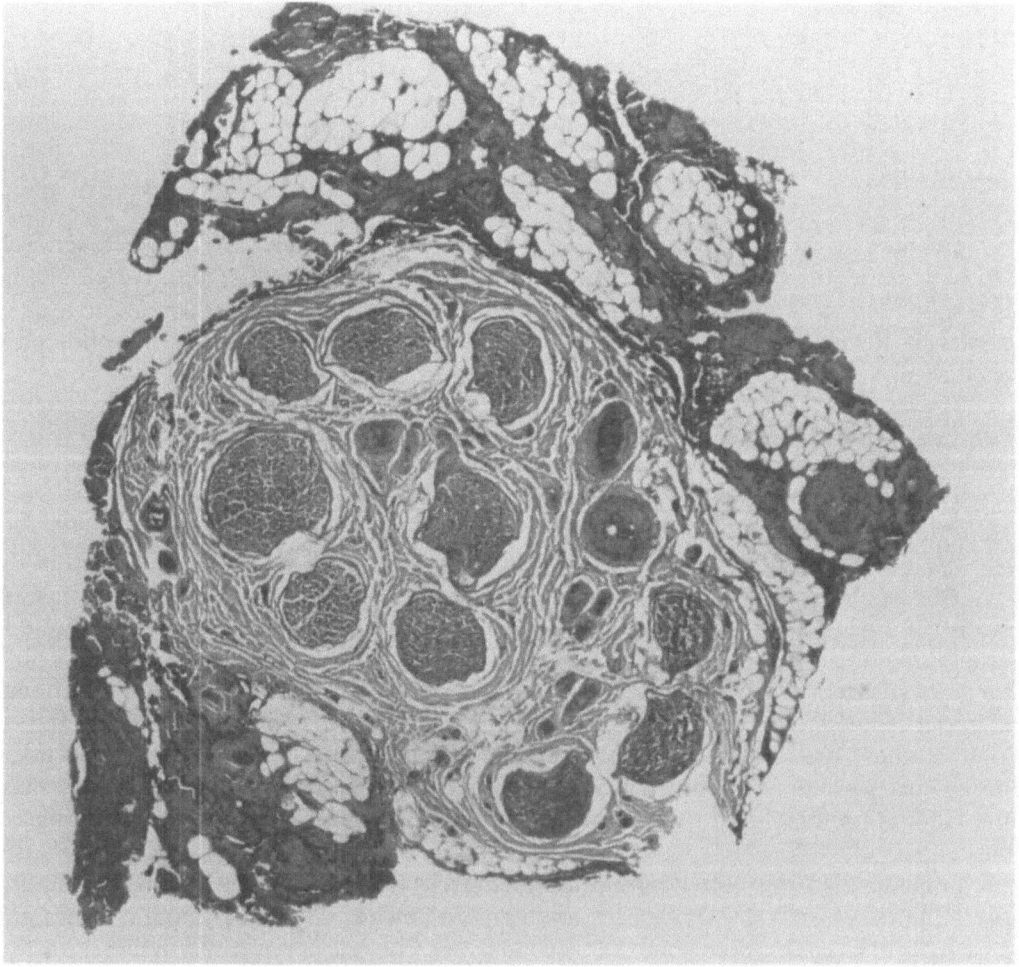

Fig. 7-1. Transverse section of normal sural nerve. Nerve fascicles, arteries and veins are embedded within the dense fibrous tissue of the epineurium (×40).

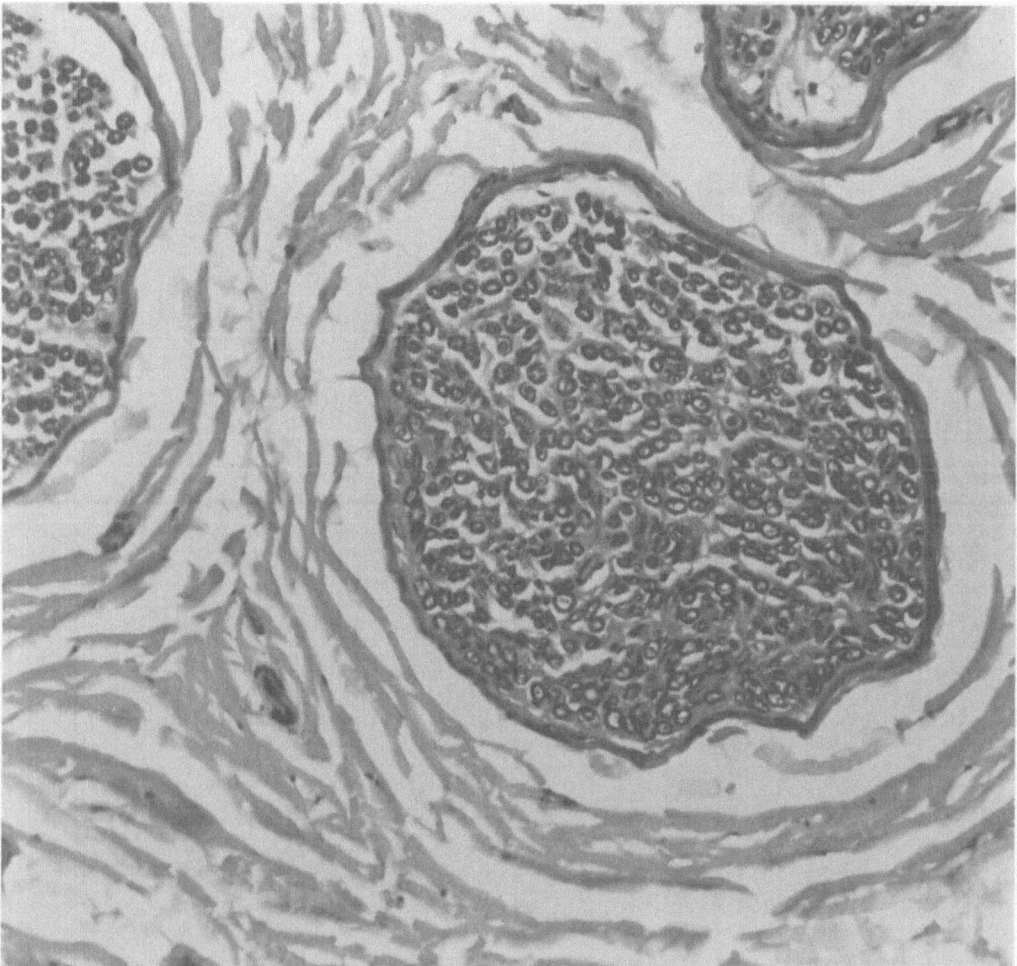

Fig. 7-2. A thin layer of perineurium delimits each nerve fascicle. The myelin sheaths are dark rings in this trichrome-stained, paraffin embedded transverse section of normal sural nerve (×210).

toxylin and eosin. Masson's trichrome method is excellent for differentially staining collagen (green) and myelin (red); Bodian's method impregnates both myelinated and unmyelinated axons. Immunohistochemistry may be done on frozen sections or paraffin-embedded nerve.[164,233] The technique of teasing single myelinated fibers and a widely used scheme for grading abnormalities in single-teased fibers are described and illustrated by Dyck et al.[66]

Normal Histology of Sural Nerve

The sural nerve consists of myelinated and unmyelinated sensory fibers and possibly some unmyelinated sympathetic efferent fibers.[39] The myelinated and unmyelinated fibers of the sural nerve are grouped into 5–15 fascicles (Fig. 7-1). The fascicles are bound together by the dense connective tissue of the epineurium, which also contains small arteries, veins, and adipose tissue. The perineurium groups the nerve fibers

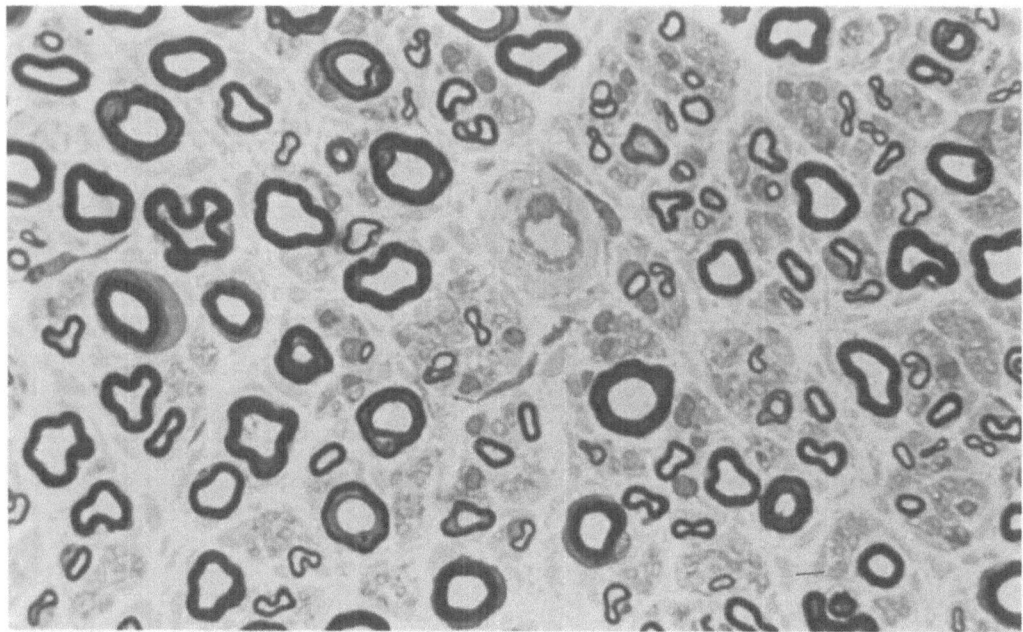

Fig. 7-3. Semi-thin (1-μm-thick) transverse section of Epon-embedded normal sural nerve reveals a population of large-diameter, thickly myelinated axons and a group of small-diameter, thinly myelinated axons. An endoneurial capillary lies just above the center of the field (Toluidine blue, ×840).

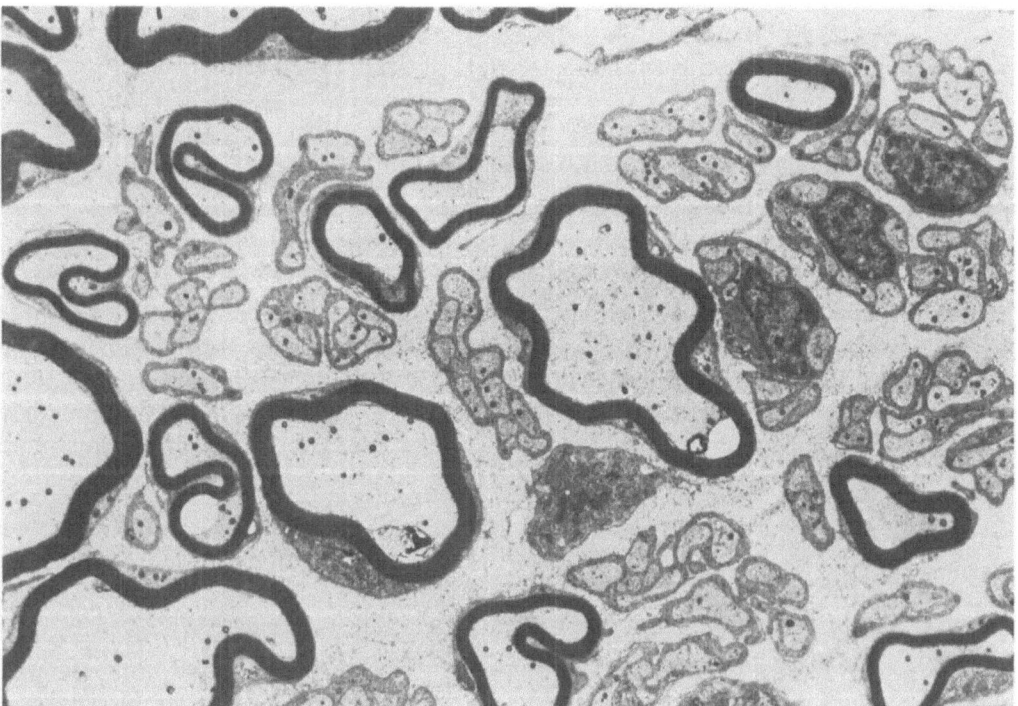

Fig. 7-4. Electron micrograph of normal sural nerve. Many small unmyelinated axons are interspersed among the myelinated axons (×3,000).

into fascicles, and is formed by multiple layers of perineurial cells (Fig. 7-2).[136] Ultrastructurally, the perineurial cells closely resemble Schwann cells and fibroblasts. Schwann cells and perineurial cells are covered by basal lamina. A distinguishing feature of perineurial cells is the large number of pinocytotic vesicles. The perineurium circumscribes the endoneurial space, which is filled with nerve fibers, collagen fibers, scattered fibroblasts and mast cells, continuous capillaries, and a few arterioles/venules (Figs. 7-3–7-8). There are no endoneurial lymphatic channels. The connective tissue within the endoneurial space is referred to as the endoneurium. Approximately 90% of the cells (and nuclei) within the endoneurial space are Schwann cells; of these, 80% are associated with unmyelinated fibers.[170]

Renaut bodies are spindle-shaped, subperineurial structures 20–200 μm wide and up to several millimeters in length. They are occasionally found in sural nerve biopsies (Fig. 7-9). These curious structures have been mistaken for focal infarcts or amyloid deposits.[23] They are more numerous at sites of nerve compression, but their function is unknown.[106]

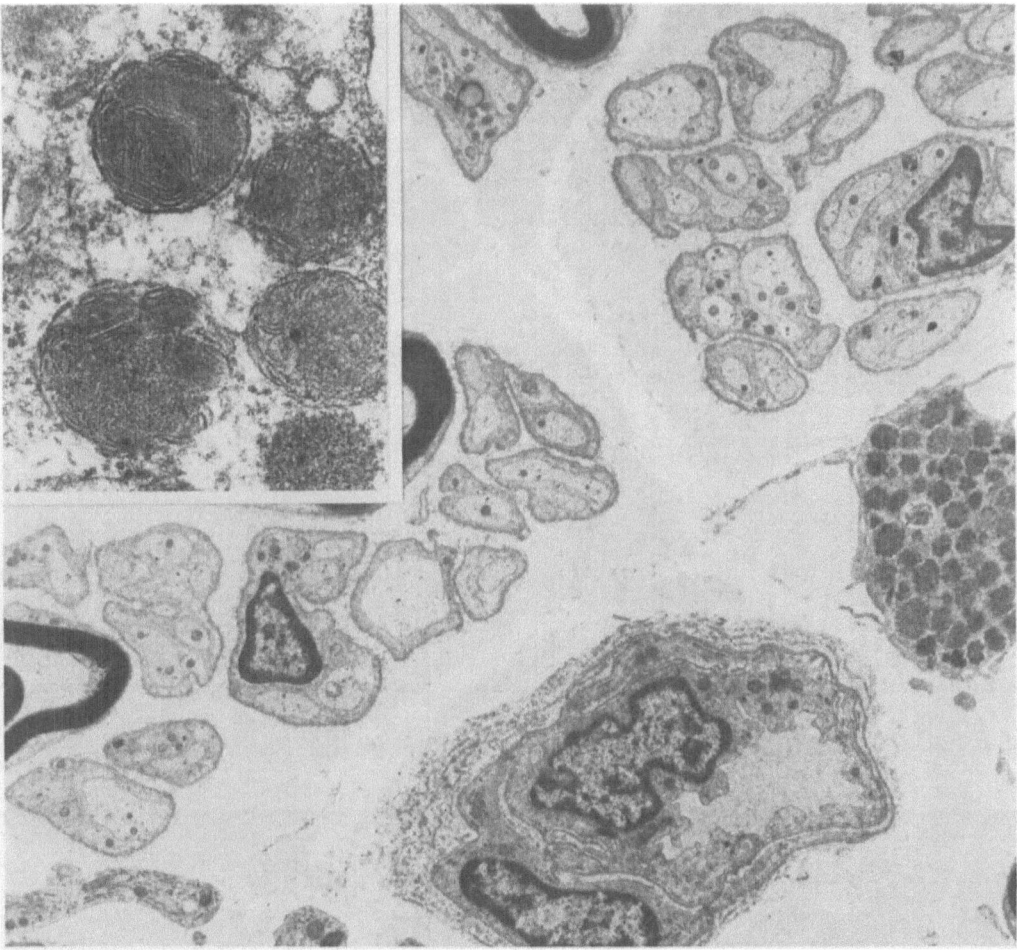

Fig. 7-5. Electron micrograph of normal sural nerve. A mast cell with several villous projections and numerous cytoplasmic granules adjoins an endoneurial capillary. At higher magnification (inset), the mast-cell granules have characteristic lamellar whorls. (×6,300; Inset, × 58,000).

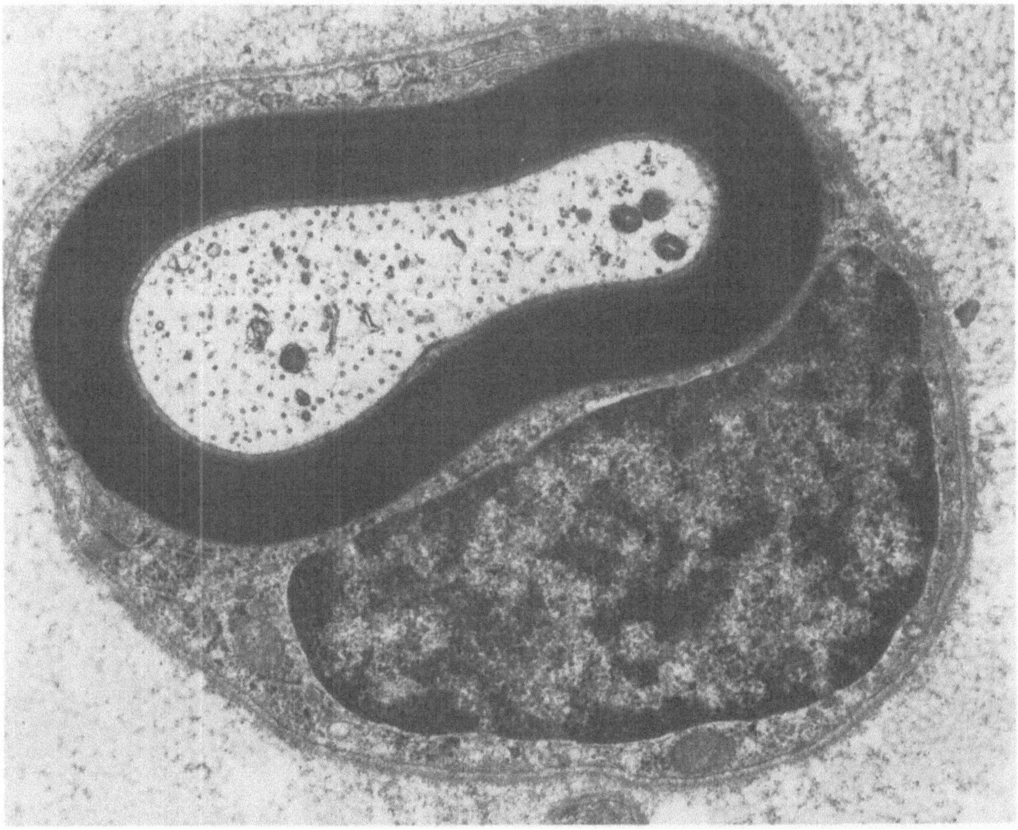

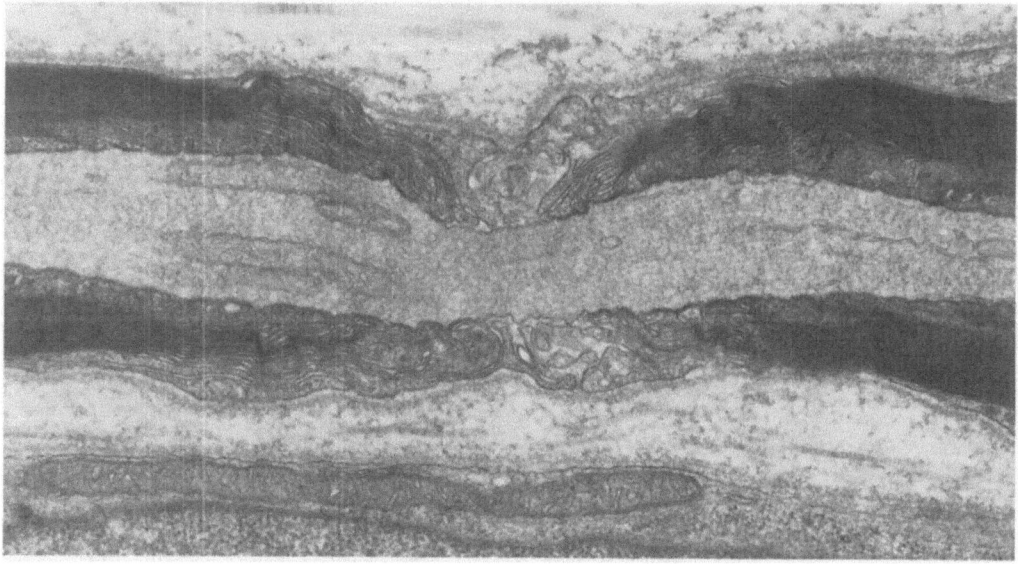

Fig. 7-6. Electron micrograph of normal myelinated axon. The transverse section is through the nucleus of the Schwann cell. The basal lamina covers the Schwann cell. (×25,300).

Fig. 7-7. Longitudinal section through node of Ranvier. Finger-like Schwann-cell processes cover the nodal axon. The basal lamina is continuous across the node of Ranvier (×30,000).

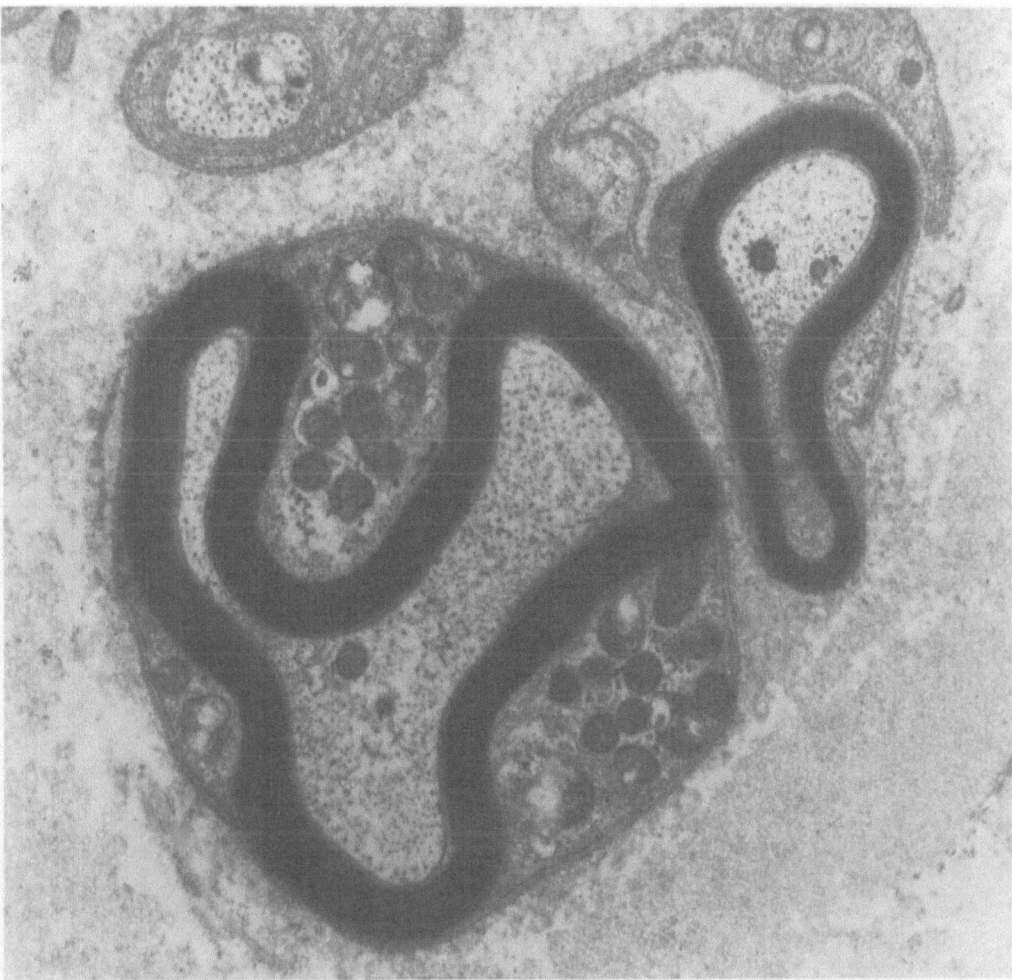

Fig. 7-8. The myelinated fiber on the left is transversely sectioned through the paranodal region. The paranodal myelin sheath of larger axons is characteristically folded; the intervening furrows of Schwann-cell cytoplasm are filled with mitochondria (×18,500).

The total number of myelinated fibers in the sural nerve of normal adults ranges from 5,000 to 10,000; the total fascicular (endoneurial) area ranges from 0.5 to 1.2 mm^2; and the density of myelinated fibers ranges from 4,000 to 12,000/mm^2.[13,17,104] The size-frequency histogram of the myelinated fibers is bimodal, with a peak between 3 and 6 μm and another peak between 9 and 12 μm. The range of fiber diameters is 1–17 μm.

Myelination of the sural nerve commences by 18 weeks of gestation, and by birth there is essentially a full complement of myelinated fibers with a median diameter similar to that of the adult population of small myelinated fibers.[75,91,104,167,212] The peak density of myelinated fibers occurs around birth and thereafter drops to reach adult values after the first decade.[75,104] A population of large myelinated fibers appears within a few months after birth, but the median large-fiber diameter does not reach adult values until 3–10 years of age.[75,91,104,167,212] The thickness of the myelin sheath is related to the diameter of the axon: larger axons have thicker myelin sheaths.[210] Similarly, in

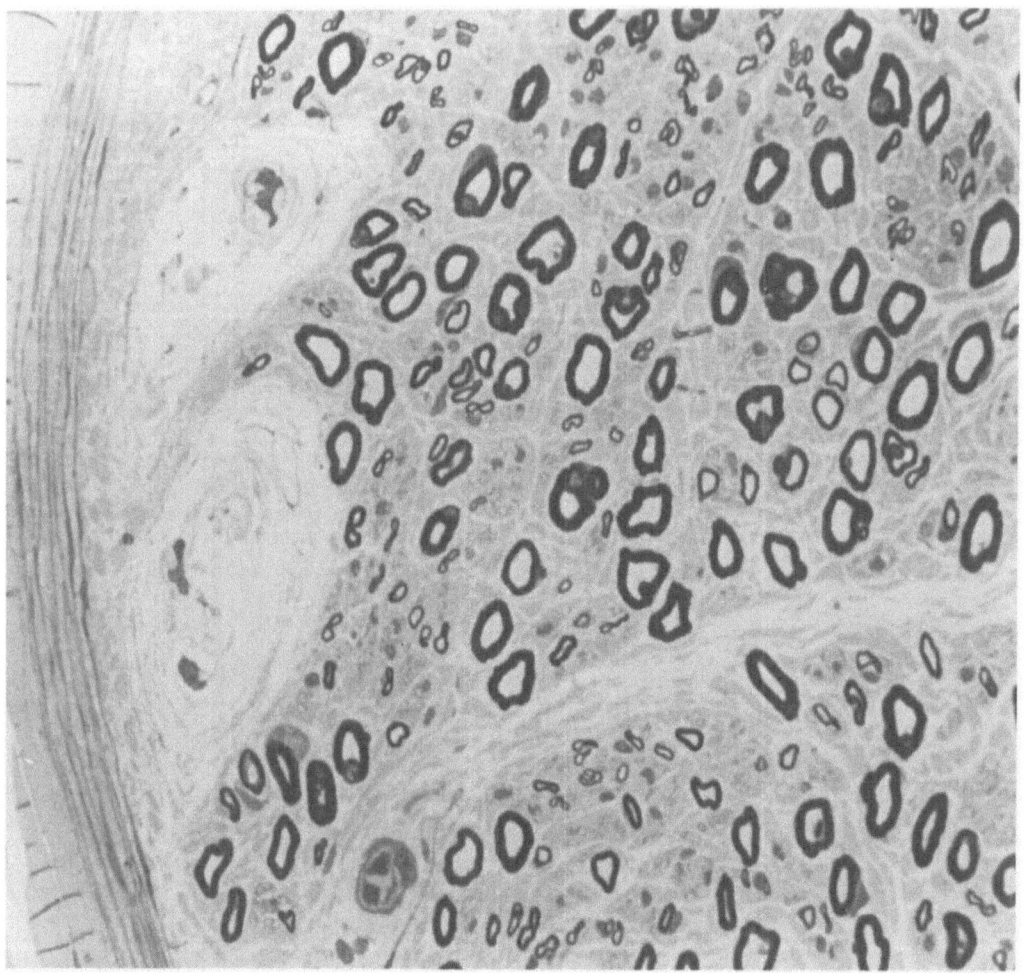

Fig. 7-9. Two Renaut bodies lie just beneath the multilayered perineurium in the left half of the field. Renaut bodies are composed of collagen fibrils, ground substance, and scattered fibroblasts. (Toluidine blue, ×550).

adult sural nerve, the internodal distance (between adjacent nodes of Ranvier) increases as the diameter of the myelinated axon increases and usually ranges from 0.15–0.2 mm in the smallest fibers to 1.0–1.2 mm in the largest fibers.[104] In the newborn, internodal distances range from 0.2 to 0.3 mm.[91,104]

Unmyelinated fibers outnumber myelinated fibers by approximately 3.7:1 in the sural nerve. The normal adult sural nerve contains between 20,000 and 38,000 unmyelinated fibers.[18,170] Unlike myelinated fibers, the size-frequency histogram of unmyelinated fibers is unimodal, with a peak between 1 and 1.6 μm and a range of diameters from 0.4 to 2.4 μm.[169] The axon diameters of the largest unmyelinated fibers overlap the axon diameters of the smallest myelinated fibers.

The Schwann cells associated with unmyelinated axons form branches (processes) that interdigitate. These interdigitating branches are collected together in small, complex structures designated as Schwann-cell subunits (Fig. 7-10).[18] Each subunit is surrounded by a basal lamina and contains an average of 1.5 unmyelinated axons.[18]

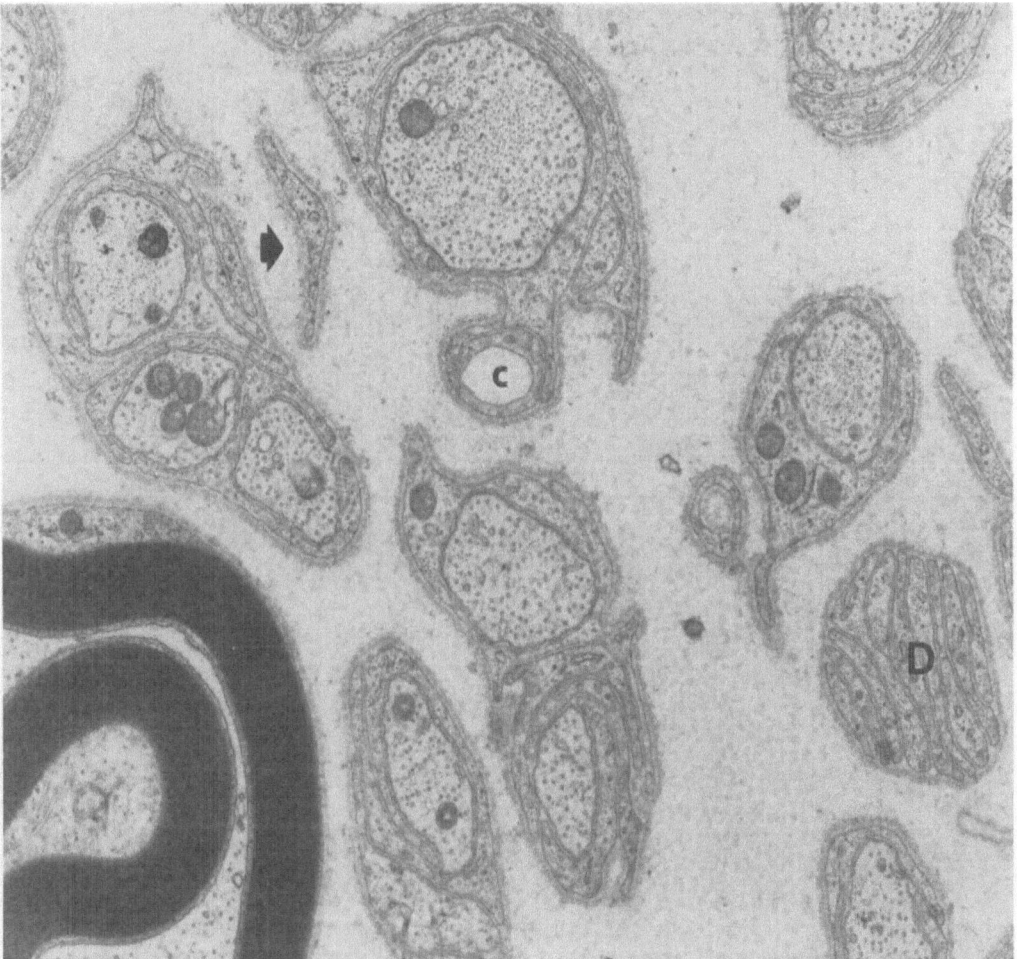

Fig. 7-10. Several Schwann-cell subunits contain from 1 to 3 unmyelinated axons. Each subunit is surrounded by basal lamina. A collagen pocket (C), a "denervated" Schwann-cell subunit (D), and an isolated Schwann-cell projection (arrow) are also present (×8,000).

Nonspecific Structural Changes in Peripheral Nerve

The peripheral nervous system (PNS) has few ways to react to injury, regardless of whether the injury is of an ischemic, traumatic, neurotoxic, metabolic, or heredodegenerative nature. Some diseases induce pathognomonic lesions in the PNS, (e.g., leprosy, systemic arteritis, certain lysosomal storage diseases, sensory perineuritis, xanthomatous neuropathy, and amyloidosis), but for many diseases the constellation of structural changes in the PNS must be correlated with an appropriate clinical history before the pathologic changes can be interpreted. The following structural features must be evaluated in sural nerve biopsies.

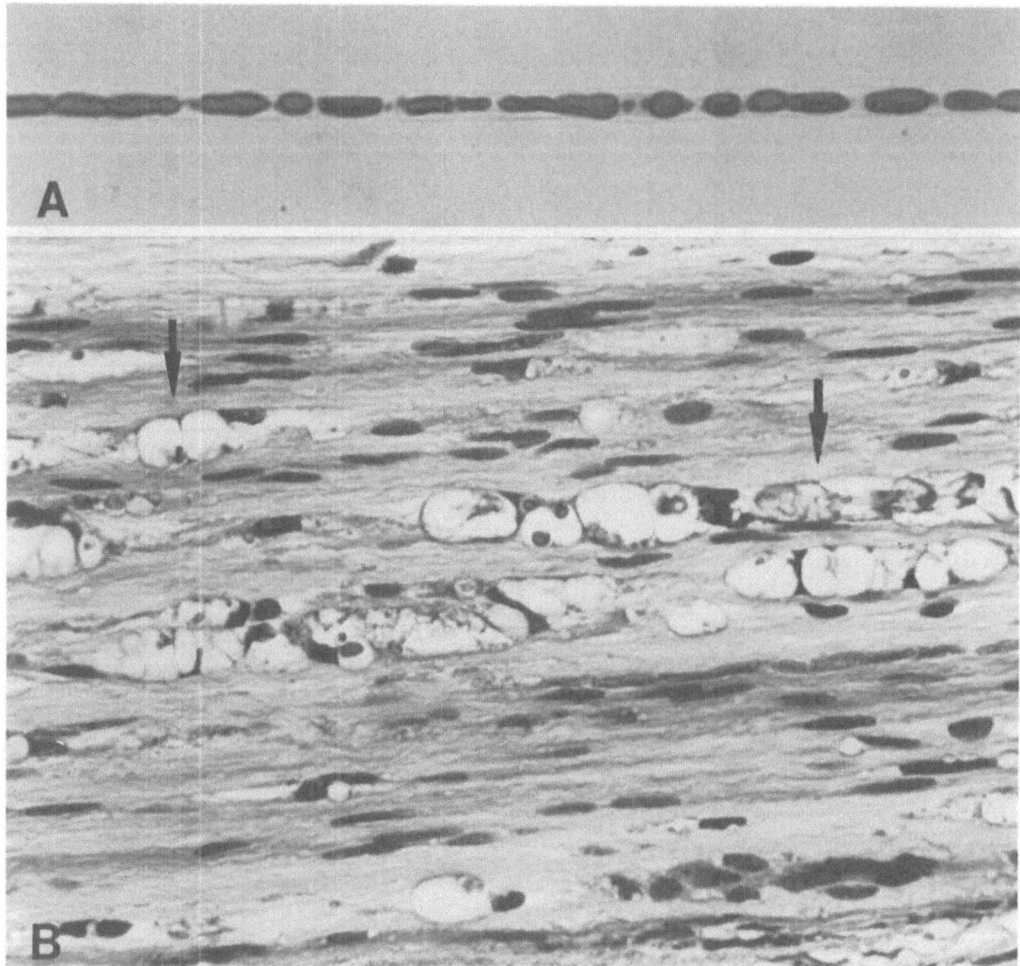

Fig. 7-11. (A) Teased myelinated fiber undergoing early axonal degeneration. The degenerating fiber has broken into myelin ovoids ("digestion chambers") of various sizes (Osmium tetroxide, ×210). (B) Longitudinal section of paraffin-embedded nerve. The myelin ovoids of axonal degeneration appear as rows of empty or debris-filled bubbles (arrows). This sural nerve is from a patient with periarteritis nodosa and a vasculitic neuropathy (Verhoeff-van Gieson, ×625).

Axonal Degeneration

A degenerating myelinated fiber is characterized by a row of myelin ovoids (Cajal's digestion chambers) (Fig. 7-11). Ultrastructurally, the evolution of axonal degeneration in a myelinated fiber is characterized by granular transformation of the neurofilaments and microtubules, disappearance of the axon, and degeneration of the myelin sheath (Fig. 7-12 and 7-13). The Schwann cells associated with the degenerating axon proliferate to form a compact column of interdigitating cells delimited by basal lamina (Büngner band) (Fig. 7-14 and 7-15). Similar ultrastructural changes occur in degenerating unmyelinated axons.[239] Myelin sheaths are degraded by both Schwann cells and macrophages.

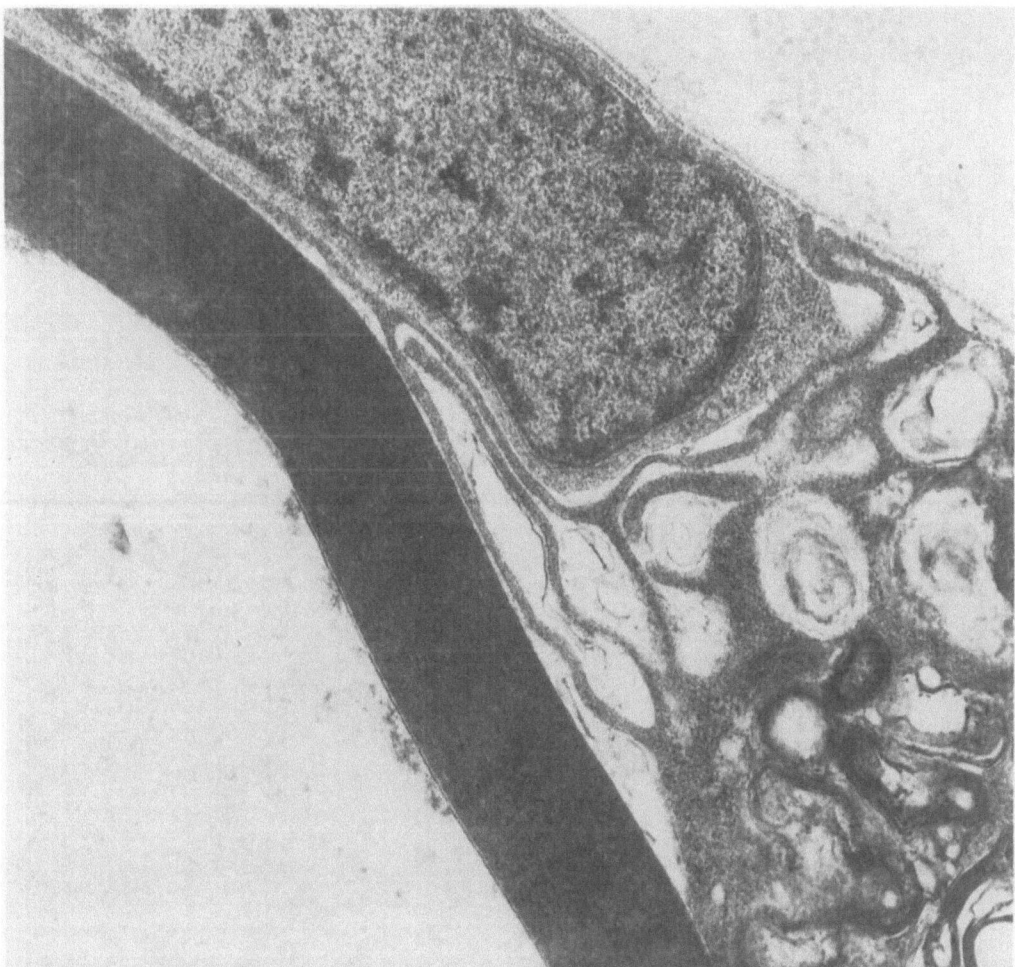

Fig. 7-12. Transverse section through a degenerating myelinated fiber from a cat. The axon has been replaced by small wisps of granular material. A macrophage with multiple villous processes is adjacent to the myelin sheath (×27,300).

The frequence of degenerating myelinated axons is 1%–2% (range of 0%–8%) in a normal sural nerve.[66] Similarly, degenerating unmyelinated fibers comprise less than 1% of all unmyelinated fibers in control sural nerve.[18]

Wallerian degeneration refers to the axonal degeneration occurring distal to a site of transection of the axon. In practice, the terms Wallerian degeneration and axonal degeneration are often used interchangeably.

Dying-back type of axonal degeneration (dying-back process, distal axonopathy) refers to axonal degeneration in which only the distal portion of the axon degenerates, leaving the proximal axon and the cell body intact.[38] This type of axonal degeneration occurs in many neuropathies. Demonstration of a dying-back neuropathy requires sampling multiple levels of the PNS.

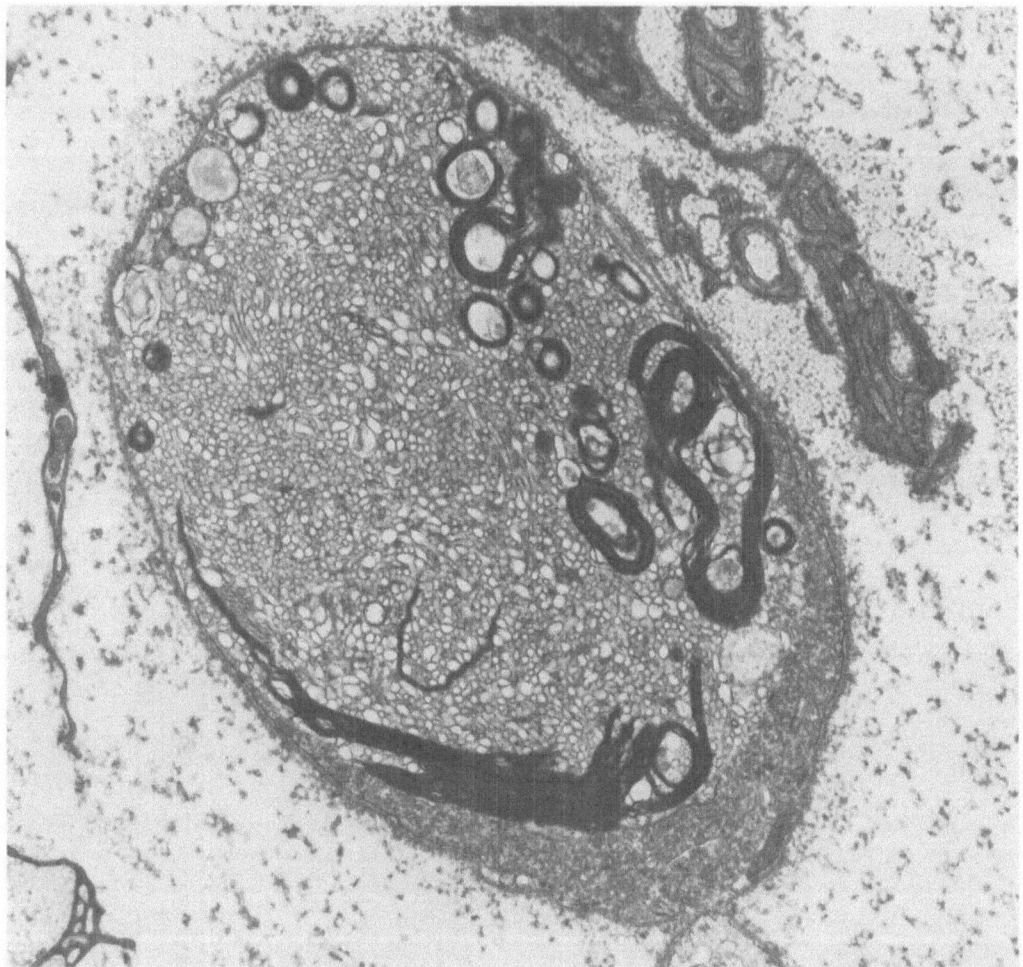

Fig. 7-13. Transverse section through a degenerating myelinated fiber. The axon has completely disappeared, and the myelin sheath is degenerating. (×8,000).

Loss of Nerve Fibers

Loss of nerve fibers is evidence of past axonal degeneration, and is best documented by morphometric studies. The methods for morphometric analysis of sural nerve are reviewed by Dyck et al.[66] Routine morphometric studies generally include total fascicular area, total number and density of myelinated fibers, a size-frequency histogram of the myelinated fibers, and the relative proportion of small and large myelinated fibers. The determination of total number of nerve fibers may be preferable to the determination of the density of nerve fibers.[17] Such studies not only quantify the degree of loss of nerve fibers, but also indicate if the large or small myelinated fibers are preferentially involved (Fig. 7-16). Because axonal regeneration may follow axonal degeneration, the occurrence of the latter in a chronic neuropathy is not inevitably evidenced by a decrease in the total number (or density) of myelinated fibers. If the axonal degeneration involves the large-diameter myelinated fibers, however, the size-frequency histogram may reveal

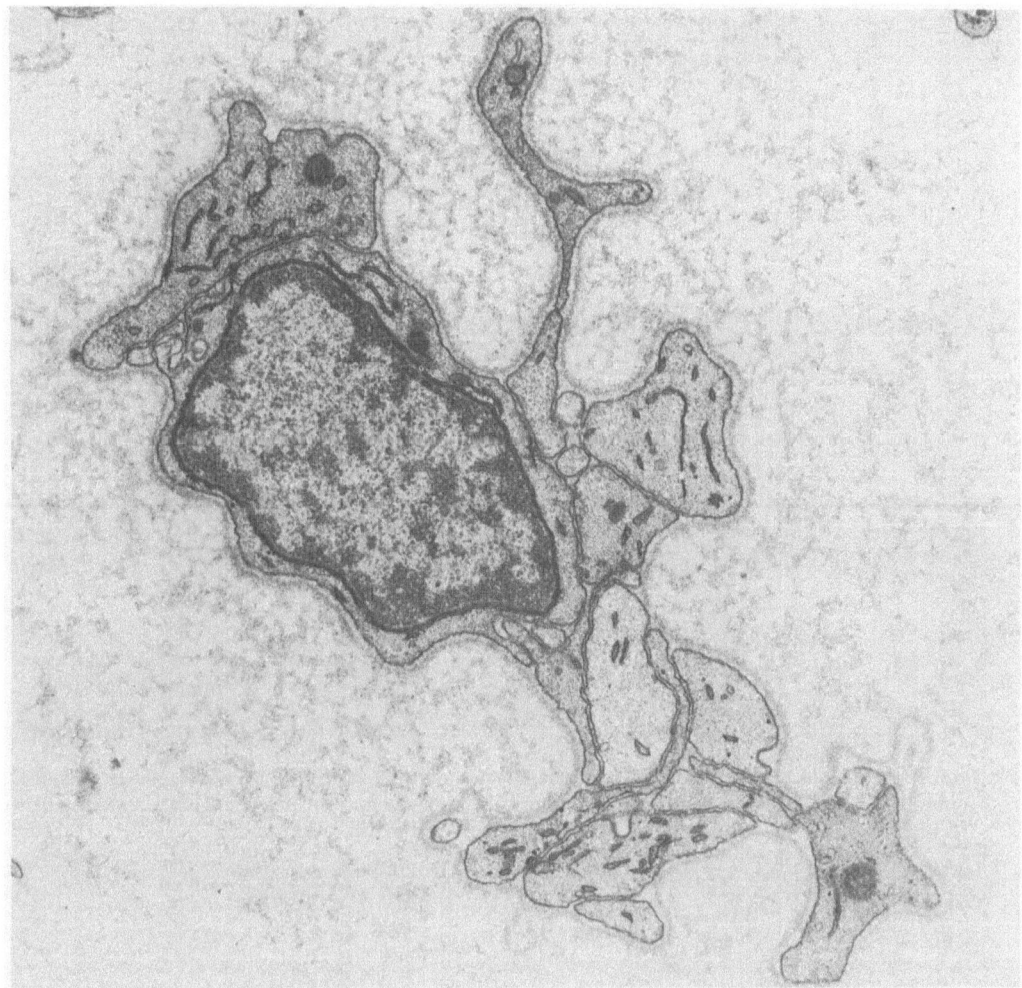

Fig. 7-14. Büngner band. Multiple Schwann-cell processes mark the site of a degenerated axon. A single basal lamina surrounds the column of proliferated Schwann cells (×20,200).

the loss of myelinated fibers even though axonal regeneration maintains the total number of myelinated fibers. In such cases, the disparity between the large diameter of the degenerated myelinated fibers and the small diameter of the regenerating myelinated fibers is such that the size-frequency histogram reveals a partial or complete loss of the large-fiber peak.

Axonal loss within unmyelinated fibers is more difficult to document by morphometric analysis. The biologic variation in the number of unmyelinated axons in a normal sural nerve makes it possible for some patients to lose many unmyelinated axons and still remain within the normal range. Furthermore, because of the strong tendency for unmyelinated axons to regenerate, the total number of axons may be within the normal range despite widespread axonal degeneration. A size-frequency histogram may detect regeneration (and thus unmyelinated fiber damage) because of the smaller size of the regenerating sprouts (miniature axons). Such an ultrastructural morphometric analysis

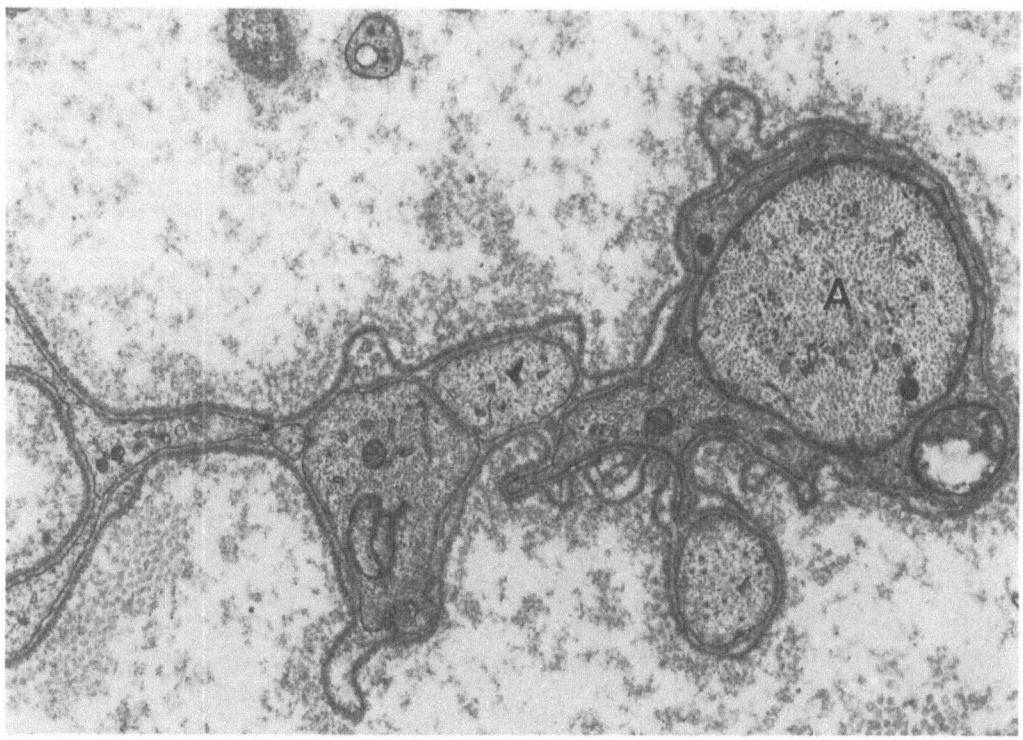

Fig. 7-15. Reinnervated Büngner band. A regenerating nonmyelinated axon (A) is enveloped by one of the numerous Schwann-cell processes in this Büngner band. Regenerating axons can usually be distinguished from Schwann-cell processes by the less electron-dense cytoplasm (×20,200).

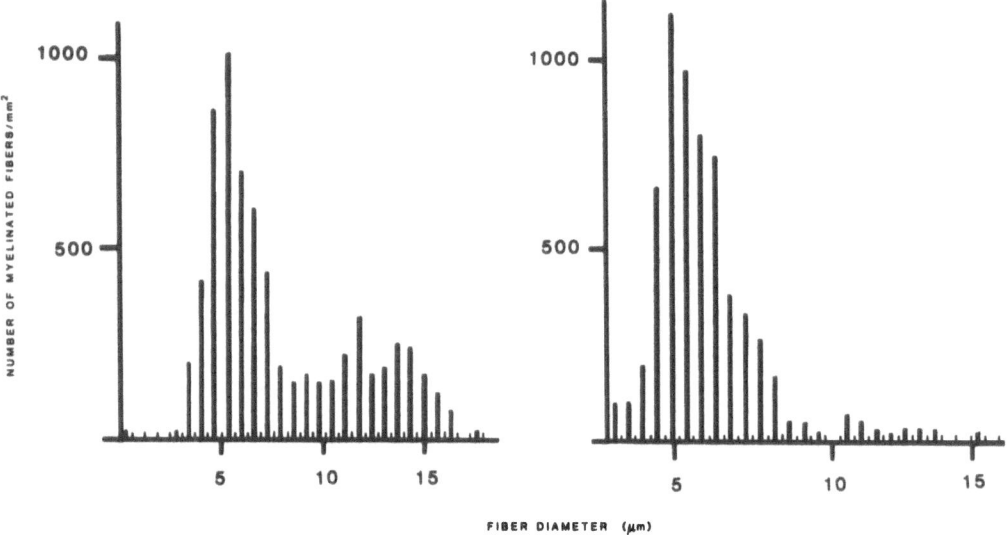

Fig. 7-16. The size-frequency histogram on the left is from a control sural nerve and shows a normal bimodal distribution of myelinated fibers. The size-frequency histogram on the right is from an 8-year-old child with a spinocerebellar degeneration clinically resembling Friedreich ataxia. Although the density of myelinated fibers in this nerve approached the range of normal, the histogram clearly shows a considerable loss of large myelinated fibers.

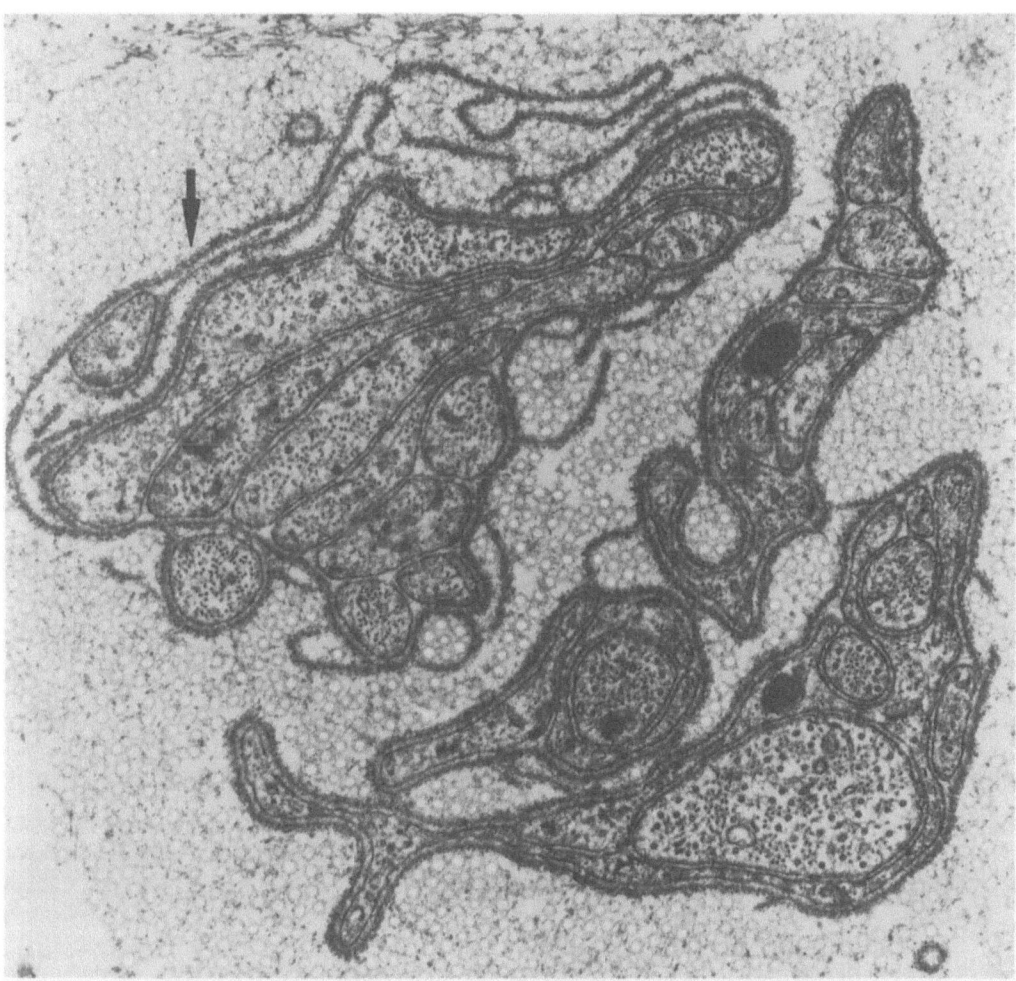

Fig. 7-17. Two denervated Schwann-cell subunits are seen in the upper half of this field. The larger subunit is surrounded by redundant basal lamina (arrow). Schwann-cell processes in denervated Schwann-cell subunits often have flattened, plate-like profiles, whereas Schwann-cell processes in Büngner bands resulting from degeneration of myelinated fibers have oval profiles (Figs. 7-14 and 7-15) (×30,200).

is not only time-consuming, but also subject to considerable error because of the difficulty in distinguishing regenerating axonal sprouts from proliferating Schwann-cell processes. For these reasons, it is best to identify and gauge the loss of unmyelinated axons by the frequency of denervated (empty) Schwann-cell subunits (Figs. 7-10 and 7-17).[18,169] An average of 14% of Schwann-cell subunits are denervated in control sural nerves.[18]

Clusters of Myelinated Fibers

Clusters of myelinated fibers indicate axonal regeneration.[161] The clusters are composed of three or more closely grouped myelinated fibers. They can easily be seen by light microscopy of 1-μm-thick, plastic-embedded transverse sections of nerve (Fig. 7-

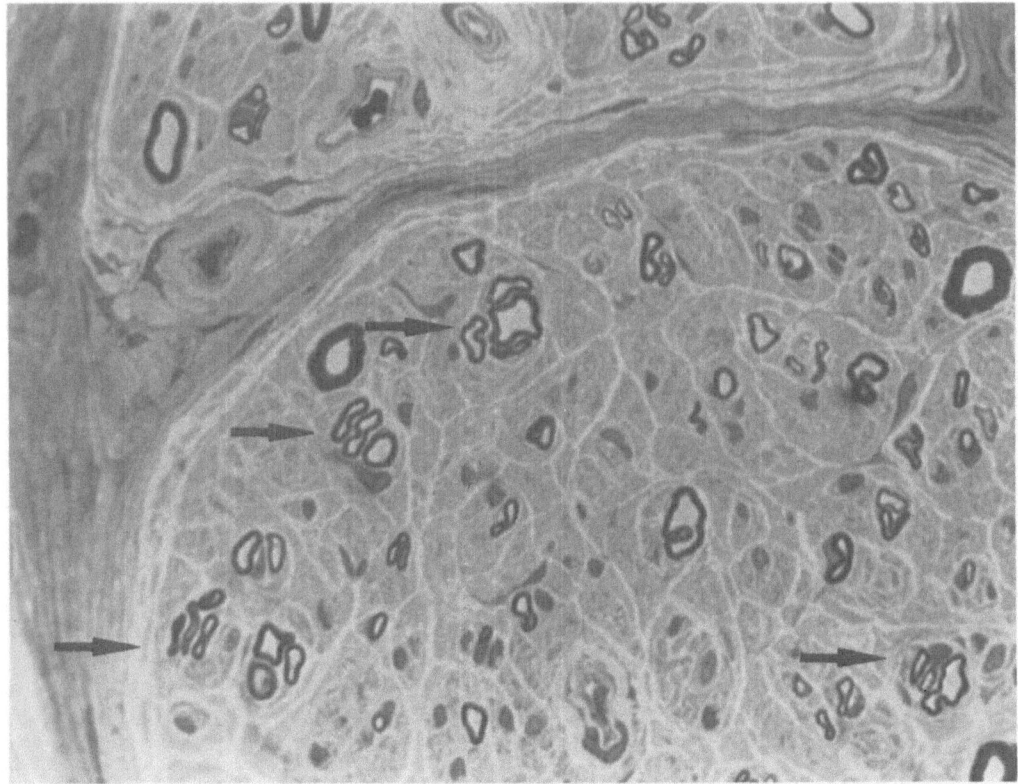

Fig. 7-18. Several clusters (arrows) of regenerating myelinated fibers are present in this semi-thin section of sural nerve from a patient with a chronic axonal neuropathy. There is also a considerable loss of both large and small myelinated fibers (Toluidine blue, ×855).

18 and 7-19). Control sural nerves usually have fewer than 5 clusters and rarely more than 10 clusters per nerve.

Segmental Demyelination

Demyelination is most easily found and quantified in preparations of teased nerve fibers (Fig. 7-20). The demyelination may be either paranodal (restricted to the paranodal bulb) or internodal (extending beyond the paranodal bulb to involve the internodal region of one or more internodes). One must be careful not to misinterpret an artifactual widening of the nodal gap for true paranodal demyelination. The term segmental demyelination is variously defined, but is used here to indicate either paranodal or internodal demyelination. The frequency of demyelinated fibers in teased-fiber preparations from normal sural nerves is in the range of 0 to 2%.

Segmental Remyelination

Remyelinated internodes indicate either previous segmental demyelination or axonal regeneration. The remyelination that follows segmental demyelination is best appreciated

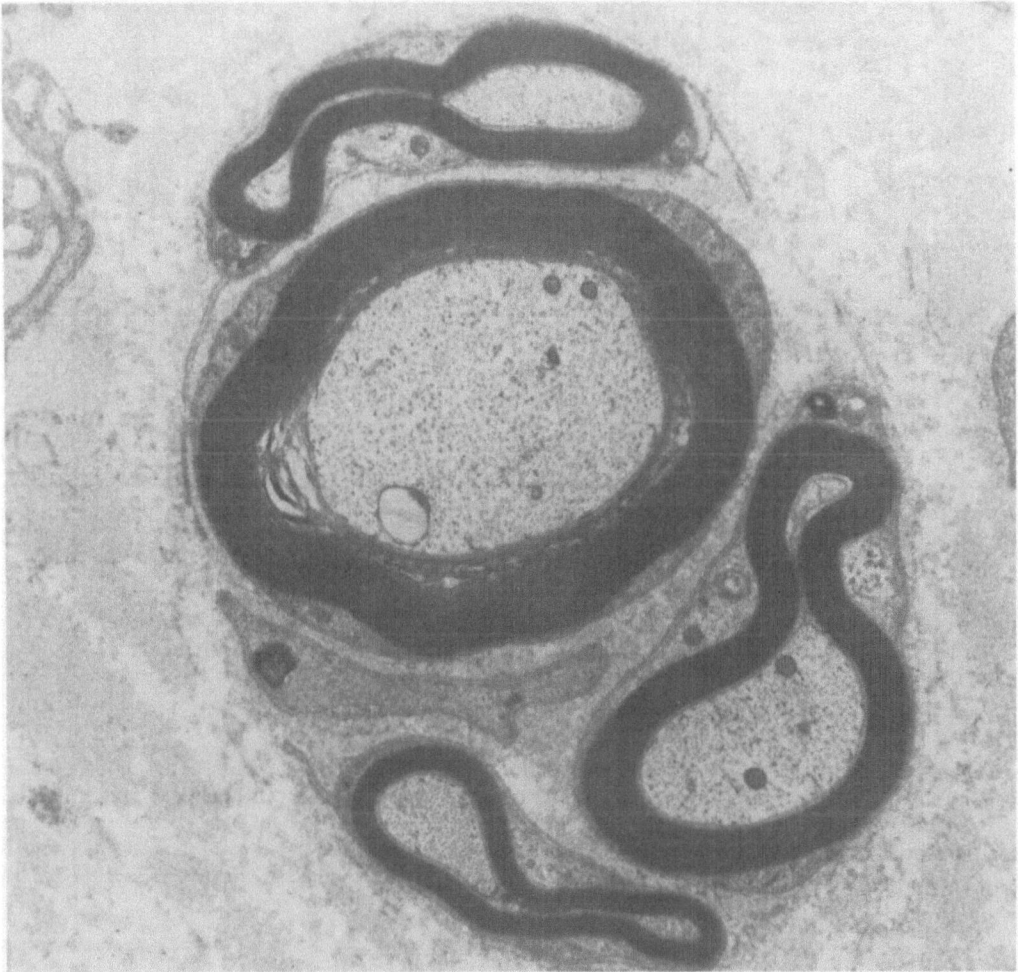

Fig. 7-19. Electron micrograph of a cluster of regenerating myelinated fibers (×18,500).

and quantified in teased nerve fibers (Fig. 7-20). The criterion suggested by Dyck et al[66] for identifying segmentally remyelinated fibers is practical. Using this criterion, a segmentally remyelinated fiber is one in which the variability of myelin sheath thickness between internodes is such that the thinnest myelin sheath is less than 50% of the thickness of the thickest myelin sheath. Remyelination following paranodal demyelination leads to a new, short, intercalated internode. Remyelination of a demyelinated segment longer than this (internodal demyelination) may lead to multiple contiguous new internodes, as new internodes rarely exceed 500 μm in length. Segmentally remyelinated axons are more common than segmentally demyelinated axons in control sural nerve. Dyck et al[66] found that the frequency of fibers showing segmental demyelination or segmental remyelination ranged from 0% to 10% (mean, 4%) among 25 healthy volunteers aged 20–47 years. In four healthy persons aged 45–54 years the frequence ranged from 2–24% (mean, 14.5%). Above age 60 years, the frequence of fibers showing segmental demyelination or remyelination in healthy persons is often above 20%.[68]

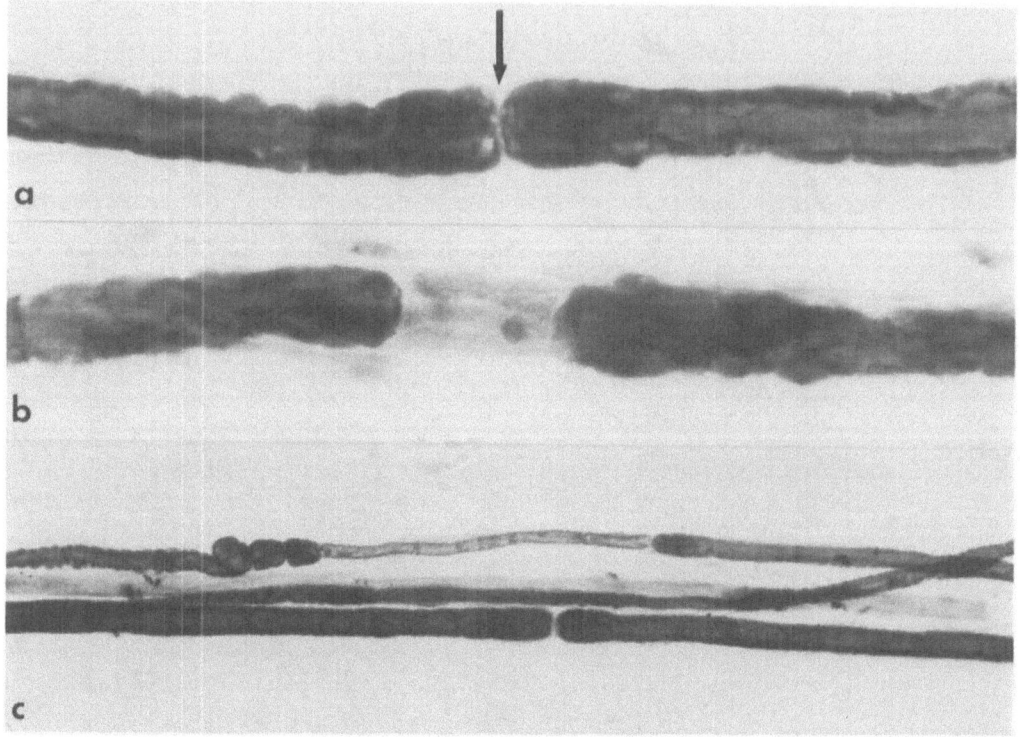

Fig. 7-20. (A) Normal teased myelinated fiber. Arrow points to the node of Ranvier (Osmium tetroxide, ×855); (B) Paranodal demyelination in a teased myelinated fiber. The demyelinated axon is not sufficiently stained by the osmium tetroxide to be recognized (Osmium tetroxide, ×855); (C) Segmental remyelination in a teased myelinated fiber. The remyelinated segment is evidenced by an inappropriately thin myelin sheath and a short internodal length. The other two myelinated fibers are unremarkable (Osmium tetroxide, ×290).

Onion Bulb Formation

When Schwann-cell processes are arranged as concentric lamellae around one or more central axons, an onion bulb is formed (Fig. 7-21). The central axon may be normally myelinated, demyelinated, or remyelinated. Occasionally, the central axon is absent because of previous axonal degeneration. The supernumerary Schwann-cell processes are covered by basal lamina and occasionally contain small nonmyelinated axons. It is not known whether these nonmyelinated axons are regenerative sprouts from the central axon or unmyelinated fibers participating in the formation of the onion bulb.[121,169]

It is generally agreed that onion bulb formations are related to successive episodes of demyelination and remyelination.[271] Other factors, as yet undefined, may also play a role in the formation of these unusual structures.[92, 193]

An occasional onion bulb may be found by electron microscopy in various neuropathies, but numerous well-formed onion bulbs are usually restricted to the small group of hereditary demyelinating neuropathies and occasional cases of diabetic neuropathy and chronic inflammatory demyelinating neuropathy. Onion bulb neuropathies are

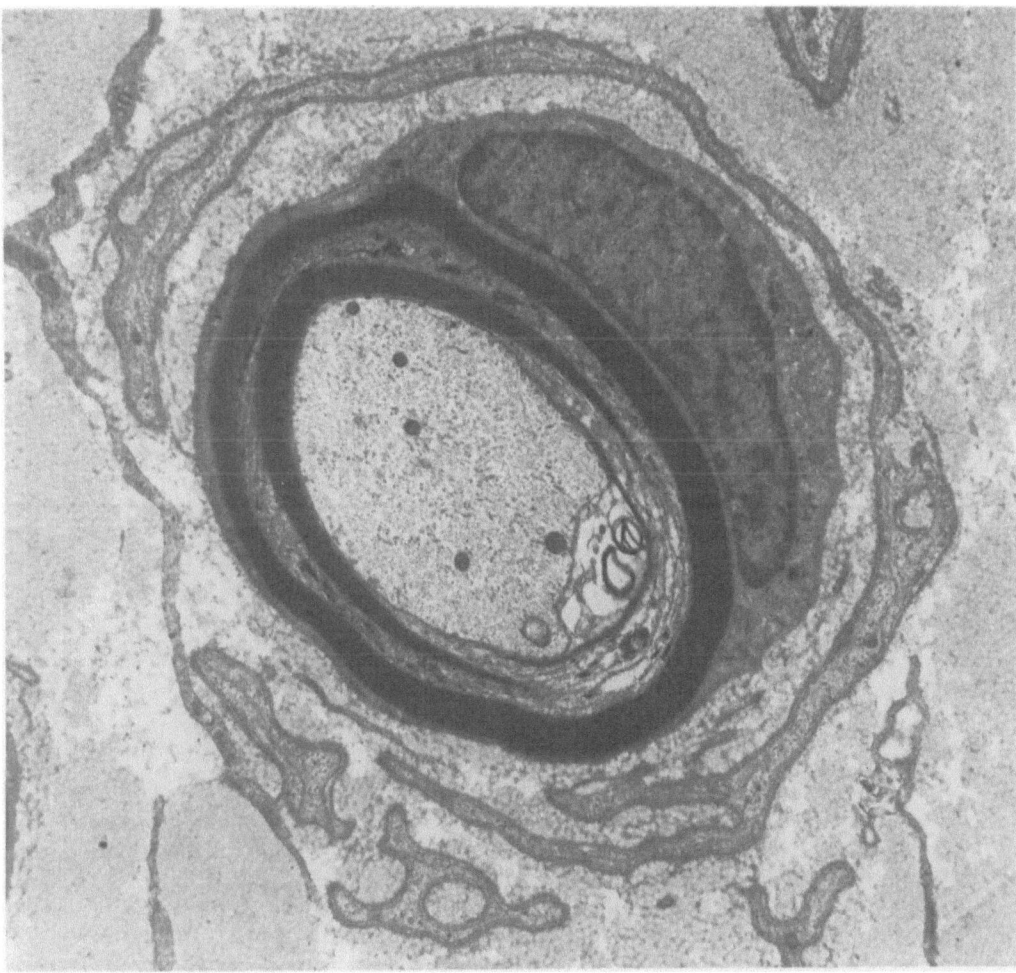

Fig. 7-21. Electron micrograph of a transverse section through an onion bulb. A myelinated axon is almost completely surrounded by a lamella of supernumerary Schwann-cell cytoplasm. The myelin sheath has been sectioned through a Schmidt-Lantermann incisure. This sural nerve is from a man with a dominantly inherited onion-bulb neuropathy (HMSN type I) (×12,000).

sometimes called hypertrophic neuropathies because the involved nerves are grossly enlarged (i.e., the total endoneurial area is greatly increased).

Other Structural Changes

Collagen pockets within Schwann-cell subunits increase with age and may be numerous in some neuropathies. (Fig. 7-10)[18,169] It was found, however, that the number of collagen pockets was increased in only a third of diseased sural nerves and was not related to either loss or regeneration of unmyelinated axons.[18]

"Budding" of the Schwann cells associated with unmyelinated axons to form either isolated projections or increased numbers of plate-like processes within Schwann-cell subunits, is the earliest morphologic evidence of damage to these unmyelinated fibers

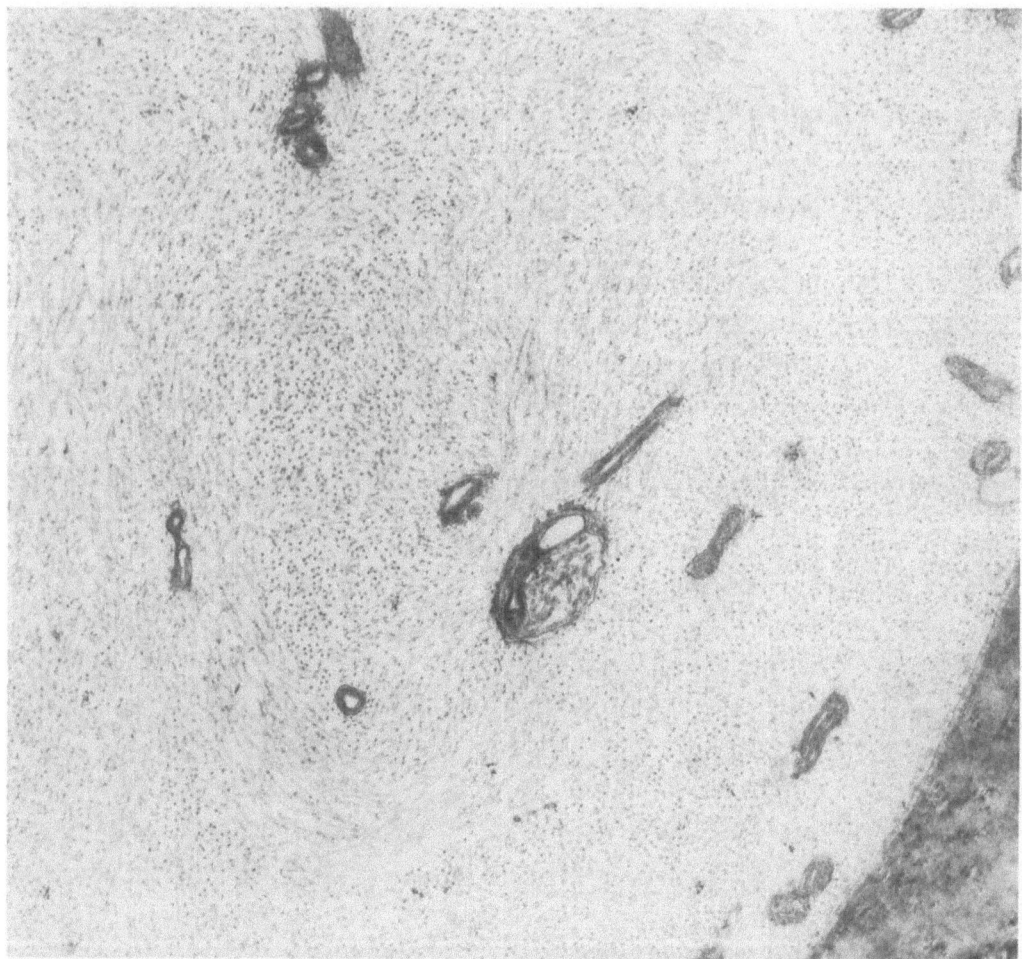

Fig. 7-22. Electron micrograph of a transverse section through an intra-axonal accumulation of neurofilaments. This nerve is from a rat with a toxicant-induced giant axonal neuropathy (×13,400).

(Figs. 7-10 and 7-17).[18] The number of plate-like processes also increases with age.[171]

Masses of whorled or interwoven neurofilaments may focally accumulate within axons to produce large axonal swellings ("giant axons") that are recognizable by both light and electron microscopy (Fig. 7-22). Such giant axons are the hallmark of hereditary giant axonal neuropathy and several toxic neuropathies.[54,125]

Pi granules (lamellar bodies, zebra bodies, pi granules of Reich) are distinctive, metachromatic granules visible by light microscopy. They are usually located in the perinuclear Schwann-cell cytoplasm of both myelinated and unmyelinated fibers. By electron microscopy, the pi granules are composed of stacks of lamellae and are of lysosomal origin (Fig. 7-23). The significance of the pi granules is unknown; they increase

Fig. 7-23. (A) Several polymorphic pi bodies are present in the Schwann-cell cytoplasm of this transversely sectioned myelinated fiber (×13,000); (B) Higher magnification of the pi bodies illustrated in Figure 7-23A reveals the characteristic internal structure. Numerous glycogen granules are also present in the Schwann-cell cytoplasm (×85,500).

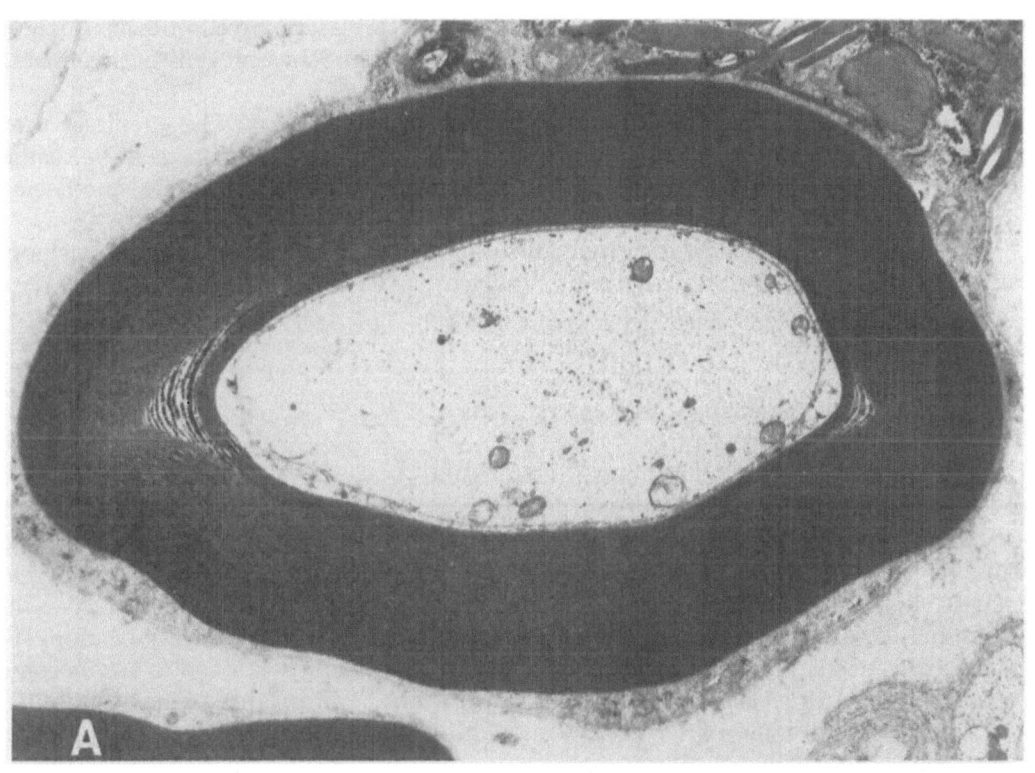

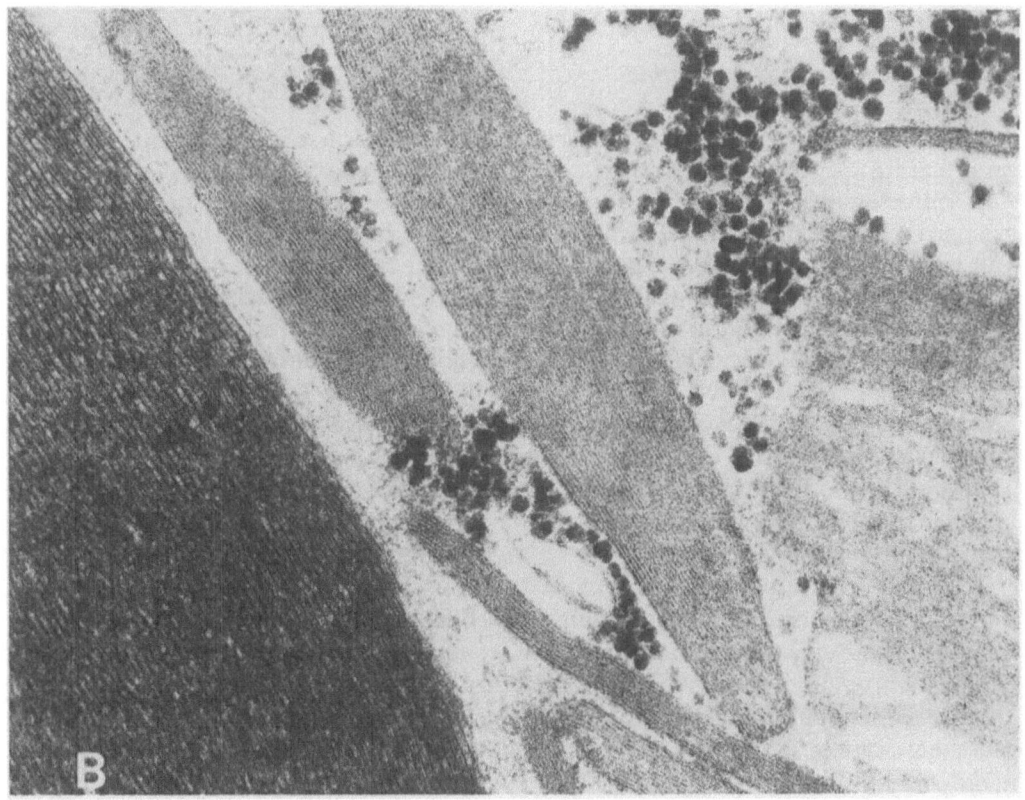

in number with age and in some neuropathies.[145] Cytoplasmic myelin ovoids (Elzholz bodies, μ granules of Reich) are also occasionally seen in Schwann cells of myelinated fibers.[66]

Endoneurial edema may be found in various neuropathies.[266] The edema is often most conspicuous in the subperineurial space. Subperineurial edema must be distinguished from artifactual contraction of the endoneurial contents, which is also reflected in an enlarged subperineurial space.

Intra-axonal corpora amylacea (polyglucosan bodies) are rarely found in nerve biopsies. The presence of multiple corpora amylacea, especially large ones, should raise the possibility of adult polyglucosan body disease.[198,264]

Age-Related Pathologic Findings in Peripheral Nerve

The density of myelinated fibers in adult sural nerve decreases with age.[68,104] The large myelinated fibers decrease proportionally more in density than the small myelinated fibers.[243] The frequency of segmental remyelination in teased fiber preparations of normal sural nerves is increased in older persons.[68,104,130] Age-related changes in the unmyelinated fibers include an increase in the number of collagen pockets, denervated Schwann-cell subunits, and plate-like Schwann-cell processes.[104,169,171] The density of unmyelinated axons decreases after age 60 years, and the size-frequency histogram may become bimodal due to an increasing number of miniature axons.[104] Mural thickening of endoneurial capillaries is common after age 50 years due to duplication of the basal lamina of endothelial and perithelial cells.[104]

Types of Peripheral Neuropathies

Peripheral neuropathies have been classified according to clinical presentation, structural features, and causative agents. A classification based on causes is best (Table 7-1). Unfortunately, neuropathies occasionally defy classification by cause even after extensive clinical study and sural nerve biopsy.[71,158] In these cases the pathologist can only offer a descriptive diagnosis that is based on the recognition of pathologic features. This descriptive diagnosis usually subsumes several disease entities.

Clinicians frequently subdivide neuropathies into axonal and demyelinating, depending on whether electrodiagnostic studies show normal or decreased nerve-conduction velocities, respectively. The pathologist does not find such an absolute division, however, because some axonal degeneration is almost always associated with demyelinating neuropathies, and demyelination frequently accompanies axonal neuropathies. The demyelination occurring with axonal neuropathies is often termed secondary demyelination. In these neuropathies, demyelination is probably secondary to the underlying axonal abnormality.[69]

McLeod et al[158] found that among 519 neuropathic patients referred for sural nerve biopsy, 27% had hereditary neuropathies, 17% had inflammatory demyelinating neuropathy, 43% had various acquired neuropathies (e.g., alcoholic, diabetic), and 13% had chronic neuropathy of unknown cause. These cryptogenic neuropathies were typically chronic axonal neuropathies morphologically. Continued follow-up revealed a possible cause (e.g., cancer, alcoholism, benign gammopathy) in 17 of 47 patients with cryptogenic neuropathy.[158]

Table 7.1.
Classification of Neuropathies

Autoimmune
    Inflammatory demyelinating neuropathy
Metabolic
    Diabetic neuropathy
    Uremic neuropathy
    Hypothyroid neuropathy
    Hepatic neuropathy
    Acromegalic neuropathy
    Neuropathy related to multi-organ failure and sepsis
Nutritional
    Alcoholic neuropathy
    Neuropathy related to vitamin deficiences
    Neuropathy related to postgastrectomy state
    Neuropathy related to celiac disease
Angiopathic
    Vasculitic neuropathy
    Neuropathy related to peripheral vascular disease
Toxic and drug-induced
Paraneoplastic
Neuropathy related to plasma cell dyscrasias
Neuropathy related to cryoglobulinemia
Amyloid
Hereditary
Infectious
    Herpes zoster
    Leprosy
    Diphtheria
    Human immunodeficiency virus
    Lyme disease
Sarcoid
Radiation-induced
Traumatic
Cryptogenic

Pathologic Changes Associated with Specific Neuropathies

Inflammatory Demyelinating Neuropathy

Inflammatory demyelinating neuropathy is an acquired demyelinating neuropathy.[8] It may be sporadic, complicate an underlying systemic disease (e.g., cancer), or follow a viral infection, mycoplasmal infection, surgery, or immunization. This neuropathy has also been associated with infection with human immunodeficiency virus.[46] The disease may have an acute, monophasic course (acute inflammatory demyelinating polyradiculoneuropathy, acute idiopathic polyneuritis, Guillain-Barré syndrome), or a chronic course characterized by either multiple relapses or a slow, continuous progression (chronic inflammatory demyelinating polyradiculoneuropathy, chronic relapsing polyneuritis, chronic demyelinating neuropathy).[149] The neuropathy is characteristically

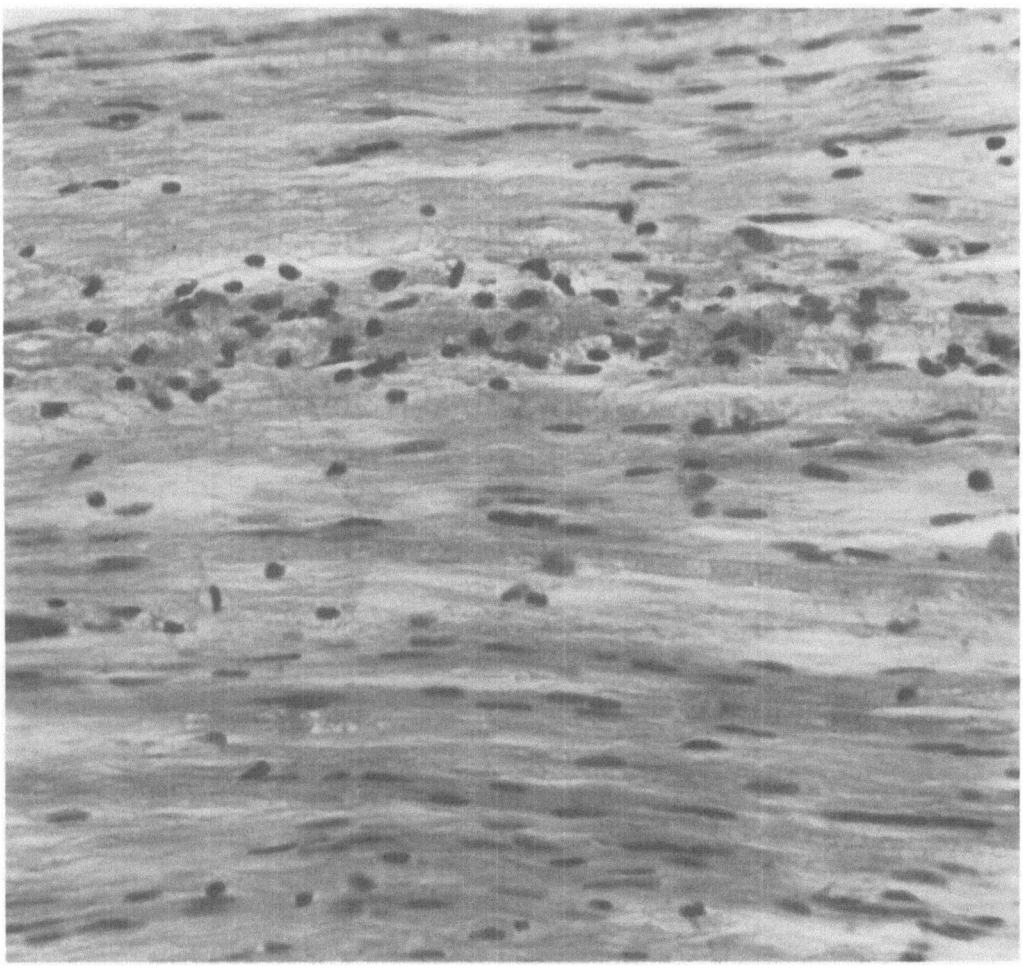

Fig. 7-24. Acute inflammatory demyelinating neuropathy. Mononuclear inflammatory cells cluster around a segmentally demyelinating axon in this longitudinally sectioned, paraffin-embedded sural nerve (×475).

associated with an elevated CSF protein, but not CSF pleocytosis. Nerve conduction is slow in about 80% of cases. Lewis et al[134] have described a variant of chronic inflammatory demyelinating neuropathy in which the presentation is that of a mononeuritis multiplex with multifocal conduction block. Autoimmune mechanisms are considered responsible for the demyelination in idiopathic polyneuritis, but it is not known if similar autoimmune mechanisms are involved in the acute and chronic forms. Of considerable interest is the association of some cases of chronic inflammatory demyelinating neuropathy with a multifocal demyelinating disease of the central nervous system resembling multiple sclerosis.[242]

The morphologic hallmarks of inflammatory demyelinating neuropathy, whether acute or chronic, are mononuclear-cell infiltrates in the endoneurium and macrophage-mediated segmental demyelination.[190] The endoneurial infiltrates consist mainly of lymphocytes and macrophages and often have a perivascular distribution, but angiitis is absent (Figs. 7-24, 7-25). The chronic inflammation is sometimes accompanied by prominent endoneurial edema. Longitudinal sections stained for myelin and axons reveal

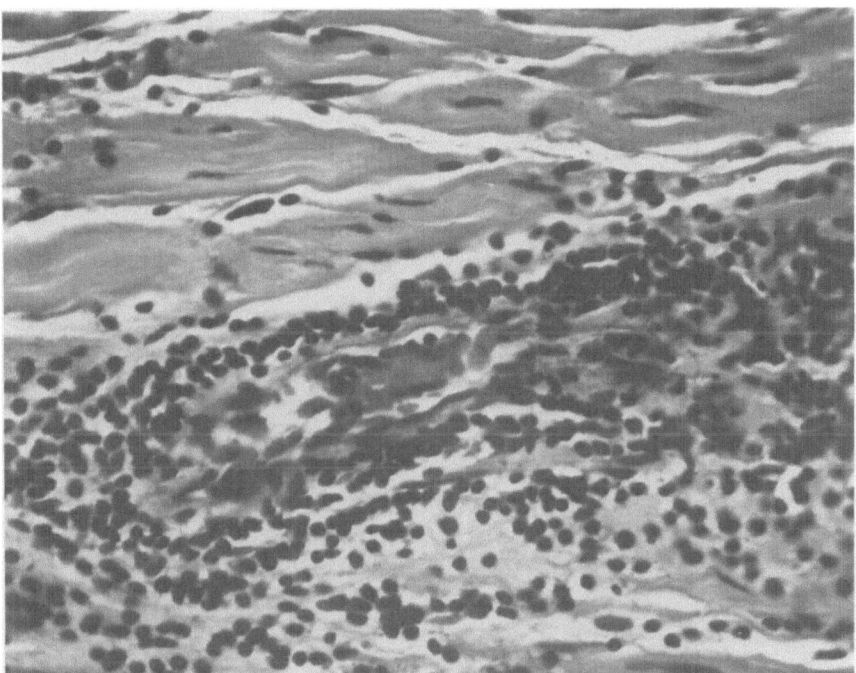

Fig. 7-25. Chronic inflammation surrounds an endoneurial capillary in a patient with chronic inflammatory demyelinating neuropathy (Courtesy of Hernando Mena, M.D., Washington, D.C.) (×500).

that the inflammatory infiltrates are associated with areas of internodal demyelination, but with relative sparing of axons. Teased fiber preparations better demonstrate the internodal demyelination and may also reveal paranodal demyelination, segmental re-myelination, and axonal degeneration. Although idiopathic polyneuritis is considered a demyelinating neuropathy, axonal degeneration is usually encountered in both the acute and chronic forms.[70,189] This alteration is reflected in the morphometric studies, which often reveal a moderate loss of myelinated fibers (Fig. 7-26). Clusters of regenerating myelinated fibers may also be present as a reflection of axonal degeneration.

Ultrastructurally, macrophage-mediated primary demyelination is the hallmark of inflammatory demyelinating neuropathy.[189,216,274] Macrophages are frequently found adjacent to degenerating myelin sheaths. The macrophages penetrate the basal lamina of the Schwann cell, push the superficial Schwann cell cytoplasm to the side, and insinuate cytoplasmic processes along the minor dense line of the myelin sheath. After stripping the superficial myelin lamellae, the macrophages phagocytose the myelin lamellae. Extracellular, vesicular degeneration of myelin in areas adjacent to the invading macrophages is less commonly found.[189] Macrophage-mediated demyelination, although characteristic of inflammatory demyelinating neuropathy, is not always found, and such demyelination has also been observed in neuropathies not thought to have an autoimmune basis.[29,142]

Well-developed onion bulb formations, often attributed to repeated episodes of demyelination and remyelination, may be numerous in chronic cases of inflammatory demyelinating neuropathy (Fig. 7-27).[70,191,216]

The lesions of inflammatory demyelinating neuropathy usually involve all levels of the PNS, including the dorsal and ventral spinal roots, dorsal root ganglia, cranial

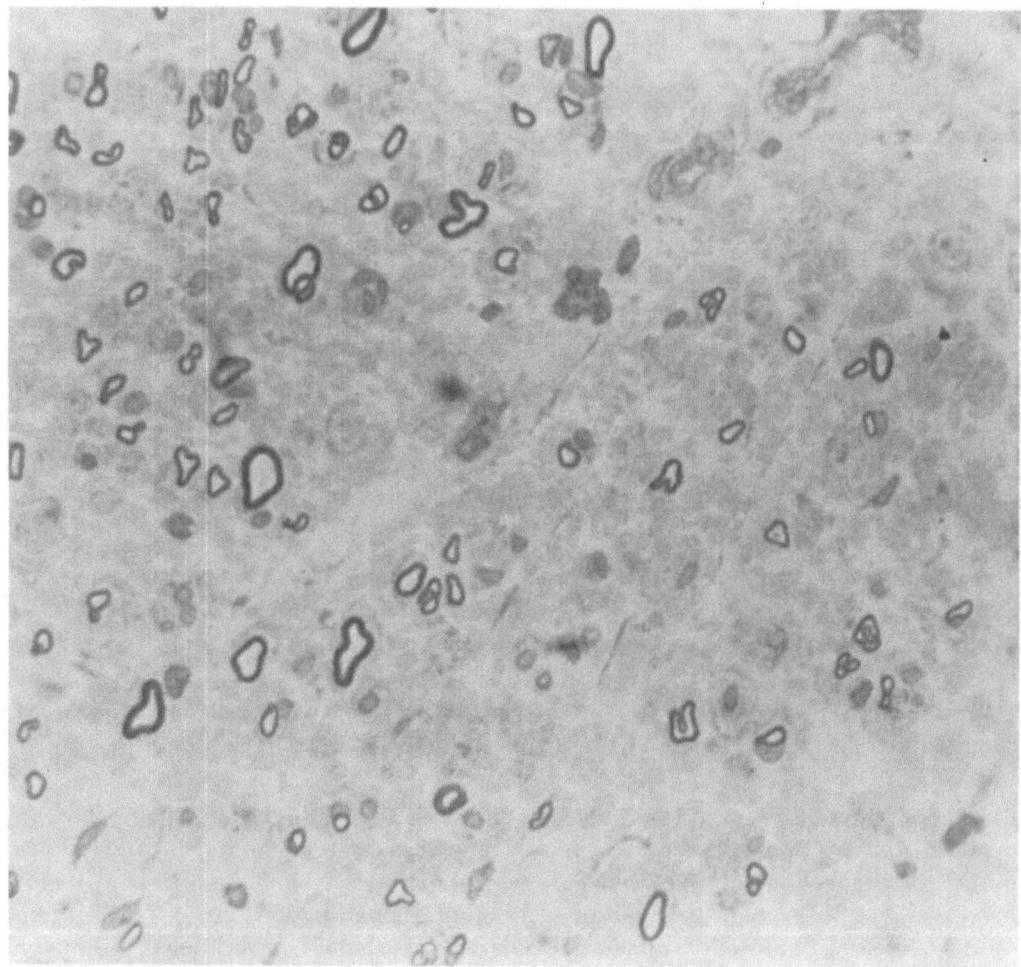

Fig. 7-26. Chronic inflammatory demyelinating neuropathy. A semi-thin transverse section of sural nerve reveals a considerable loss of myelinated fibers (Toluidine blue, ×840).

nerves, and autonomic nervous system.[9] The neural involvement is patchy, hence a sural nerve biopsy may be free of the characteristic structural changes. In an analysis of sural nerve biopsies derived from 65 patients with a clinical diagnosis of acute inflammatory-demyelinating neuropathy, electron microscopy revealed demyelinated fibers in 63 nerves and macrophage-mediated demyelination in 32 nerves.[29] Only 5 of the 57 nerves examined by light microscopy had endoneurial inflammation. In another series, only 6 of 26 sural nerve biopsies from patients with chronic inflammatory demyelinating neuropathy had endoneurial inflammation.[70]

Vasculitic Neuropathy

An ischemic neuropathy may complicate a vasculitis, chronic peripheral vascular disease, arterial embolism, arterial trauma, or diabetes mellitus.[7,72,260] Sural nerve biopsy is generally restricted to those patients suspected of having a systemic vasculitis.

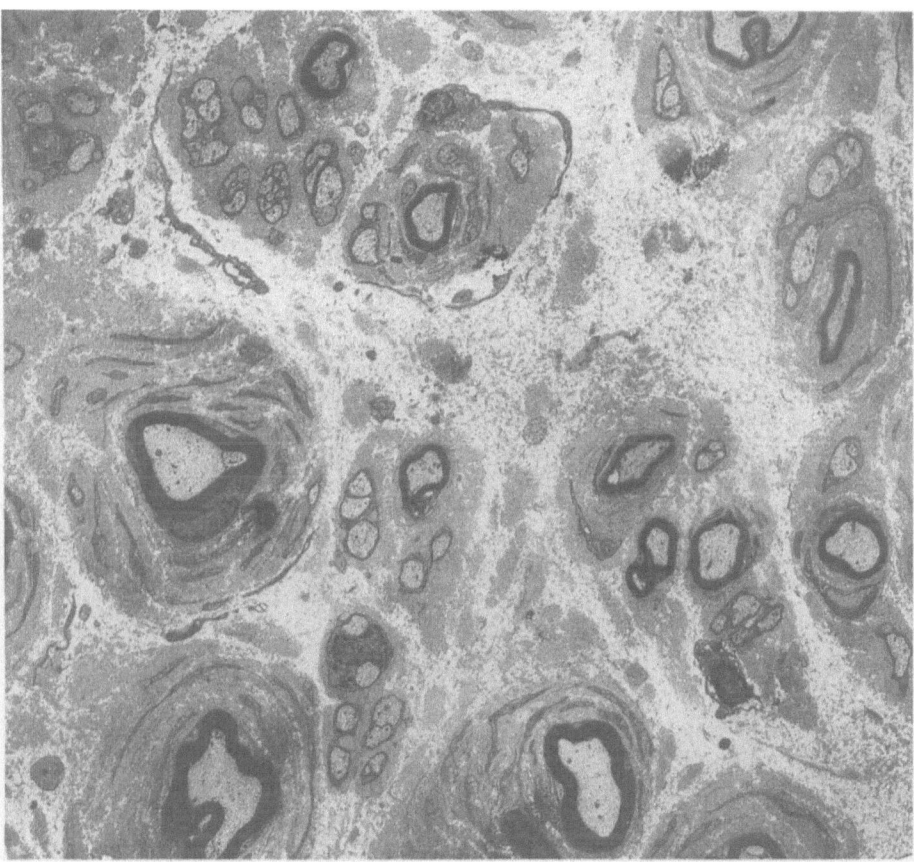

Fig. 7-27. Supernumerary Schwann-cell processes surround most of the myelinated axons in this cross-section of nerve from a patient with chronic inflammatory demyelinating neuropathy and an onion-bulb neuropathy (Courtesy of Hernando Mena, M.D., Washington, D.C.) (×3,000).

Involvement of the vasa nervorum by vasculitis may lead to an ischemic neuropathy, characteristically presenting as a mononeuropathy multiplex. The vasculitis may be restricted to the PNS (nonsystemic vasculitic neuropathy) or may be one aspect of a systemic vasculitis associated with periarteritis nodosa, allergic granulomatosis, hypersensitivity angiitis, rheumatoid arthritis, progressive systemic sclerosis, systemic lupus erythematosus, Sjögren syndrome, Wegener granulomatosis, cryoglobulinemia, amphetamine abuse, lymphomatoid granulomatosis, or hepatitis B.[9,35,40,62,100,111,123,223,249] Only a portion of the cases of neuropathy associated with systemic lupus erythematosus, rheumatoid arthritis, progressive systemic sclerosis, or Sjögren syndrome are secondary to vasculitis.[150,244] A vasculitic neuropathy may also be associated with carcinoma or human immunodeficiency virus infection.[51,62,111]

The vascular lesions in a vasculitic neuropathy are almost always in the small muscular arteries of the epineurium. A leukocytoclastic vasculitis involving the microvasculature may accompany the epineurial arteritis, but rarely is leukocytoclastic vasculitis the only identifiable lesion. An epineurial phlebitis may accompany the arteritis in exceptional cases.[268] The histologic features of the epineurial arteritis are similar, regardless of the underlying disease.[63] The sine qua non of an arteritis is inflammation of all

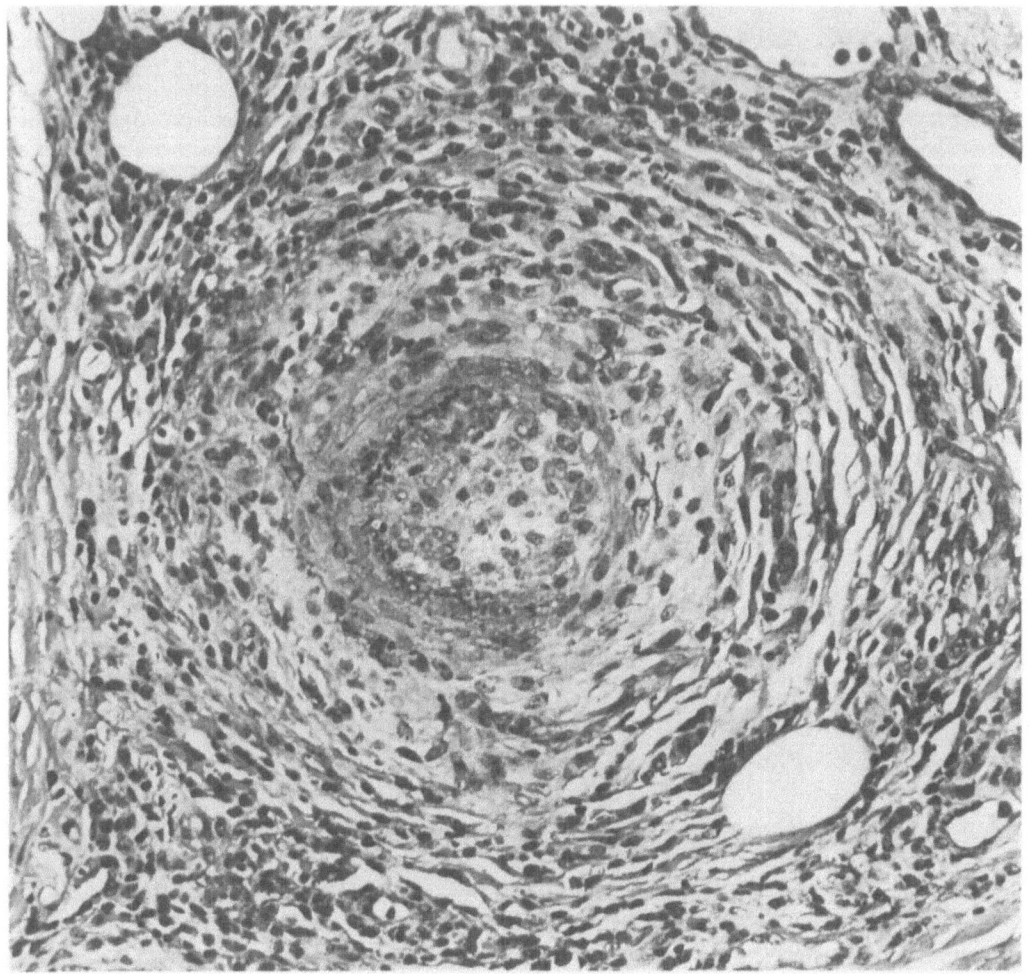

Fig. 7-28. Vasculitic neuropathy. Transmural inflammation and occlusion of an epineurial artery in a patient with periarteritis nodosa and a mononeuropathy multiplex (Verhoeff-van Gieson, ×300).

layers of the arterial wall (Fig. 7-28). The infiltrate is composed of mononuclear cells and variable numbers of neutrophils and eosinophils. The intima is thickened, initially by the infiltrate and later by proliferation of myointimal cells and fibrosis; the internal elastica is often fragmented. Fibrinoid necrosis may be focal in the media or involve large areas of the media and intima. Thrombi, either mural or occlusive, often complicate the arteritis. In the resolving stage of an arteritis, granulation tissue replaces the foci of fibrinoid necrosis, and the arterial wall is severely fibrotic. Transverse sections from multiple levels of the nerve must be examined histologically because the arterial lesions in an angiitis are segmental.

The nerve in ischemic neuropathy shows loss of myelinated and unmyelinated fibers secondary to axonal degeneration (Fig. 7-11). The fiber loss may be focal, multifocal, or diffuse.[62,108] Infarcts of the endoneurial contents are rare; in this regard, care must be taken not to misinterpret Renaut bodies as infarcts.[63] Ultrastructural examination reveals degenerating axons and occasional swollen axons.[256] The swollen axons are filled with tubulovesicular structures, filaments or abnormal mitochondria.[256] Teased fiber preparations reveal variable amounts of demyelination and remyelination.[63]

Focal or multifocal myelinated fiber loss, proliferating epineurial capillaries, and the separation and proliferation of smooth muscle cells from epineurial vessels suggest an angiopathic process, but are not diagnostic of vasculitic neuropathy.[108,209]

Diabetic Neuropathy

The symmetric polyneuropathy associated with diabetes mellitus is generally considered to be of ischemic or metabolic origin; the cranial mononeuropathies and at least some of the multiple mononeuropathies are considered to be ischemic.[7,67,108,186,215,277,68] The clinical and morphologic criteria for the diagnosis and staging of diabetic neuropathy have been discussed by Dyck et al.[65]

Behse et al[19] analyzed the histologic findings in sural nerve biopsies from 12 diabetic patients with symptomatic peripheral neuropathy. Ten of the 12 nerves had decreased myelinated fibers; in 7, the loss involved both large and small myelinated fibers. In 3, however, the small myelinated fibers were preferentially lost (Fig. 7-29). Nine nerves had an increased frequence of clusters of regenerating myelinated fibers. Ten to 40% of teased fibers displayed segmental remyelination, but active demyelination was rarely observed. Electron microscopy demonstrated frequent Büngner bands, especially in patients with neuropathy of short duration. Three nerves had less unmyelinated fibers, 4 had an increased number of degenerating unmyelinated axons, and 6 had numerous denervated Schwann-cell subunits. The size distribution and mean diameter of the unmyelinated axons were not altered, however. Half the endoneurial vessels had abnormal thickening of the perivascular space or more concentric layers of basal lamina; these changes were not considered diagnostic, however, because similar changes occurred in 25% of vessels from nerves with other types of acquired neuropathy. The basal lamina of the perineurial cells is also thickened in diabetic neuropathy.[107]

In another study, Dyck et al[68] examined sural nerve biopsies in 32 diabetic patients with neuropathy. Focal, multifocal, or diffuse loss of myelinated fibers and axonal degeneration were the major pathologic abnormalities. Myelinated fibers of all sizes were lost, although occasionally there was preferential loss of the large- or small-diameter fibers. Mural thickening and lumenal closure of endoneurial capillaries and arteriosclerosis of epineurial arteries appeared more frequent in diabetic nerves than in control nerves. Teased fiber preparations revealed that 22 of the 32 nerves from diabetics had an increased frequency of axonal degeneration, but only 7 had an increased frequency of segmental demyelination and remyelination.

Recent studies indicate that the demyelination associated with diabetic neuropathy is secondary to underlying axonal abnormalities.[67,108,68] Repeated episodes of demyelination and remyelination in diabetic neuropathy may lead to numerous onion bulb formations.[236,240]

Brown et al[32] reported that a painful diabetic neuropathy associated with preservation of large-fiber sensory modalities was reflected in a preferential loss of small myelinated and large unmyelinated axons, an increased number of small, unmyelinated axons (regenerating sprouts), and few demyelinated and remyelinated fibers. Said et al[205] also noted a severe involvement of small fibers in cases of diabetic neuropathy with dissociated sensory loss. Other authors have not found such a strong clinicopathologic correlation and report that the structural changes in sural nerve are similar, whether

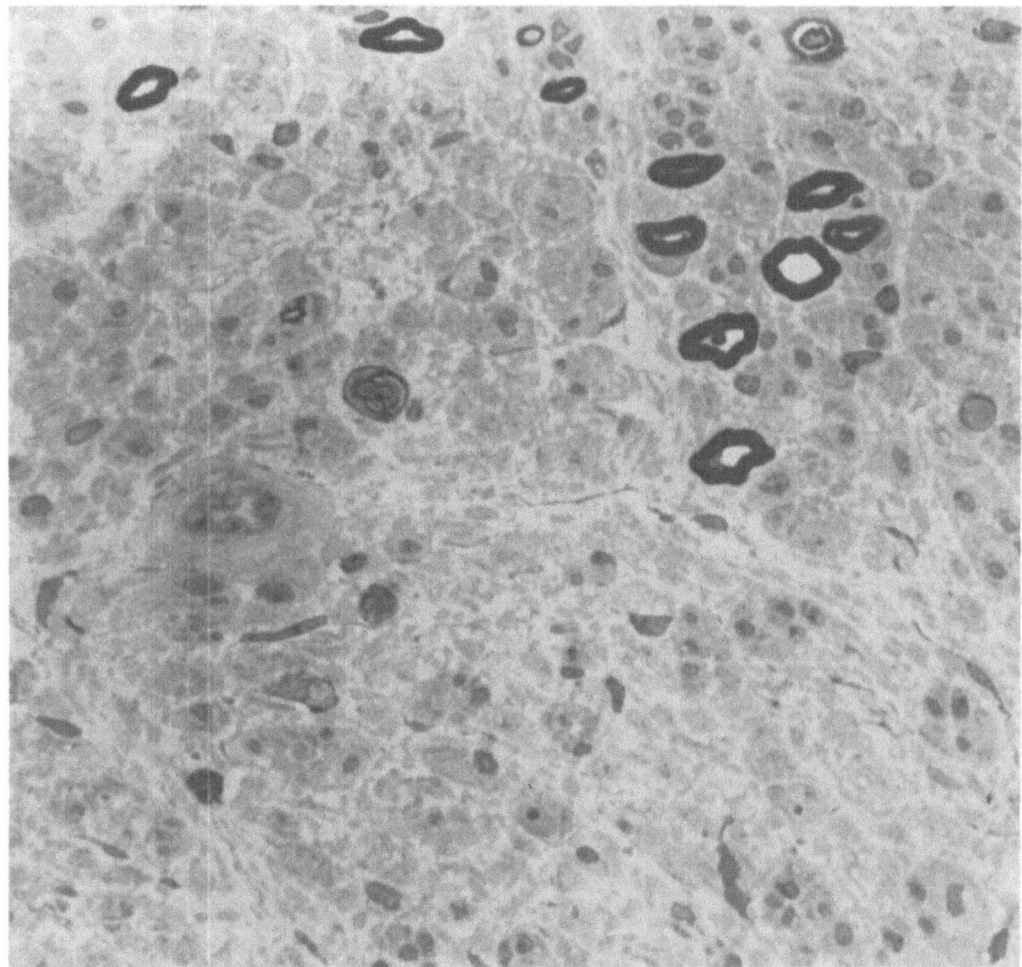

Fig. 7-29. Diabetic neuropathy. A semi-thin transverse section of sural nerve shows a severe loss of myelinated fibers. The small-diameter myelinated fibers are more severely involved than the large-diameter fibers (Toluidine blue, ×820).

the patient has predominantly a symmetric sensory neuropathy, a symmetric sensorimotor neuropathy, or a mononeuropathy multiplex.[19]

Preferential involvement of small fibers is not limited to diabetes. A small-fiber neuropathy may also be found in amyloidosis, Fabry disease, acute pandysautonomia, Tangier disease, and certain rare hereditary sensory neuropathies.[137]

Uremic Neuropathy

Uremic neuropathy is a distal, symmetric, sensorimotor neuropathy characterized by both axonal degeneration and demyelination. Morphologic studies indicate the axonal degeneration is the dying-back type, and the demyelination is secondary to axonal atrophy, which precedes the degeneration of the axon.[64] The metabolic defect responsible for the neuropathy is unknown. Not all neuropathies in uremic patients are secondary to uremia.[26]

Thomas et al[237] reported the pathologic findings in sural nerve biopsies from six patients with uremic neuropathy. Five of the six nerves had loss of myelinated fibers, usually of large diameter. An increased frequency of demyelination (predominantly paranodal) and remyelination was evident in teased fibers, but these changes were overshadowed by the loss of myelinated fibers. Electron microscopy reveals a decreased density of unmyelinated fibers and nonspecific degenerative changes in myelinated and unmyelinated axons.[3,64]

Nutritional and Alcoholic Neuropathies

Neuropathy as evidenced by pathologic changes in sural nerve may complicate thiamine deficiency (beriberi neuropathy), vitamin B_{12} deficiency, vitamin E deficiency, megavitamin doses of pyridoxine, and the postgastrectomy state.[1,14,148,206]

It is not clear whether alcoholic neuropathy is related solely to malnutrition or also involves a direct toxic effect of ethanol on the PNS. The sural nerve in cases of alcoholic neuropathy shows a loss of myelinated fibers, particularly those of large diameter. Unmyelinated fibers are also usually lost. Teased fiber preparations reveal axonal degeneration and occasionally a slightly increased frequency of demyelination or remyelination. Ultrastructural studies reveal only nonspecific axonal degeneration. The intra-axonal accumulations of smooth membranes found in beriberi neuropathy do not occur in alcoholic neuropathy.[14,176,203]

Amyloid Neuropathy

Amyloid neuropathy is associated with both hereditary systemic amyloidosis and the nonhereditary (acquired) systemic amyloidosis associated with immunocyte dyscrasias.[84,101,147,224] Amyloid neuropathy does not complicate the reactive systemic amyloidosis (secondary amyloidosis) associated with chronic infection, chronic inflammatory disease, or neoplasia. The neuropathy is typically a distal sensorimotor polyneuropathy. Amyloidosis may also be associated with a carpal tunnel syndrome caused by amyloid deposition in the flexor retinaculum.[20]

Amyloid neuropathy, whether hereditary or acquired, is characterized histologically by the deposition of amyloid in the endoneurium (Fig. 7-30).[78,238] The endoneurial deposits may be nodular or diffuse, often are perivascular, and have apple-green birefringence after staining with Congo red. One must be cautious in interpreting Congo red-stained sections of sural nerve, because false-positive staining and green birefringence may occur due to retention of excess dye.[37] Infiltration of vessel walls with amyloid is frequent and may be severe. Amyloid is also often found in the epineurium. The endoneurial deposits are usually accompanied by a moderate to severe loss of myelinated and unmyelinated fibers.

In some cases, unmyelinated and small myelinated fibers are preferentially lost; this change correlates with the frequent clinical finding of involvement of pain and temperature sensation, and severe autonomic dysfunction. Teased fiber preparations reveal that demyelination and remyelination often accompany the loss of myelinated and unmyelinated fibers.

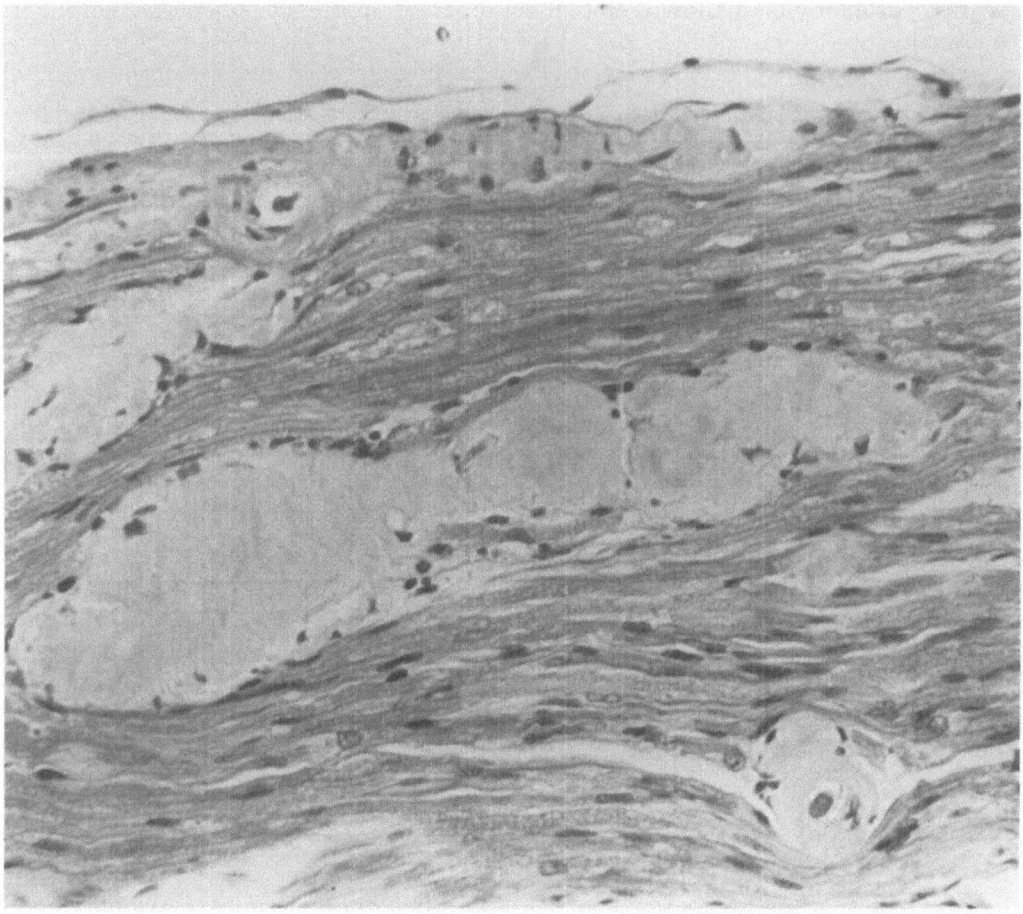

Fig. 7-30. Amyloid neuropathy. Nodular accumulations of amyloid are present within the endoneurium of a longitudinally sectioned sural nerve from a patient with systemic amyloidosis secondary to an immunocyte dyscrasia (×310).

Clusters of regenerating myelinated fibers may be increased in number. Ultrastructurally, aggregates of linear, nonbranching fibrils of 7.5–10 nm diameter are diagnostic of amyloid. As emphasized by Vital and Vallat,[261] it is important not to misinterpret Renaut bodies or immunoglobulin deposits as amyloid deposits by electron microscopy. Postulated mechanisms of nerve fiber damage in amyloid neuropathy include ischemia secondary to amyloid infiltration of vessel walls, direct injury of nerve fibers or their ganglion cells by large endoneurial deposits of amyloid, or a remote (paraneoplastic) effect of the immunocyte dyscrasia.[238,248,255]

Paraneoplastic Neuropathy

Neuropathy, as a remote effect of cancer, occurs with many different types of cancer but especially in cases of small cell carcinoma of the lung. Three clinico-pathologic types of paraneoplastic neuropathy are generally recognized.[9]

PARANEOPLASTIC SENSORIMOTOR NEUROPATHY

This symmetric, mixed, distal neuropathy is characterized by loss of myelinated fibers, axonal degeneration, and a variable amount of demyelination and remyelination.[47] Perineurial deposits of immunoglobulin M have been reported,[178] but the pathogenesis of the neuropathy remains unknown.

PARANEOPLASTIC SUBACUTE SENSORY NEUROPATHY (DORSAL ROOT GANGLIONITIS)

This sensory neuropathy is characterized by loss of dorsal root ganglion cells and chronic inflammation of these ganglia. There may be an associated paraneoplastic encephalitis. Loss of dorsal root ganglion cells is reflected in the sural nerve in loss of myelinated fibers, active axonal degeneration, and a variable amount of demyelination and remyelination.[47,98] A microangiitis may also be present.[111] No structural changes were found in the sural nerve biopsy from one patient with a paraneoplastic subacute motor neuropathy.[208]

INFLAMMATORY DEMYELINATING NEUROPATHY

An acute or chronic idiopathic polyneuritis may be associated with cancer and especially with Hodgkin's disease. The structural features of inflammatory demyelinating neuropathy are described elsewhere in this chapter.

Neuropathy Associated with Plasma Cell Dyscrasias

Peripheral neuropathy unrelated to nerve compression or direct invasion has been associated with all types of plasma cell dyscrasias, including benign monoclonal gammopathy, multiple myeloma, osteosclerotic myeloma, Waldenström macroglobulinemia, and heavy chain disease.[116,155,160] The neuropathy may be any of the three clinicopathologic types of paraneoplastic neuropathy, a distinctive chronic demyelinating neuropathy, or an amyloid neuropathy.[78,117,217]

The chronic demyelinating neuropathy is usually associated with an IgM monoclonal protein in the context of a benign monoclonal gammopathy or Waldenstrom macroglobulinemia. The chronic demyelinating neuropathy is characterized morphologically by segmental demyelination and remyelination, a variable number of onion bulbs, axonal degeneration, and in some cases, widening of the myelin lamellae owing to separation of the intraperiod line.[112] This distinctive myelin alteration, which has also been reported in inflammatory demyelinating neuropathy, should be distinguished from the uncompacted myelin lamellae also occasionally occurring in dysglobulinemic and other neuropathies (Fig. 7-31).[22,122,174,259] Immunofluorescent studies often reveal deposition of the M protein on myelin sheaths.[102,110,165,217,225,233] Evidence is accumulating to implicate these myelin-binding M proteins in the pathogenesis of the chronic demyelinating neuropathy.[225]

The demyelination found in the paraneoplastic sensorimotor neuropathy associated with osteosclerotic myeloma and multiple myeloma may be secondary to underlying axonal abnormalities.[172]

Cryoglobulinemic Neuropathy

A subacute symmetric sensorimotor neuropathy or an acute mononeuropathy occurs in 7%–15% of patients with cryoglobulinemia.[40] The cryoglobulinemia is usually mixed,

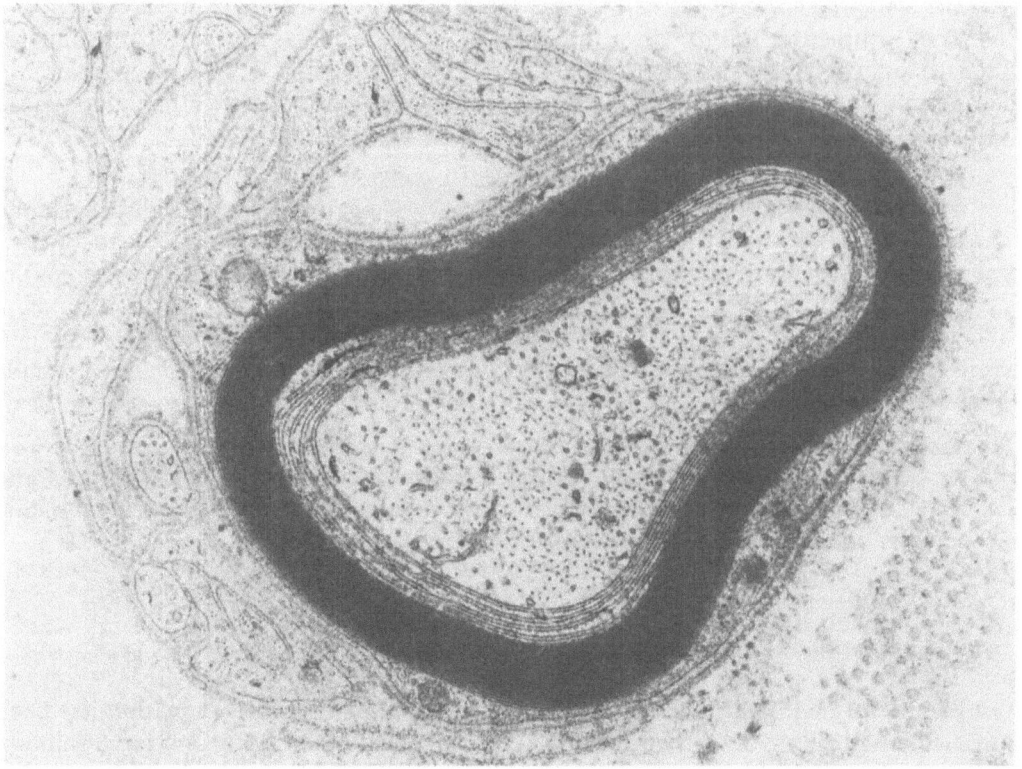

Fig. 7-31. Electron micrograph of a transversely sectioned myelinated axon. Several inner spirals of the Schwann-cell are not compacted to form myelin lamellae. Such uncompacted lamellae may be found in various neuropathies. (Original magnification, ×35,300).

but a neuropathy has also been associated with the monoclonal cryoglobulinemia of a plasma cell dyscrasia.[253]

The findings in sural nerve biopsies from patients with cryoglobulinemic neuropathy are variable.[163] Of the 7 biopsies reviewed by Chad et al.,[40] 2 revealed demyelination and perivascular mononuclear cells, 2 had axonal degeneration and demyelination, and 3 showed angiitis and axonal degeneration. In one biopsy, cryoglobulin precipitates were identified by electron microscopy in the endoneurium and within vessel walls and lumens.[253] A perineuritis, histologically similar to that of sensory perineuritis, may also accompany the cryoglobulinemic vasculitis.[126]

The pathogenesis of cryoglobulinemic neuropathy is not established.[135] In those cases showing angiitis of the epineurial arteries, a reasonable speculation is that the nerve fiber damage is secondary to ischemia.[163] The mechanism of the demyelination and axonal degeneration in those cases without angiitis is not clear.

Hereditary Motor and Sensory Neuropathies (HMSN)

The hereditary motor and sensory neuropathies (HMSN) are heterogeneous diseases characterized by involvement of both lower motor neurons and primary sensory neurons. Autonomic neurons may also be involved in HMSN. Unfortunately, the molecular

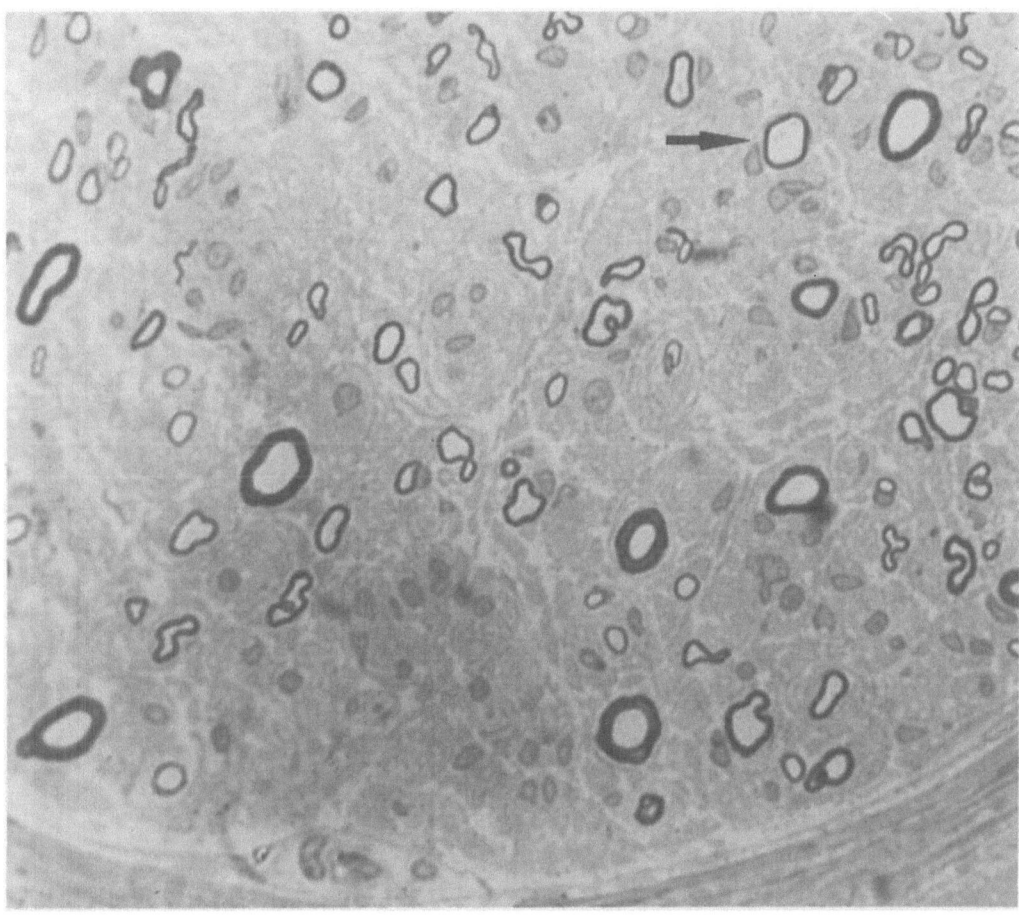

Fig. 7-32. Dominantly inherited onion-bulb neuropathy (HMSN type I). A transverse, semi-thin section of sural nerve reveals moderate loss of myelinated fibers. An arrow indicates one of several remyelinated fibers, characterized by large-diameter axons with inappropriately thin myelin sheaths (Toluidine blue, ×840).

abnormalities underlying the various HMSN are, with few exceptions, not known. Therefore, classification must be based on a combination of clinical, genetic, electrodiagnostic, and morphologic criteria. Such a classification has drawbacks, including the possibility of genetic heterogeneity within a clinicopathologic disease entity.[24] HMSN are characterized by either an onion-bulb neuropathy or an axonal (neuronal) neuropathy. HMSN type I is the prototypical hereditary onion-bulb neuropathy and HMSN type II is the prototypical hereditary axonal neuropathy. The clinicopathologic classification proposed by Dyck[61] is widely used.

HMSN TYPE I (HYPERTROPHIC FORM OF CHARCOT-MARIE-TOOTH DISEASE)

This relatively common form of HMSN usually has an autosomal dominant mode of inheritance.[93] HMSN type I is characterized by an onion-bulb (hypertrophic) neuropathy. The sural nerve biopsy reveals increased total fascicular area, slight to severe loss of myelinated fibers with preferential loss of the large myelinated fibers, and only rare clusters of regenerating myelinated fibers (Fig. 7-32).[13,138,142] Onion bulbs may be inconspicuous by light microscopy, especially in very young patients, but are easily

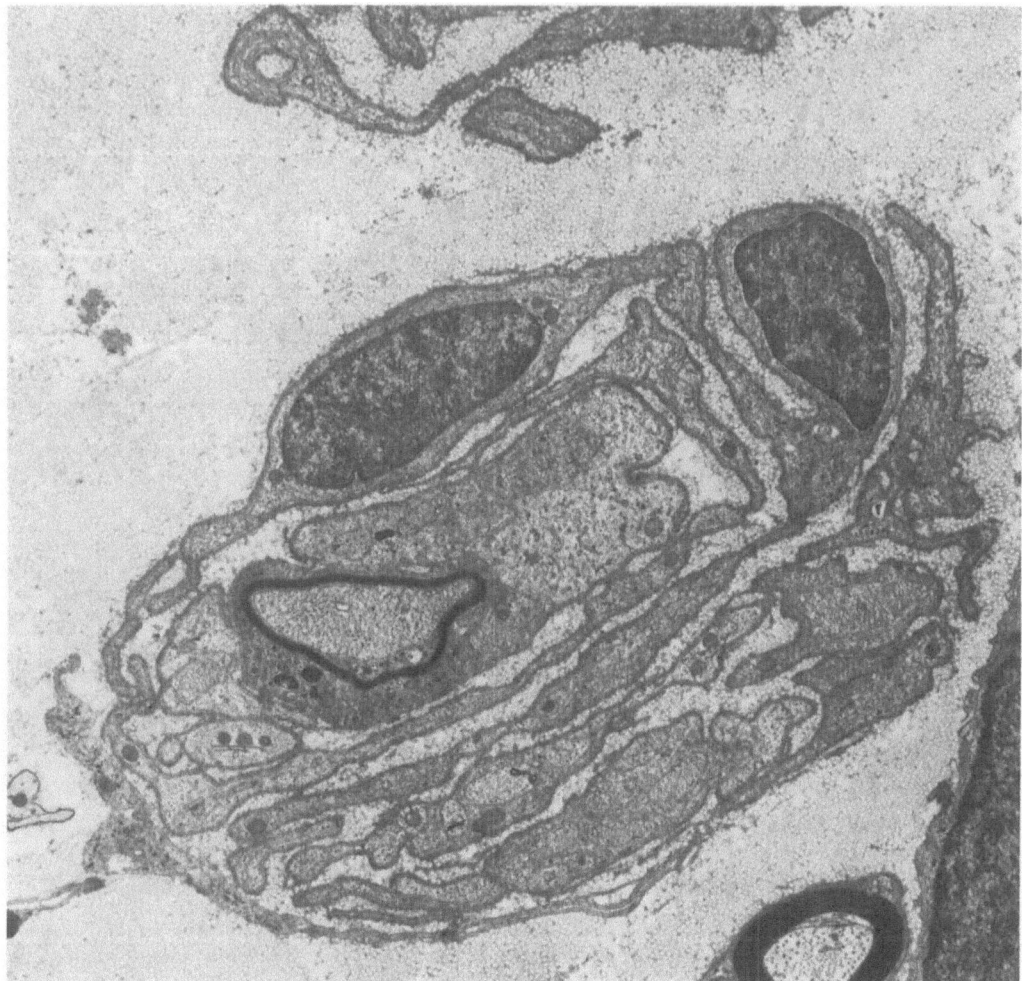

Fig. 7-33. Electron micrograph of a transverse section through a large onion bulb reveals numerous Schwann-cell lamellae around a myelinated axon. The myelin sheath of the axon is inappropriately thin, indicating remyelination. The patient has HMSN type I (×8,800).

found by electron microscopy.[138] Many myelinated fibers have one or more supernumerary Schwann-cell lamellae (Figs. 7-33, 7-34). Electron microscopy may also reveal occasional axons with inappropriately thick myelin sheaths, suggesting axonal atrophy.[13,166] Loss of unmyelinated fibers is reflected in increased numbers of denervated Schwann-cell subunits. The density of unmyelinated fibers may be increased, normal, or decreased; small-diameter, regenerating unmyelinated fibers may be increased. Onion-bulb formations are not discernible in routinely prepared teased fiber preparations, but demyelination and remyelination are typically present in 30%–100% of the teased fibers.

Onion bulb neuropathy is not restricted to HMSN type I. A neuropathy with similar pathologic features is present in HMSN type III, HMSN type IV, and a few unclassified, but apparently phenotypically unique, HMSN. Recessively inherited HMSN type III (Dejerine-Sottas disease) is distinguished morphologically from the more common HMSN type I by a greater loss of large myelinated fibers, greater frequency of onion

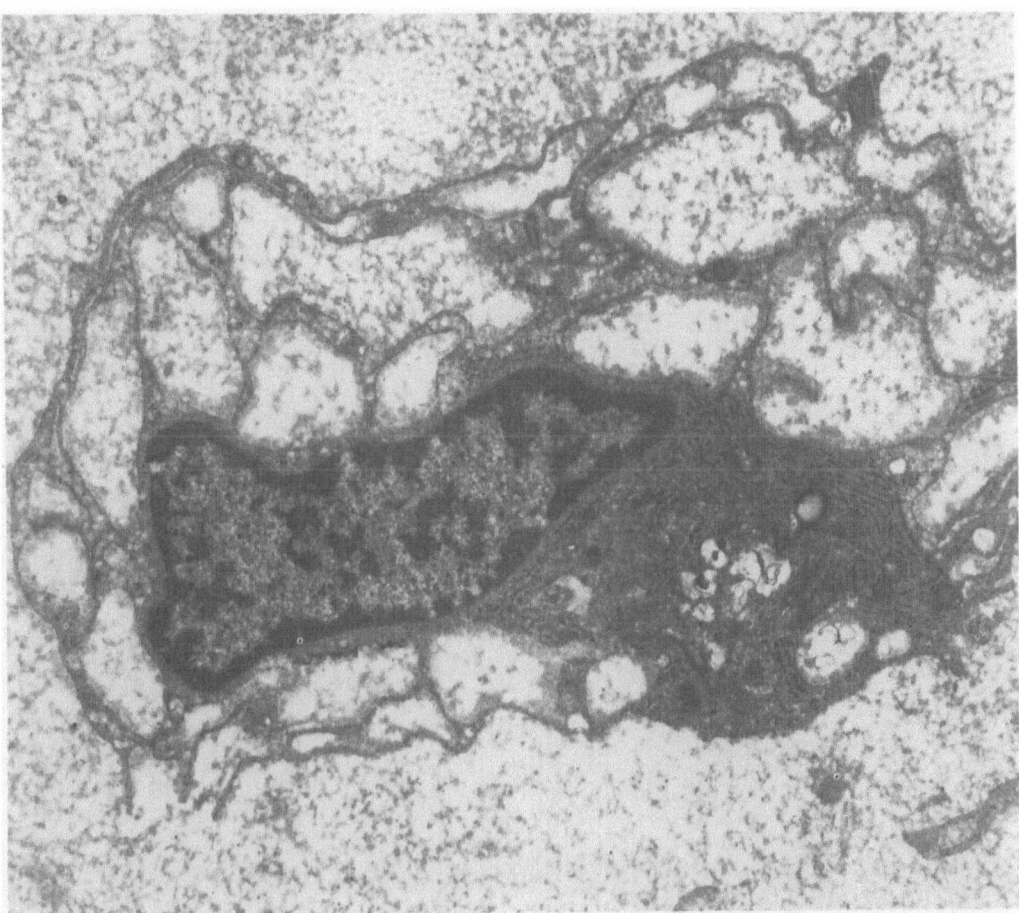

Fig. 7-34. This endoneurial fibroblast has many large cytoplasmic vacuoles. Vacuolated fibroblasts were first
   described in hereditary sensory neuropathy, but similar cells may also be found in hereditary onion-
   bulb neuropathy and other neuropathies (×12,500).

bulbs, more numerous onion-bulb lamellae, and a higher ratio of mean axon diameter
to fiber diameter.[180] The diagnosis of HMSN type IV (Refsum disease, phytanic acid
storage disease) rests on the finding of an elevated phytanic acid level in serum. A
hereditary, steroid-responsive onion-bulb neuropathy has also been described.[61]

Numerous onion-bulb formations are not limited to the hereditary demyelinating
neuropathies. They may also be found in several acquired chronic neuropathies, including diabetic neuropathy,[240] chronic idiopathic polyneuritis (Fig. 7-27),[70] and acromegalic
neuropathy.[55]

HMSN TYPE II (NEURONAL FORM OF CHARCOT-MARIE-TOOTH DISEASE)

This entity usually has an autosomal-dominant mode of inheritance.[93] The neuropathy is categorized as an "axonal" ("neuronal") neuropathy because the loss of axons
is not accompanied by demyelination and onion bulbs. The total fascicular area of the
sural nerve is normal or only slightly increased. The density of myelinated fibers ranges
from normal to severely decreased; the size-distribution histogram is often unimodal
with preferential loss of the large myelinated fibers (Fig. 7-35).[13,21,142,153] Clusters of

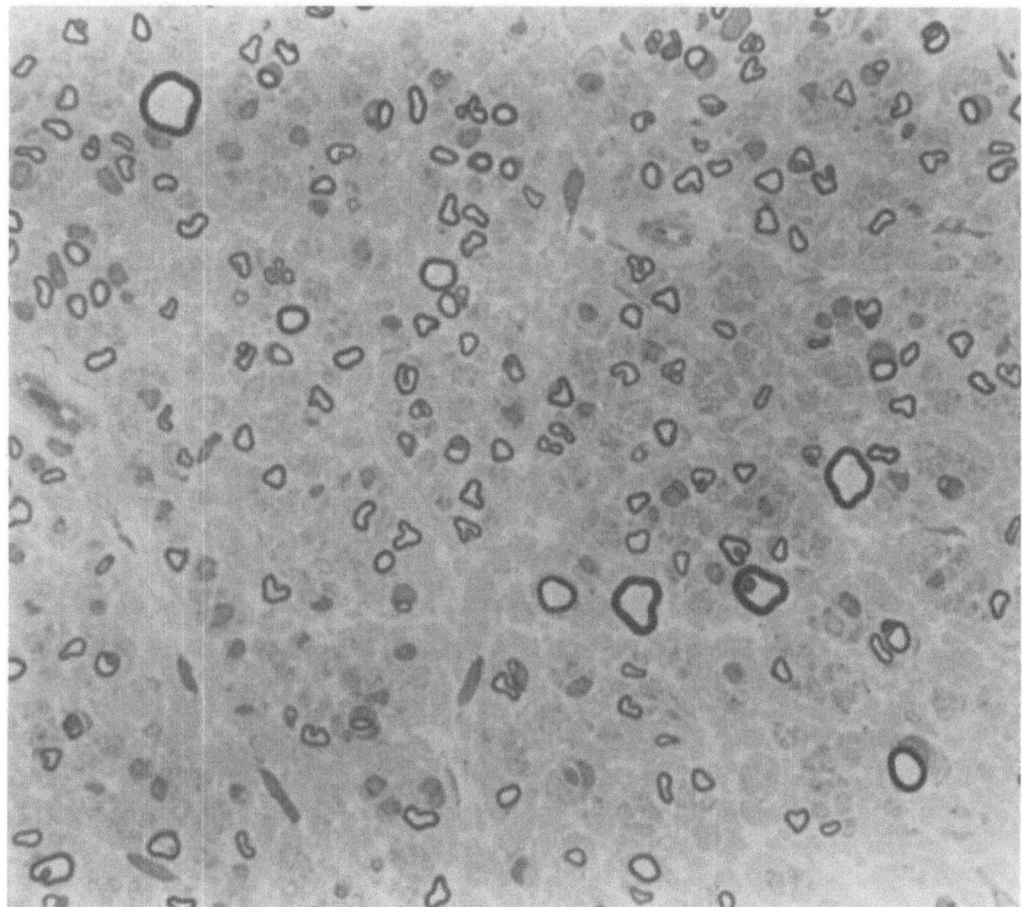

Fig. 7-35. Friedreich ataxia. Semi-thin transverse section of sural nerve reveals a preferential loss of the large-diameter myelinated fibers (Toluidine blue, ×800).

regenerating myelinated fibers are commonly present (Fig. 7-36). Ultrastructurally, the remaining myelinated fibers are normal except for an infrequent, small, onion bulb. The number of unmyelinated fibers may be increased, normal, or decreased, but the presence of denervated Schwann-cell subunits attests to a loss of unmyelinated fibers. Teased fiber preparations are either unremarkable or show only a slightly increased frequency of demyelination and remyelination.

An axonal neuropathy with a preferential loss of large myelinated fibers is not limited to HMSN type II. A neuropathy with similar structural changes (in sural nerve) is found in cases of Friedreich ataxia, hereditary spastic paraplegia, abetalipoproteinemia (Bassen-Kornzweig disease), and several less well-defined hereditary conditions in which a peripheral neuropathy is part of a widespread multisystem degeneration involving both the CNS and PNS.[13,151,159,204,245,272] An axonal neuropathy with a loss of small as well as large myelinated fibers may occur in hereditary spinocerebellar degenerations other than Friedreich ataxia.[152]

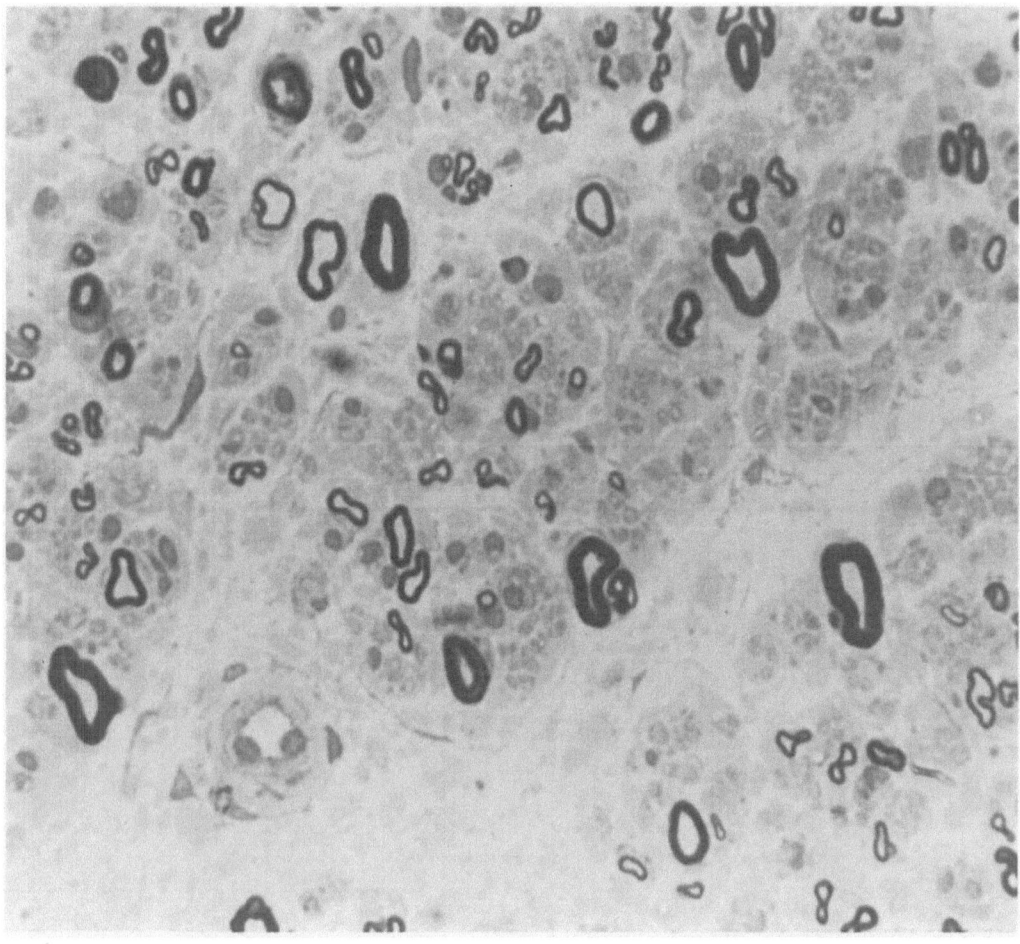

Fig. 7-36. Moderate loss of myelinated fibers and several clusters of regenerating myelinated fibers are noted in this sural nerve from a patient with a dominantly inherited axonal neuropathy (HMSN type II) (Toluidine blue, ×855).

Hereditary Sensory Neuropathies

The classification, clinical presentation, and morphological features of these rare neuropathies are discussed by Dyck[60] and Donaghy et al.[57]

Werdnig-Hoffman Disease and Amyotrophic Lateral Sclerosis

Werdnig-Hoffmann disease (WHD) is usually considered a disease of spinal and bulbar motor neurons, but recent studies indicate that primary sensory neurons are also frequently affected. In one series, an increased frequency of axonal degeneration was consistently present in sural nerve biopsies from seven patients with typical WHD.[36] Sural nerve biopsy may be especially helpful diagnostically in cases in which the young age of the patient makes interpretation of the muscle biopsy difficult.

An atypical WHD (infantile neuronal degeneration), which clinically resembles WHD

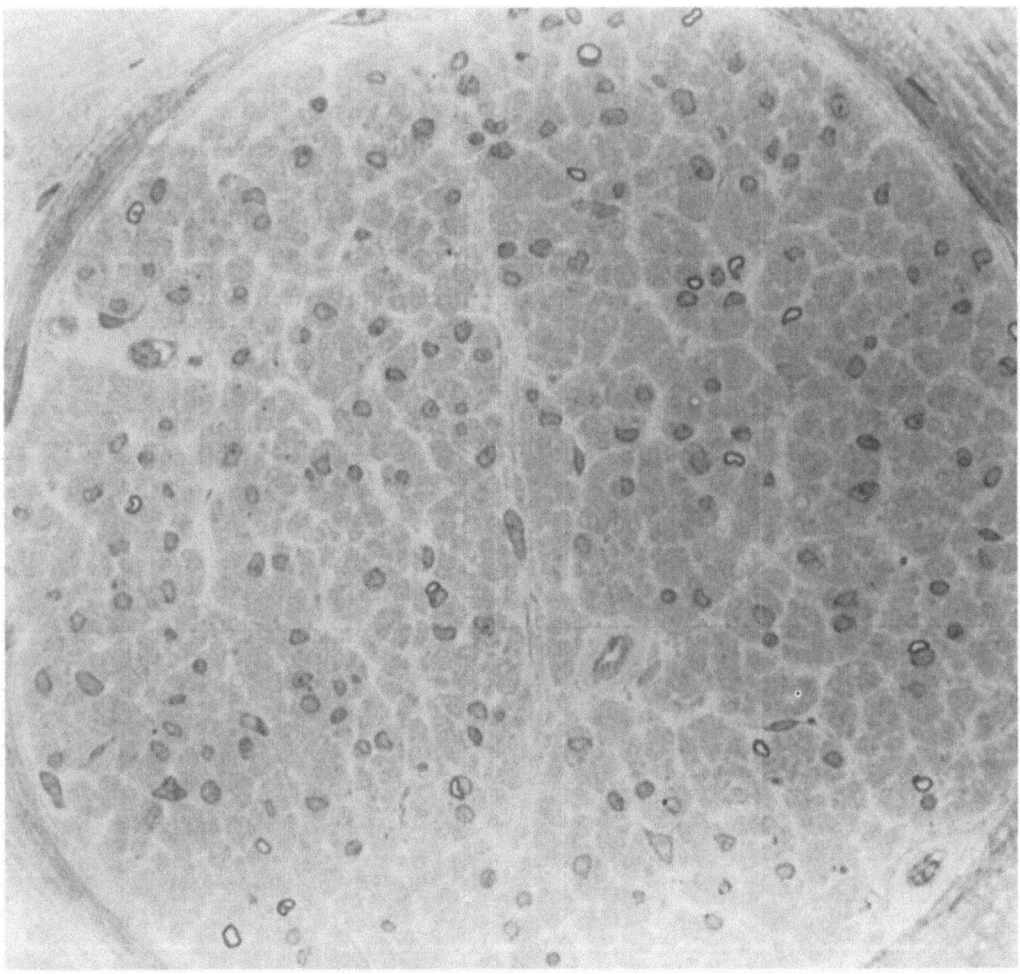

Fig. 7-37. Congenital motor and sensory neuropathy. This semi-thin transverse section reveals an almost total absence of myelinated fibers in this sural nerve from a 10-month-old child with a severe congenital neuropathy. Electron-microscopic studies revealed that the lack of myelin was related to axonal degeneration rather than hypomyelination or primary demyelination (Toluidine blue, ×800).

but is a multisystem degeneration affecting all levels of the nervous system, is reported in association with a demyelinating neuropathy.[227]

Amyotrophic lateral sclerosis (ALS) also frequently involves sensory neurons. Bradley et al[28] found a 30% reduction in myelinated fibers and an increased number of denervated Schwann-cell subunits in sural nerve biopsies from 10 patients with ALS. The loss of myelinated fibers involves both small- and large-diameter fibers, with the loss of large fibers predominating.[56] Personal experience indicates that sural nerve biopsy does not always reveal a detectable loss of myelinated fibers in patients with ALS.

Congenital Neuropathies

Several diseases, including HMSN type I, HMSN type III, Krabbe disease, and metachromatic leukodystrophy, may present as a symptomatic neuropathy at birth.

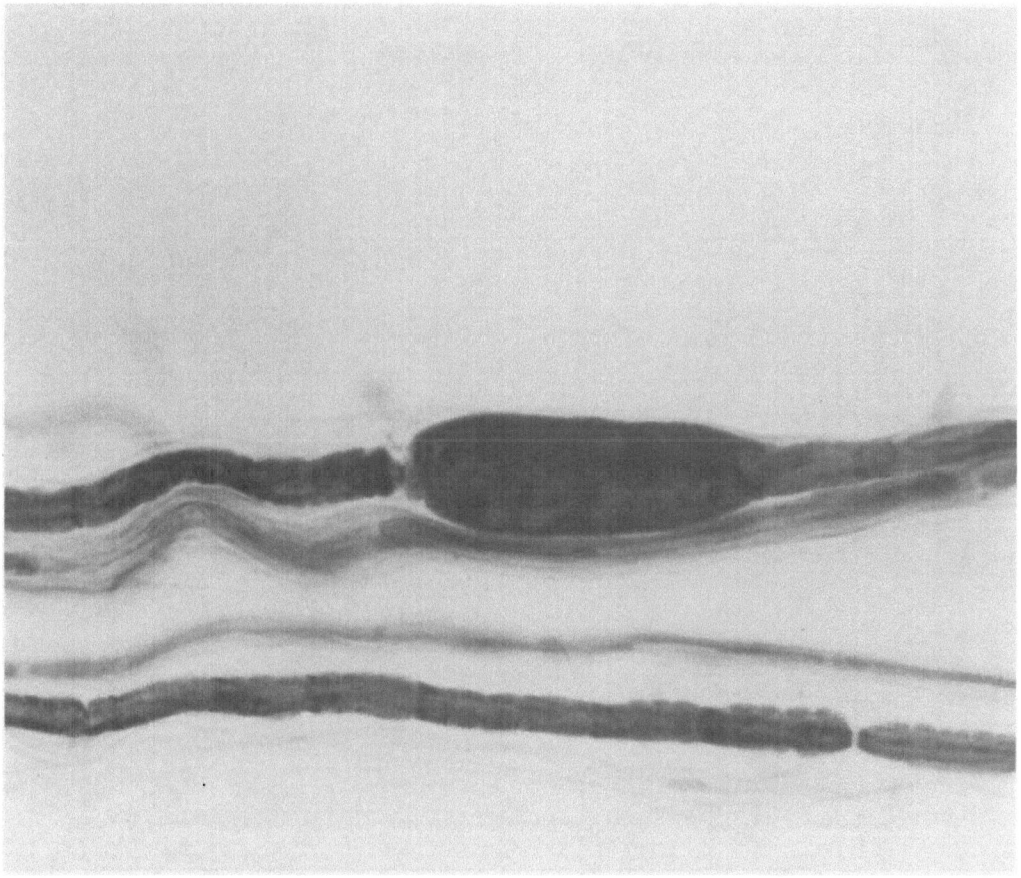

Fig. 7-38. Tomaculous neuropathy. A sausage-shaped swelling is present in the paranodal region of one of the two teased myelinated fibers. (Osmium tetroxide, ×500).

Congenital hypomyelination neuropathy, an onion bulb neuropathy, congenital motor and sensory neuropathy, an axonal neuropathy, and congenital absence of peripheral myelin are also described (Fig. 7-37).[42,86,119,179,250,257]

Hereditary Pressure-Sensitive Neuropathy

A "tomaculous" (tomaculum, Latin = sausage) or "sausage-body" neuropathy is the structural substrate of this dominantly inherited clinical syndrome of increased susceptibility to pressure palsies.[16,141] The distinctive and striking abnormality in tomaculous neuropathy is the presence of numerous sausage-like swellings (tomacula) on many of the myelinated fibers. The localized swellings are related to an abnormally thick myelin sheath rather than a swollen axon. They are easily seen in both plastic-embedded 1.0 μm thick sections and in teased fibers (Figs. 7-38, 7-39). In teased-fiber preparations, the tomacula range from 40 to 250 μm in length and may be twice the diameter of the uninvolved portion of the fiber. The sausage-like swellings are found in both paranodal and internodal areas and in remyelinated internodes. In the six cases of tomaculous neuropathy reported by Behse et al,[16] about one-fourth of the

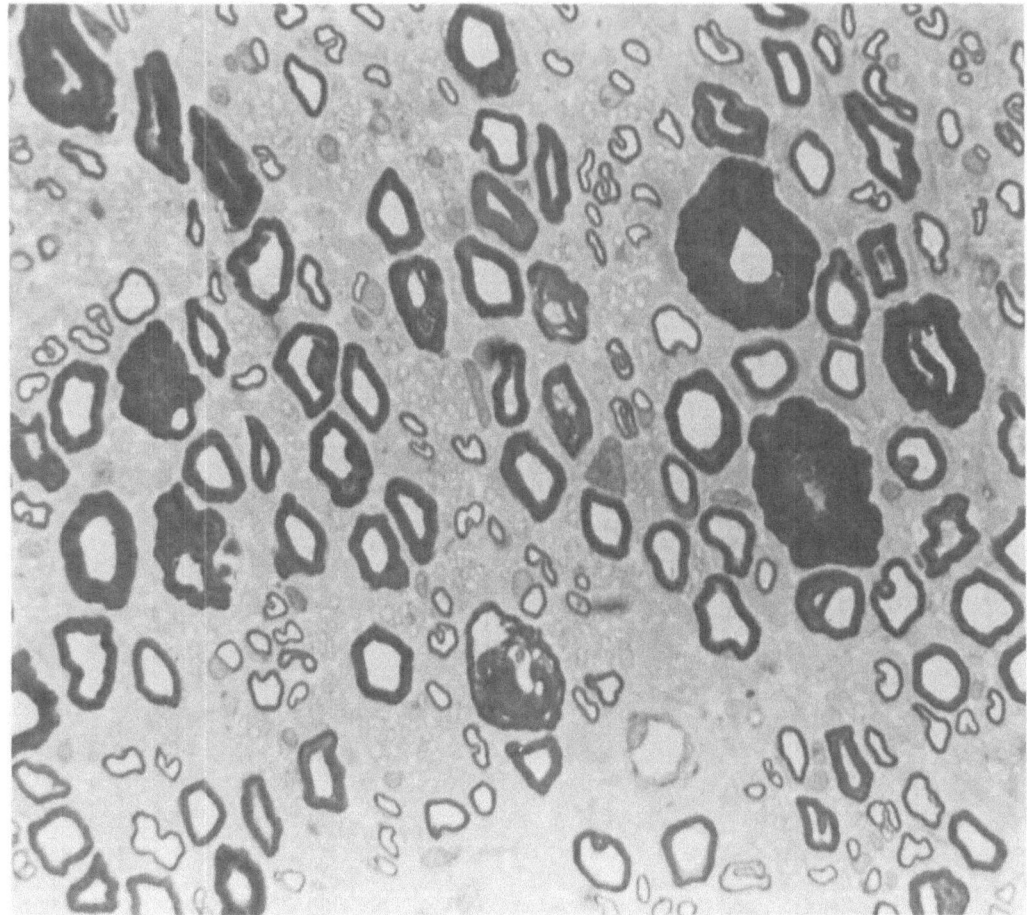

Fig. 7-39. Tomaculous neuropathy. Semi-thin transverse section reveals several axons with abnormally thick myelin sheaths. This sural nerve is from a patient with an inherited susceptibility to pressure palsies. (Toluidine blue, ×840).

internodes contained tomacula. The density of myelinated fibers is normal to moderately decreased, with preferential loss of large myelinated fibers. A variable amount of demyelination and remyelination is present in teased fibers.

Electron microscopy confirms that the swellings are related to an abnormally thick myelin sheath (Fig. 7-40). These sheaths may be induced by various mechanisms, including hypermyelination, wrapping of axons by redundant myelin loops, branching and duplication of the mesaxon, transnodal myelination, and localized degeneration of the myelin sheath.[141] The axon within the tomaculum is often constricted and has increased numbers of neurofilaments and microtubules. An occasional onion bulb may be present. Unmyelinated fibers are not affected.

Sausage-body neuropathy has also been reported in a familial exercise-related mononeuropathy with abdominal colic, in a recurrent brachial plexus neuropathy, in a congenital neuropathy, and in a chronic senscrimotor neuropathy primarily affecting the upper limbs.[27,246,254] Recent studies suggest that tomaculous neuropathy is not the pathologic substrate of hereditary brachial plexus neuropathy.[6]

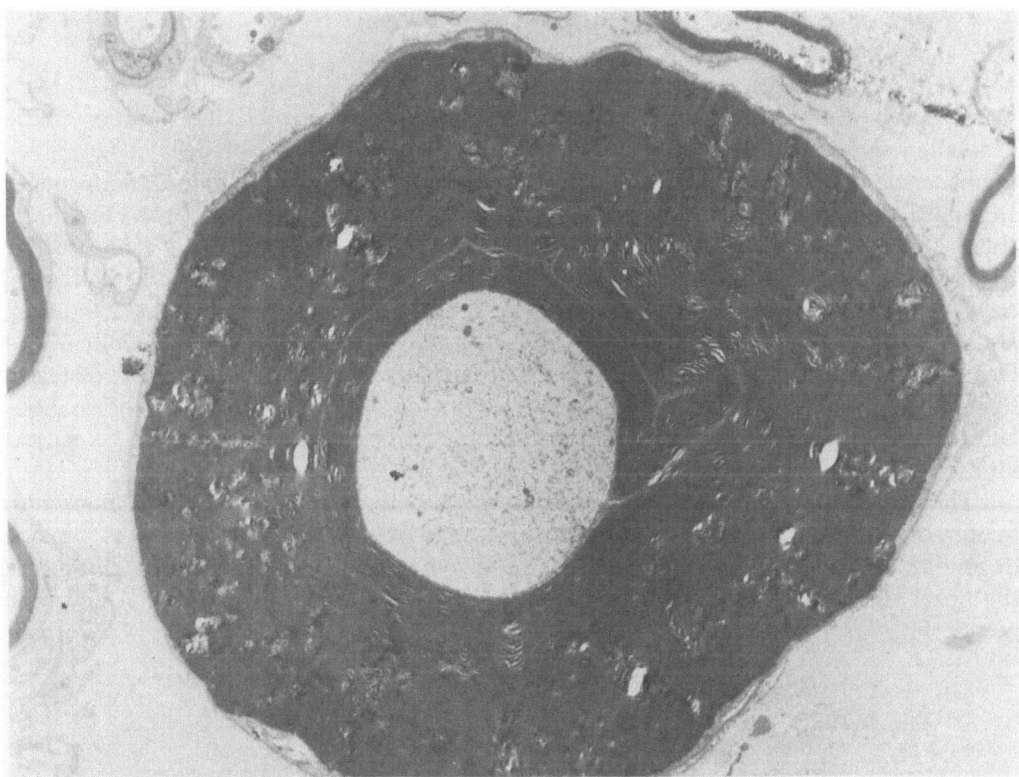

Fig. 7-40. Tomaculous neuropathy. Electron micrograph of a sausage-shaped swelling demonstrates the severely thickened myelin sheath (Original magnification, ×5,600).

Metabolic Storage Diseases

The advent of enzymatic assays has reduced the use of sural nerve biopsy as a diagnostic procedure in the study of metabolic storage diseases. Storage material has been found within Schwann cells in several metabolic diseases, including metachromatic leukodystrophy,[25] Krabbe disease,[207] type II and type III glycogenosis,[85,187] neuronal ceroid lipofuscinosis,[10] Niemann-Pick disease,[90,129] sialidosis type I,[228] Farber disease,[261] Wolman disease,[33] I-cell disease,[143] and Tangier disease.[124] In Fabry disease, storage material is prominent in perineurial cells, endothelial cells, and perithelial cells, but not in Schwann cells.[173] Fabry disease is also of interest because of the selective involvement of small myelinated and unmyelinated fibers.

A peripheral neuropathy characterized by axonal loss and demyelination may be associated with cerebrotendinous xanthomatosis and adrenoleukodystrophy (adrenoleukomyeloneuropathy).[144,177,188,262] The distinctive cytoplasmic clefts characterizing adrenoleukodystrophy are inconstantly found in Schwann cells.[144,177,188] A demyelinating neuropathy with a variable number of onion bulbs and occasional Schwann-cell inclusions is described in Cockayne syndrome.[263] Peripheral neuropathy has also been described in patients with mitochondrial myopathies. The abnormal mitochondria may be found in Schwann cells.[184,278]

Toxic Neuropathies

Many drugs and industrial chemicals may produce a toxic neuropathy (Table 7-2).[9,222] Most of these toxic neuropathies induce nonspecific axonal degeneration, hence a detailed account of the changes associated with each neurotoxin will not be given. Diphtheritic neuropathy is unique, being a predominantly demyelinating neuropathy. In general, the sural nerve biopsy shows a loss of myelinated fibers (Fig. 7-41). Frequently, there is a preferential involvement of large myelinated fibers; Kepone (chlordecone) neuropathy is remarkable because of the involvement of unmyelinated and small myelinated fibers.[145] Unless several weeks have elapsed between exposure to the neurotoxicant and nerve biopsy, a variable amount of active axonal degeneration is also usually found. Demyelination and remyelination, if present, usually involve less than 15% of teased fibers and are generally considered secondary to the underlying axonal abnormalities. Ultrastructural studies may reveal increased pi bodies and dense bodies of various kinds, but such findings are nonspecific (Fig. 7-42).[145,157]

The neuropathies caused by perhexiline, sodium cyanate, gold, and Buckthorn toxin are characterized by significant demyelination as well as axonal degeneration.[114,175,202] The neuropathies caused by acrylamide, carbon disulfide, and the hexacarbon solvents are distinguished by accumulations of intra-axonal neurofilaments (Fig. 7-22).[54]

Table 7.2.
Drugs and Toxicants Associated with Neuropathy

I. DRUGS	*II. ENVIRONMENTAL TOXICANTS*
Almitrine	Acrylamide
Amiodarone (Cordarone)	Arsenic
Amytriptyline	Buckthorn toxin (Coyotillo fruit)
Chloramphenicol	Carbon disulfide
Chloroquine	Chlordecone (Kepone)
Cisplatinum	2,4-Dichlorophenoxy acetic acid (2,4-D)
Colchicine	Dimethylaminopropionitrile
Dapsone	Diphtheria toxin
Diphenylhydantoin (Phenytoin)	Ethylene oxide
Disulfiram (Antabuse)	n-Hexane, Methyl n-butyl ketone, 2,5-Hexane-
Ethyl alcohol	dione
Glutethimide	Lead
Hydralazine	Mercury
Isoniazid (INH)	Methyl bromide
Lithium carbonate	Organophosphorous compounds
Misonidazole and Metronidazole (Flagyl)	Polybrominated biphenyls (PBB's)
Nitrous oxide	Tetrachlorobiphenyl (TCB)
Nitrofurantoin	Thallium
Organic gold compounds	Trichloroethylene
Perhexiline maleate (Pexid)	
Pyridoxine (Vitamin B_6)	
Sodium cyanate	
Thalidomide	
Vincristine	

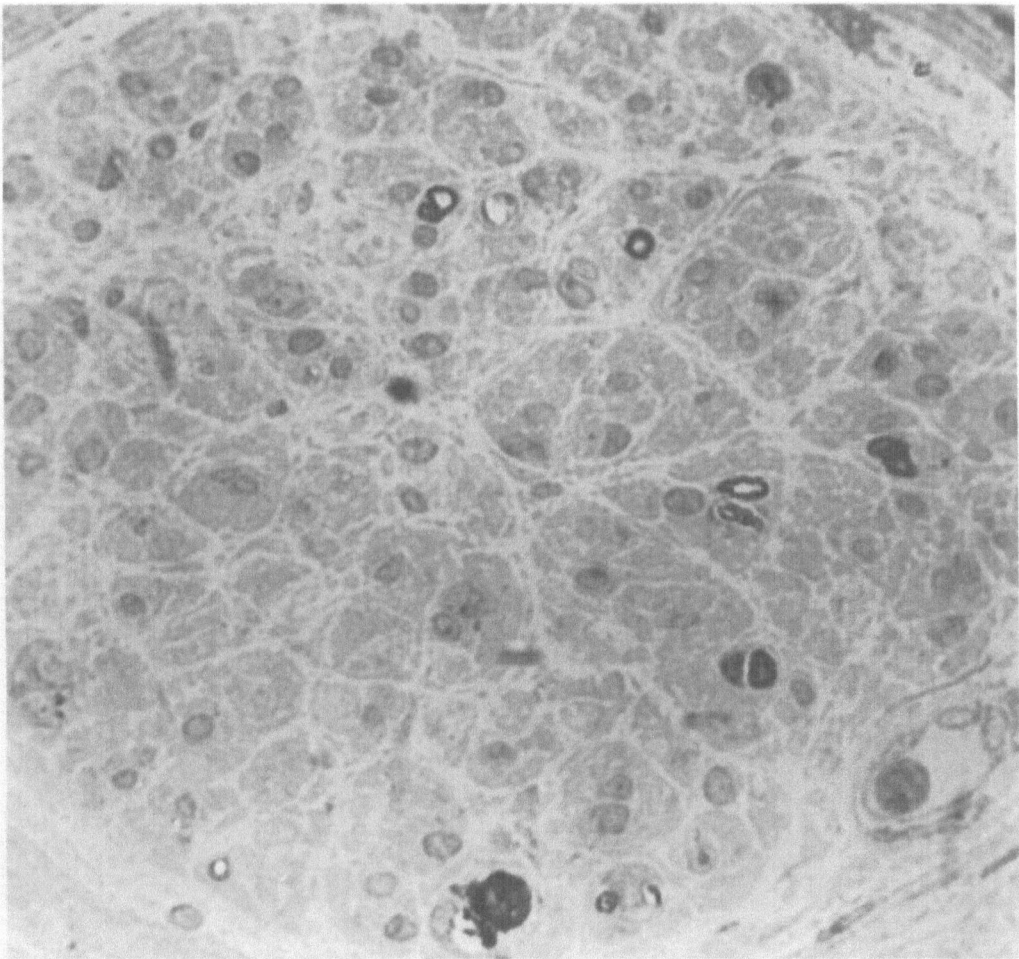

Fig. 7-41. Vincristine neuropathy. There is a severe loss of myelinated fibers in this semi-thin section of sural nerve. An actively degenerating myelinated fiber is present at 6 o'clock (Toluidine blue, ×855)

Traumatic Neuropathies

NEUROMA-IN-CONTINUITY

Acute compression, contusion, stretching, injection injury, gunshot wound, or partial laceration of a nerve trunk may produce significant nerve fiber damage without complete division of the nerve trunk and a consequent terminal bulb neuroma. The localized lesion, referred to as a neuroma-in-continuity, is characterized by various amounts of demyelination and Wallerian degeneration.[99] There is an associated fibrosis of the endoneurium, perineurium, and epineurium. Scattered siderophages or a foreign body reaction may be present in the surrounding connective tissue. If the trauma is sufficient to interrupt the perineurium of one or more fascicles, a "lateral neuroma," composed of regenerating axonal sprouts, will develop at the site of the break.[231]

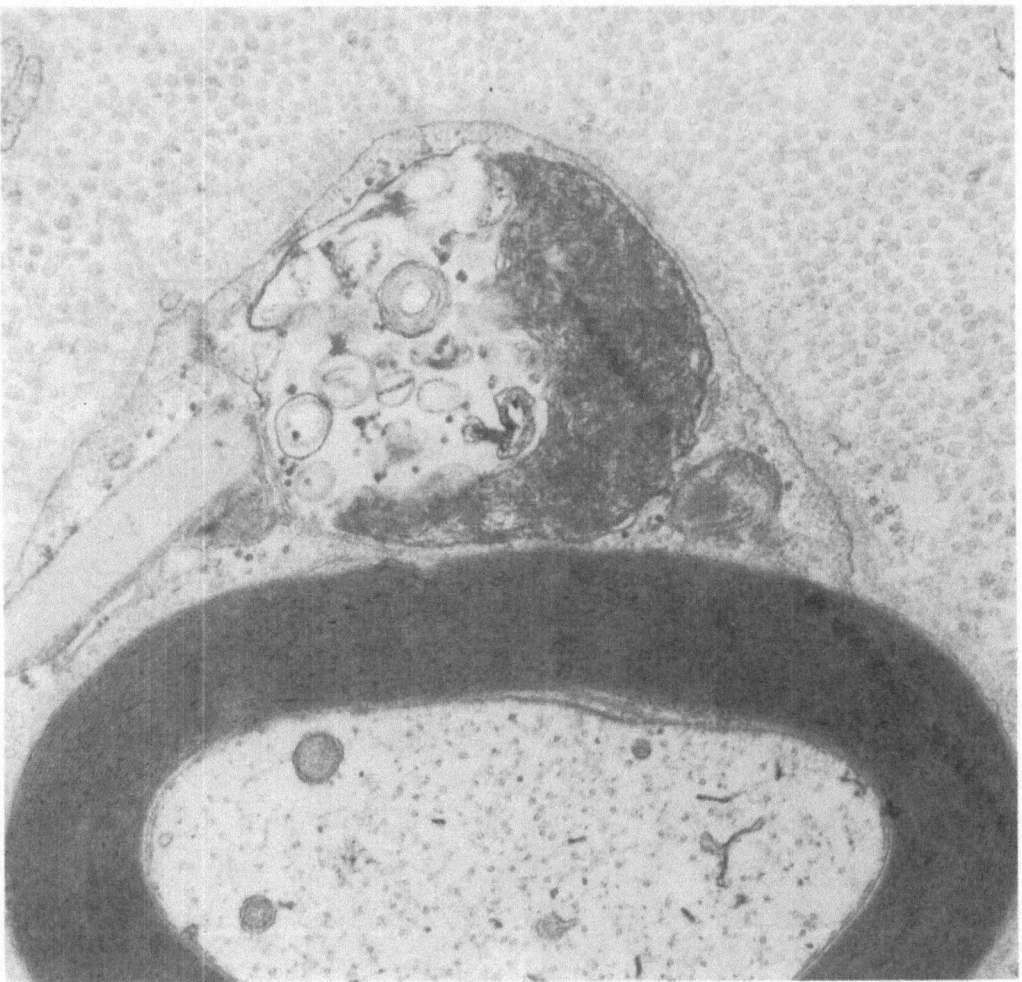

Fig. 7-42. Electron micrograph of the sural nerve from a patient who developed a neuropathy after commencing treatment with amiodarone. Polymorphic dense bodies are present in the Schwann-cell cytoplasm (×37,000).

PLANTAR NEUROMA (MORTON'S TOE, MORTON'S METATARSALGIA)

Plantar neuroma is most likely caused by chronic entrapment of the plantar digital nerve between the second and third, or less commonly, third and fourth, metatarsal bones in the region of the metatarsophalangeal joints.[131,168]

Grossly, the plantar neuroma is a sausage-shaped swelling of the plantar digital nerve. The intermetatarsal bursa is usually firmly adherent to the swelling. Microscopy reveals that the "neuroma" is actually a pseudoneuroma (i.e., the swelling noted grossly is related to proliferation of fibrous tissue rather than the proliferation of regenerating axons found in a true neuroma) (Fig. 7-43).[131,154,194] The digital nerve shows loss of myelinated and unmyelinated fibers and endoneurial fibrosis. Paranodal demyelination and polarized paranodal swellings of the myelin sheath have also been found in teased fiber preparations.[168] The endoneurium may contain foci of myxoid degeneration or hyalinized nodules, and the walls of endoneurial blood vessels are frequently strikingly

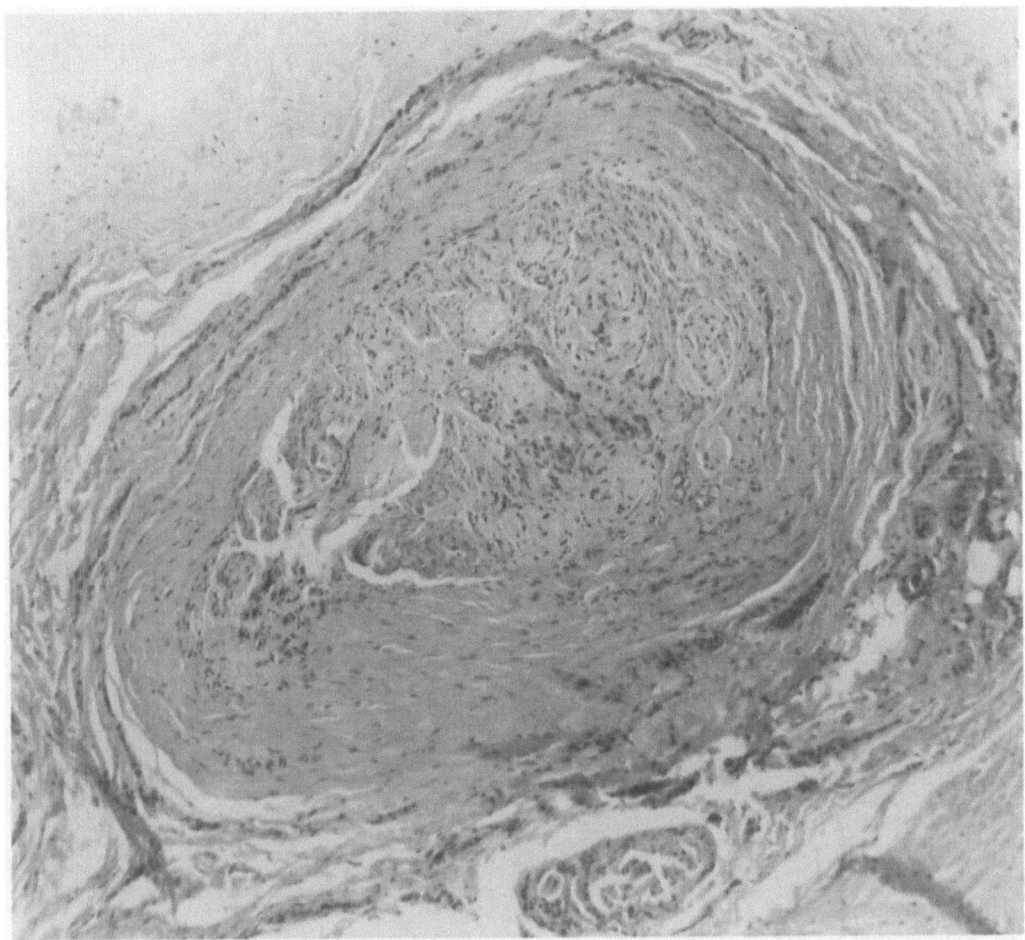

Fig. 7-43. Plantar (Morton's) neuroma. There is severe fibrosis of the perineurium and endoneurium in this nerve fascicle from the plantar digital nerve (×105).

hyalinized (Fig. 7-44). The perineurium is thickened and often merges imperceptibly with the greatly thickened and fibrotic epineurial tissues.

The surrounding epineurium and fibroadipose tissue range from a dense, hyalinized fibrous tissue to a loose, myxoid fibrous tissue. Foci of fibrinoid degeneration are common in the fibrous tissue, and rheumatoid nodules may be present if the patient has rheumatoid arthritis.[252] A large amount of epineurial inflammation is uncommon. Elastosis of the fibroadipose tissue may be prominent.[194] The intermetatarsal artery typically shows intimal fibrosis, which sometimes completely occludes the lumen. The wall of the intermetatarsal bursa may be thick, with focal areas of fibrinoid material on the synovial surface.

TRAUMATIC NEUROMA (TERMINAL BULB NEUROMA)

Complete division of a nerve trunk may be related to trauma or amputation. There is Wallerian degeneration in the distal segment of nerve trunk, and replacement of the myelinated fibers by Büngner bands. If the distal segment is not reinervated, the Büngner bands shrink progressively until they are only 2–3 μm in diameter.[231] Although

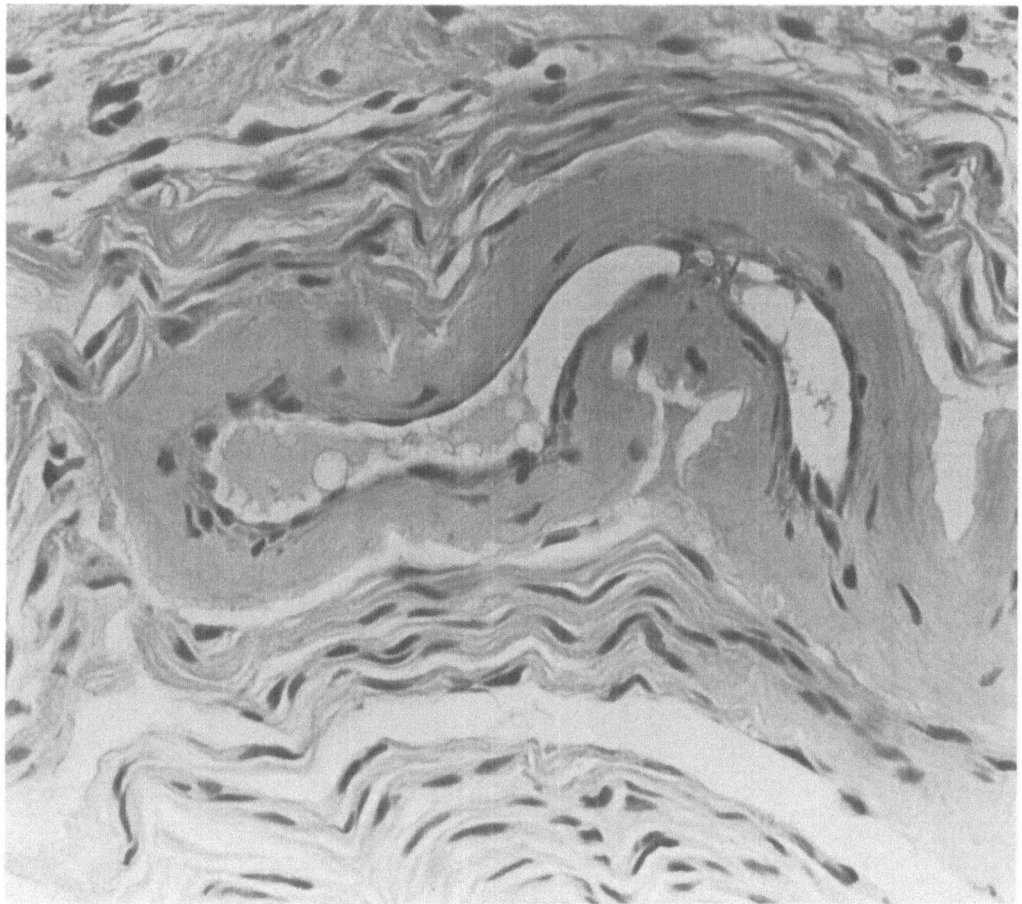

Fig. 7-44. Striking hyalinization of the walls of endoneurial blood vessels is a frequent finding in plantar neuromas (×500).

there is a concomitant increase in endoneurial fibrous tissue, the net effect is a progressive decrease in the total fascicular area of the distal segment (nerve trunk atrophy).

A fibrous scar invariably forms at the cut ends of the nerve trunk because of the hemorrhage, inflammation, and cellular reaction associated with severance of the nerve. This scar becomes an insurmountable obstacle for many of the regenerating axonal sprouts growing toward the Büngner bands of the distal segment. These sprouts arise from the terminal ends of the axons in the proximal segment and carry with them ensheathing Schwann cells. Passage to the distal segment is blocked, hence the regenerating axons grow haphazardly within the scar tissue to form a bulbous swelling known as a traumatic neuroma (Fig. 7-45) (amputation neuroma, true neuroma, terminal bulb neuroma).[221,231]

Histologically, a traumatic neuroma is composed of many small bundles of myelinated and unmyelinated axons traveling in various directions through a dense fibrous stroma (Fig. 7-46). Often, the nerve fibers are organized into miniature fascicles replete with a perineurium. Traumatic neuromas must be distinguished histologically from schwannomas, neurofibromas, cutaneous neuromas, and the mucosal neuromas found

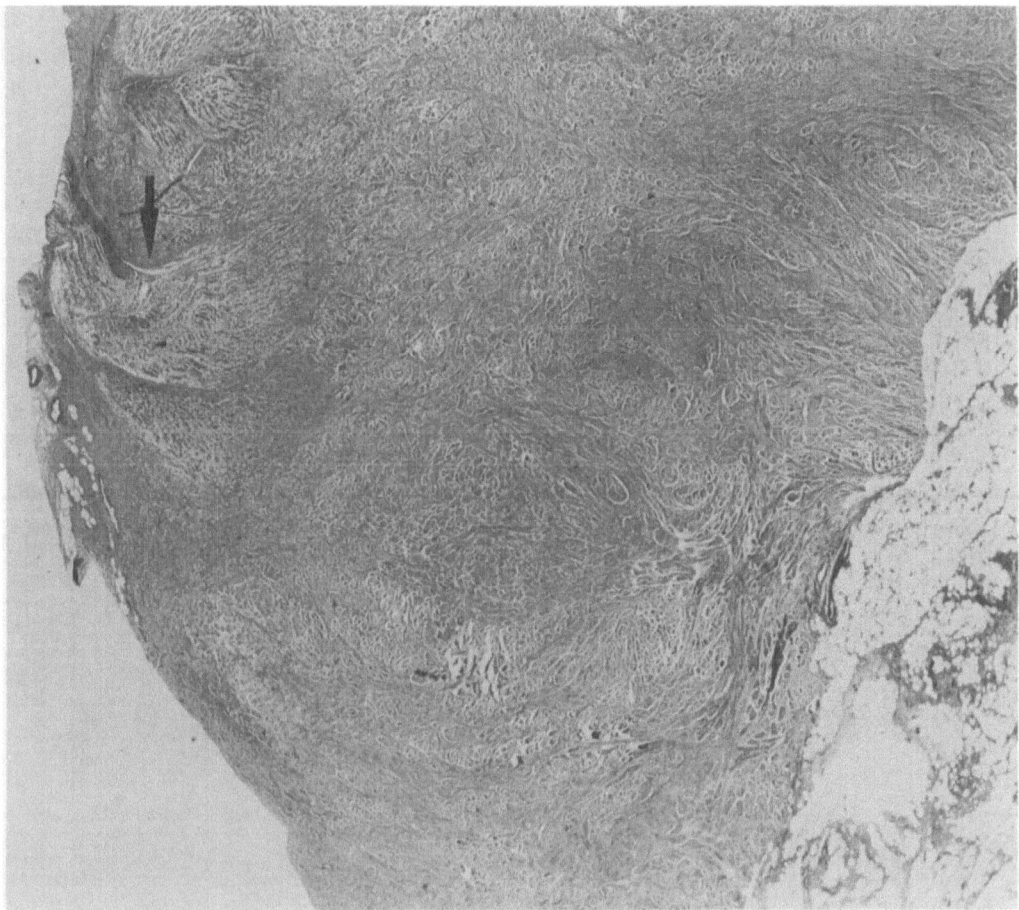

Fig. 7-45. Traumatic neuroma. A nerve fascicle (arrow) loses its identity in a disorganized mass of scar tissue and proliferating nerve fibers (×13).

in cases of the multiple mucosal neuroma syndrome. A silver impregnation for axons readily identifies the tangles of axons in the traumatic neuroma and excludes neurofibroma and schwannoma (Fig. 7-47). The location of the neuroma and the clinical history may be essential for distinguishing between a traumatic neuroma and a cutaneous or mucosal neuroma.[97,195,270]

Leprous Neuritis

Invasion of peripheral nerve by Mycobacterium leprae occurs in all cases of leprosy.[201] The changes in the peripheral nerve are variable and are greatly determined by the immunologic responsiveness of the patient. Recent reviews of leprosy include those of Dastur,[53] Sabin and Swift,[201] and Asbury and Johnson.[9]

In tuberculoid leprosy, the type of leprosy associated with a strong host response, the tissue reaction is identical to that of tuberculosis. The normal architecture of the nerve is destroyed by the granulomatous inflammatory reaction, which includes giant

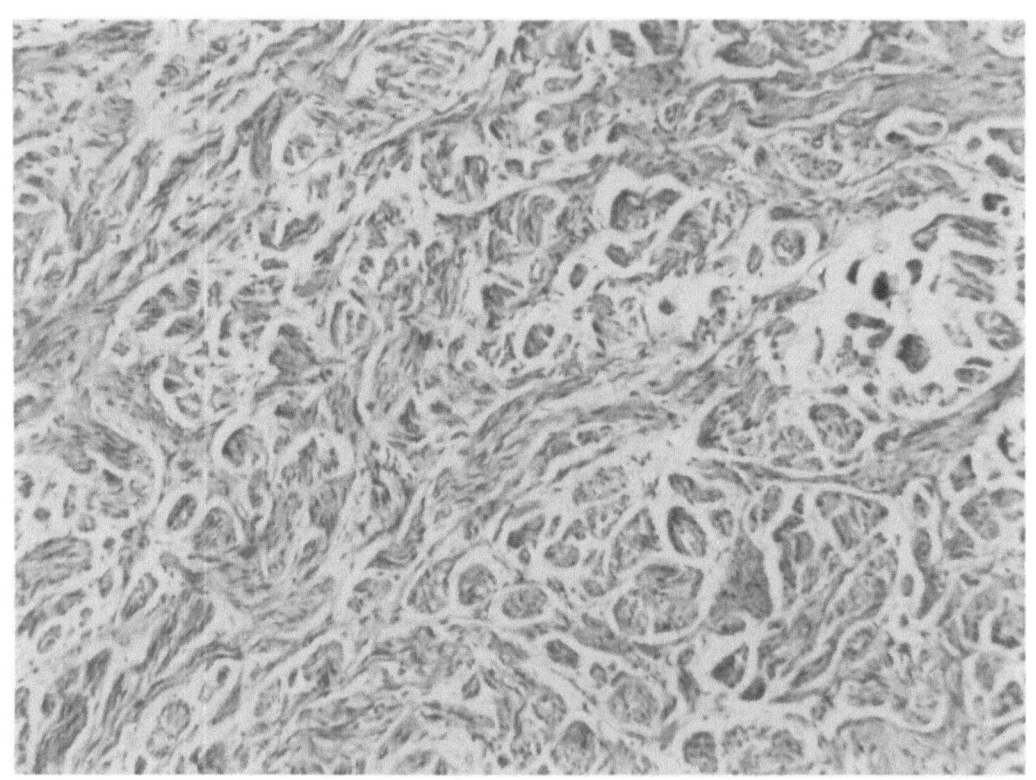

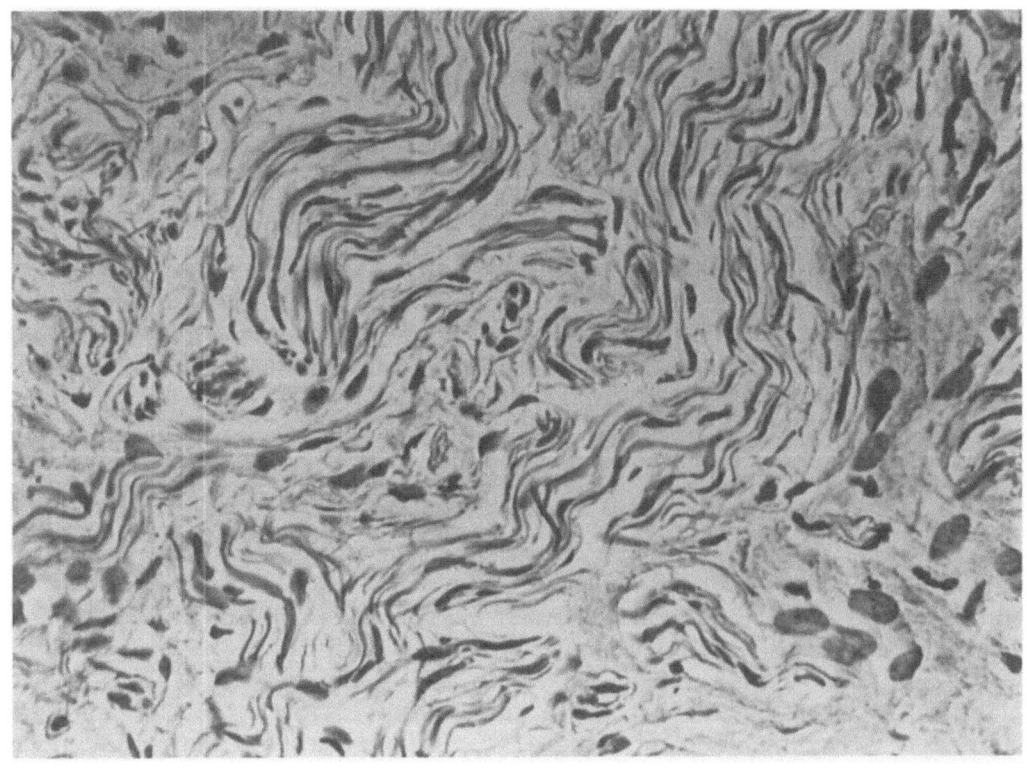

Fig. 7-46. Traumatic neuroma. Small fascicles of regenerating nerve fibers course haphazardly through collagenous stroma (×110).

Fig. 7-47. The presence of many thin, regenerating axons distinguishes this traumatic neuroma from a schwannoma or neurofibroma (Bodian, ×500).

cells, tubercles, and occasional caseous necrosis (Fig. 7-48). Accompanying the inflammatory reaction is a slight to complete loss of myelinated and unmyelinated fibers, endoneurial fibrosis, and disruption and fibrosis of the perineurium. Bacilli are rarely encountered either by light or electron microscopy.

Lepromatous leprosy, the type of leprosy associated with a minimal host response, is characterized by innumerable acid-fast bacilli within the affected nerves. Bacilli are found within Schwann cells, macrophages, endothelial cells, perineurial cells, and axons. Macrophages distended by phagocytosed bacilli are often termed foam cells, lepra cells, or Virchow cells (Fig. 7-49). Acid-fast masses of bacilli within macrophages are termed globi. Demyelination and axonal degeneration accompany the bacillosis of the nerve.[105,211] Endoneurial and perineurial fibrosis and scattered chronic inflammation

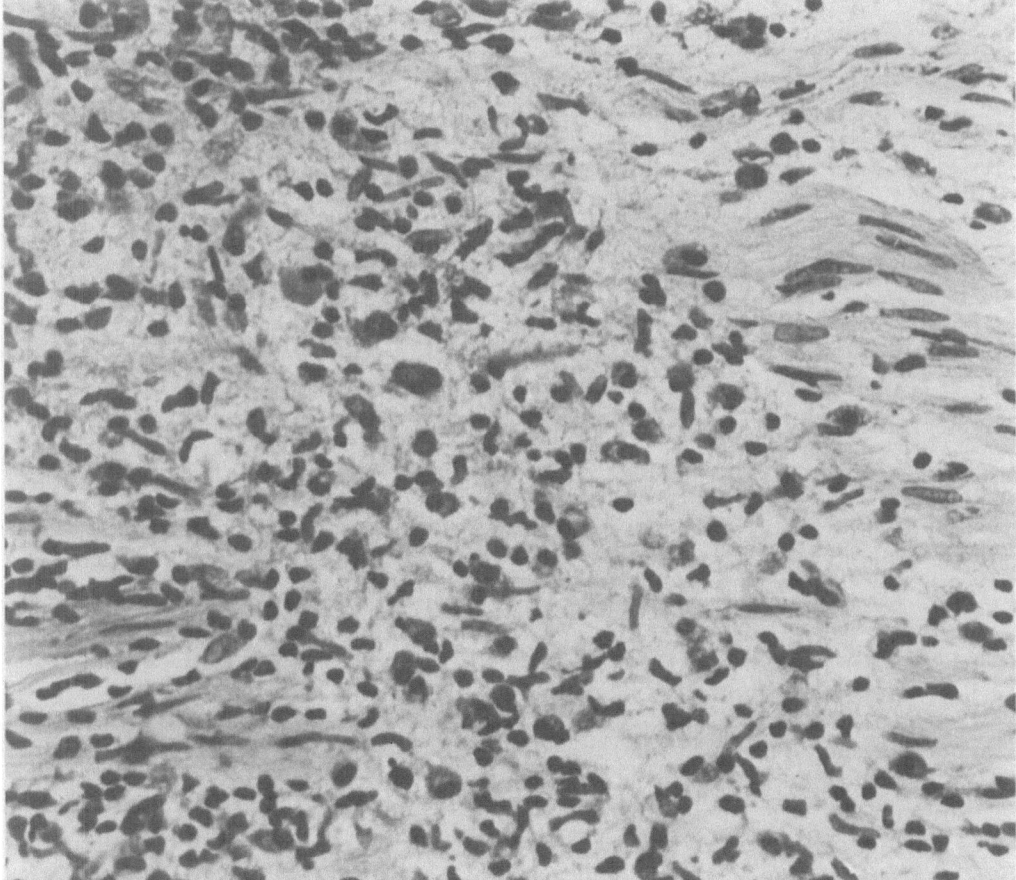

Fig. 7-48. Leprous neuritis. Granulomatous inflammation focally obliterates the normal endoneurial contents (Courtesy of Uriel Sandbank, M.D., Tel Aviv, Israel) (×500).

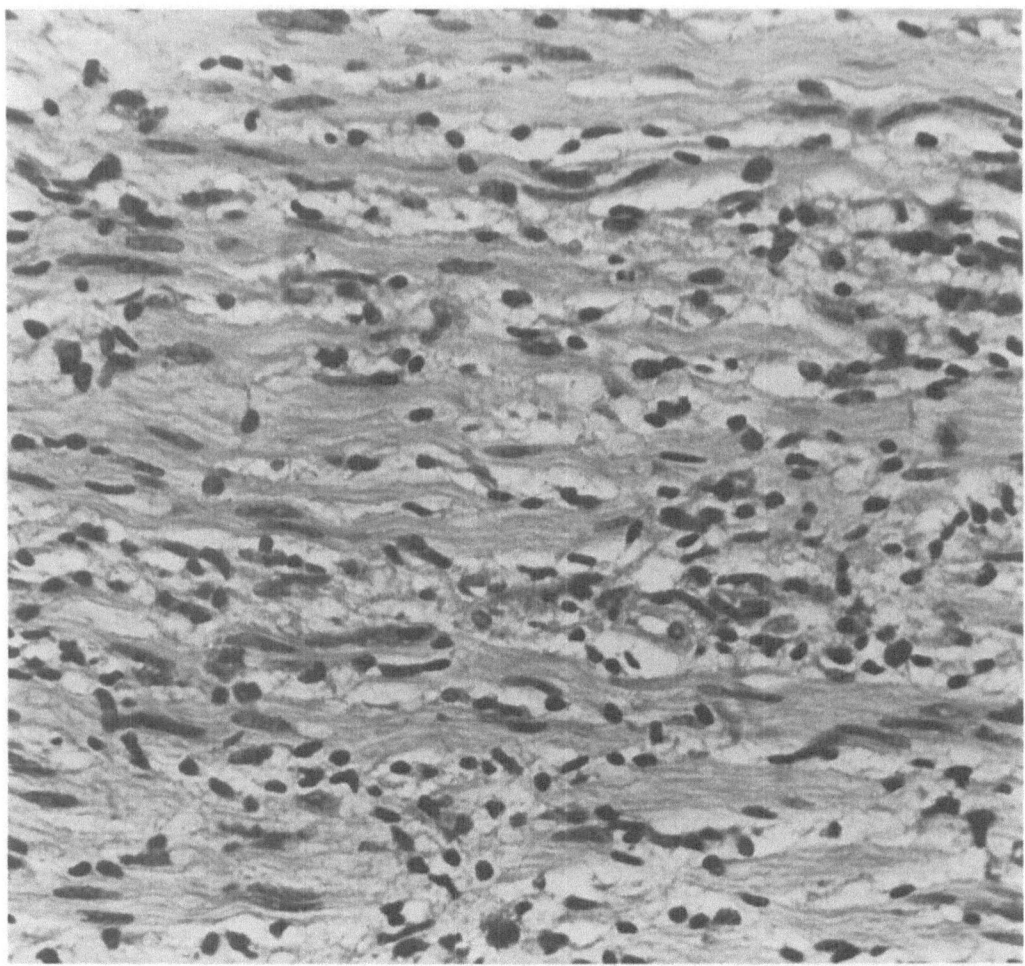

Fig. 7-49. Leprous neuritis. Numerous foam cells are present in the endoneurium (Courtesy of Uriel Sandbank, M.D., Tel Aviv, Israel.) (×500).

are found. A granulomatous neuritis with well-formed noncaseating granulomas may also be found in cases of sarcoidosis (Fig. 7-50).[81,258]

Miscellaneous Neuropathies

Peripheral neuropathy is becoming increasingly recognized in patients with human immunodeficiency virus infection.[46,51,181] The neuropathy may take a wide variety of clinico-pathologic types. Neuropathy is also found in Lyme disease.[77]

Structural changes in sural nerve may occur in instances of hypothyroidism,[156,162] acute infective hepatitis or cirrhosis,[41,44] primary biliary cirrhosis,[43,241] acute intermittent porphyria,[4] and acute panautonomic neuropathy.[132] A "xanthomatous neuropathy" characterized by subperineurial collections of foam cells occurs in a few patients with chronic liver disease.[140] Attention has recently been drawn to a "critical illness neuropa-

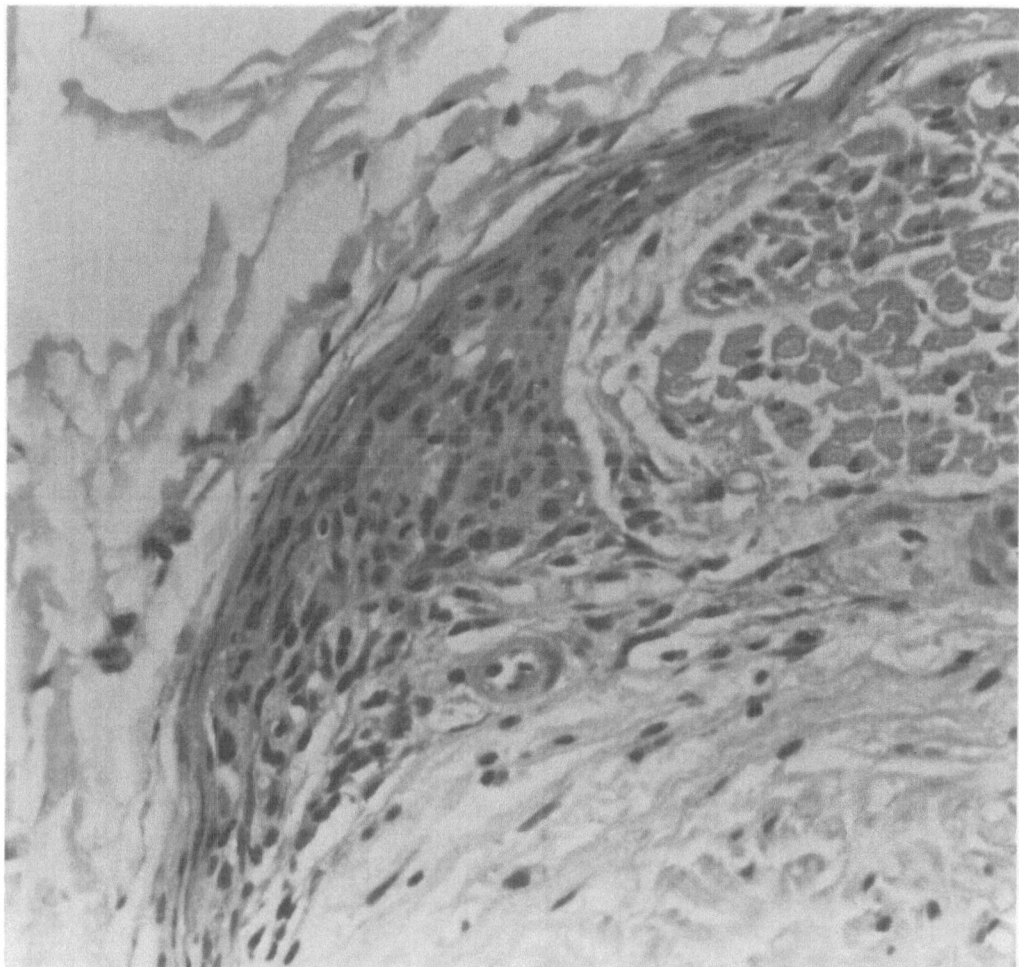

Fig. 7-50. Sarcoid neuropathy. In the center of the field is a small noncaseating granuloma within the perineurium. This sural nerve is from a patient with sarcoidosis and a mononeuropathy multiplex. Involvement of the endoneurium, epineurium, and epineurial arteries also occurs in sarcoid neuropathy (×500).

thy" complicating sepsis and multiple organ failure.[279] The neuropathy is characterized morphologically by axonal degeneration.

Tumors of the Nerve Sheath

Schwannoma (Neurilemmona, Neurinoma)

Schwannoma is a neoplasm arising from Schwann cells found on cranial nerves, spinal nerve roots, or peripheral nerves. Rare examples of intracerebral and intramedullary schwannomas have also been reported; the latter must be distinguished from intramedullary peripheral neuromas, which are perivascular traumatic neuromas associated with old destructive lesions in the spinal cord or brain stem.[2,82,232] Solitary or multiple

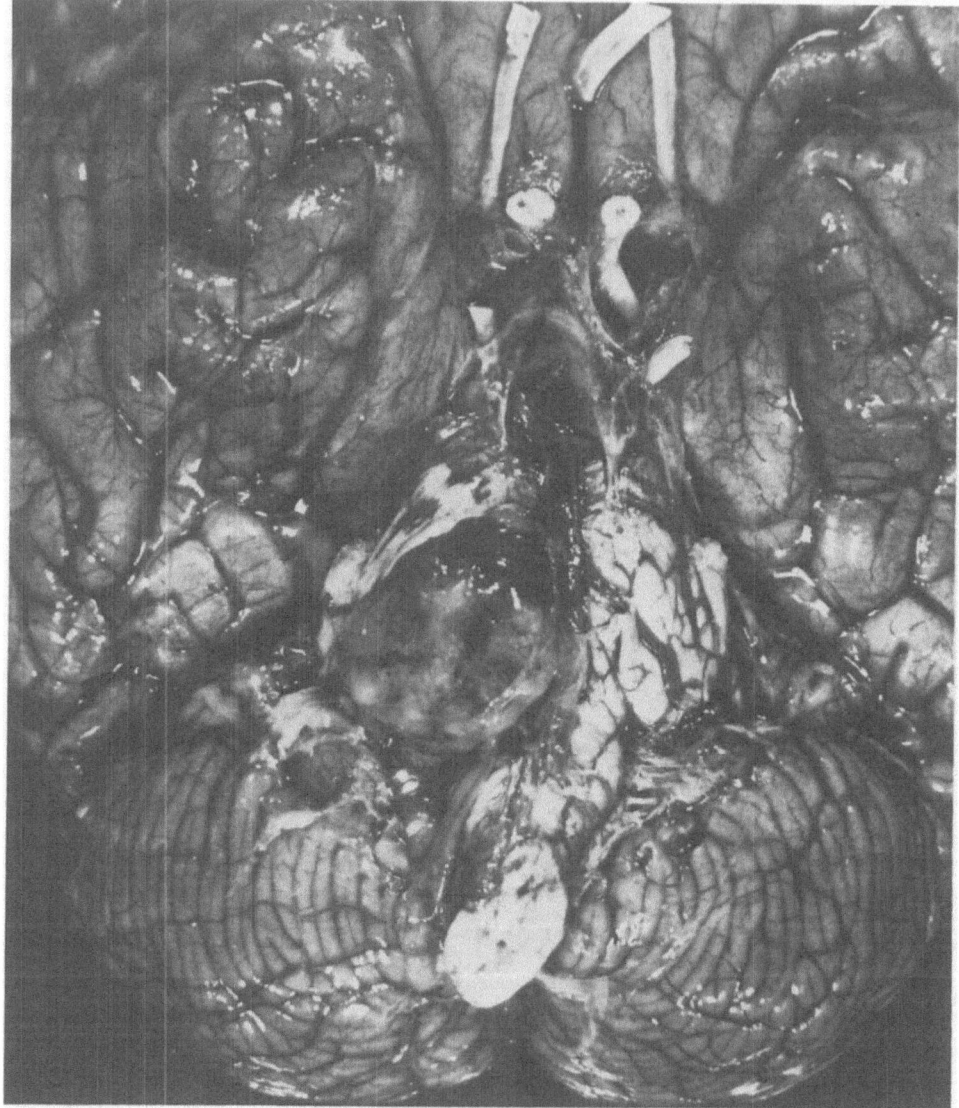

Fig. 7-51. Acoustic schwannoma. The oval, encapsulated neoplasm is in the right cerebellopontine angle.

schwannomas may be a manifestation of neurofibromatosis, but most solitary schwannomas are not associated with von Recklinghausen disease.

Intracranial schwannomas constitute about 8% of all intracranial tumors, one-third of all posterior fossa tumors, and 60% of all schwannomas.[270] Two-thirds of these tumors occur in patients older than 40 years; they are more common and tend to be of larger size in women than men.[113] Most intracranial schwannomas arise on the eighth cranial nerve (acoustic schwannoma, acoustic neuroma); they occasionally arise on the fifth cranial nerve or its ganglion, but rarely on other cranial nerves.[5,76] Schwannomas never occur on the first or second cranial nerves; these nerves are tracts of the CNS and do not contain Schwann cells.

Acoustic schwannomas arise between the glial-Schwann cell junction and the labyrinth; the neoplasm does not preferentially arise at the glial-Schwann cell junction.[229] For unknown reasons, the vestibular branch of the eighth nerve is more frequently the site of origin than the cochlear branch.[229] The Schwann-cell ensheathment of the eighth nerve does not commence until the nerve is either near the internal auditory meatus or within the internal auditory canal. Most schwannomas are, therefore, located at the meatus or within the canal.[30] The tumor grows slowly, and usually enlarges the meatus. Taking the course of least resistance, it grows medially into the cerebellopontine angle rather than laterally within the internal auditory canal (Fig. 7-51). The eighth cranial nerve is progressively compressed and destroyed by the tumor. As the tumor enlarges, it may also compress one or more of the adjacent cranial nerves (V, VII, IX, X, XI), the brain stem, and the cerebellum. The enlarging mass eventually leads to increased intracranial pressure, hydrocephalus, and cerebellar herniation. Tumors of this large size are encountered infrequently since the improvement of tests of auditory function. Currently, the brain stem auditory-evoked response (BAER) allows detection of tumors still in the internal auditory meatus.[96] The presence of bilateral acoustic schwannomas and cafe-au-lait spots is diagnostic of acoustic neurofibromatosis, an entity distinct from peripheral (typical) neurofibromatosis.[146,196] Unilateral acoustic schwannomas may occur in cases of peripheral neurofibromatosis.

Intraspinal schwannomas are intradural, extramedullary tumors usually arising from the posterior (sensory) spinal roots (Fig. 7-52). They occur mainly in adults and eventually grow in size to compress the cord. In some instances, the neoplasm may extend through the intervertebral foramen to form a dumbbell-shaped (hourglass) tumor.

Peripheral schwannomas may arise on any peripheral nerve. They are found at all ages, and there is no sex predilection.[200] Most commonly, the tumors arise in the large nerves of the extremities, in the posterior mediastinum, or in the retroperitoneum. Intradermal schwannomas are rare.[95]

Grossly, schwannomas are oval, discrete, encapsulated tumors ranging in diameter from a few millimeters to several centimeters. Very rarely, peripheral schwannomas may have a plexiform or multinodular growth pattern.[103] The nerve of origin can often be identified in the capsule of the neoplasm. The cut surfaces are usually firm, rubbery, white to gray, and whorled. Foci of necrosis, recent or old hemorrhage, and xanthomatous or cystic degeneration may be present, especially in the larger tumors.

Characteristically, schwannoma has a biphasic histologic pattern (Fig. 7-53). One pattern, designated type A by Antoni, is produced by interwoven fascicles of elongated cells with indistinct cytoplasmic borders, acidophilic cytoplasm, and spindle-shaped nuclei (Fig. 7-54). The stroma is acidophilic and finely fibrillar. In some tumors, the spindle-shaped nuclei focally palisade to form structures termed Verocay bodies (Fig. 7-55). Occasionally, the spindle cells form whorls resembling those found in meningiomas, or isolated, wavy fascicles similar to those occurring in neurofibromas.

The second pattern, designated type B, is characterized by an edematous stroma and numerous microcysts (Fig. 7-56). Within the loose stroma are cells with indistinct cytoplasm and oval, often pyknotic nuclei.

Degenerative changes are common in schwannomas and include foci of foam cells, recent hemorrhage, collections of siderophages, cysts, focal necrosis, lymphocytic or plasmacytic infiltrates, zones of dense fibrosis, and hyalinized blood vessels (Figs. 7-53 and 7-57). Calcification is infrequent, and psammoma bodies are also rare. Metaplastic foci of bone and cartilage are occasionally present. Rarely, focal glandular differentiation or melanin pigment produced by the neoplastic Schwann cells is found.[139,275]

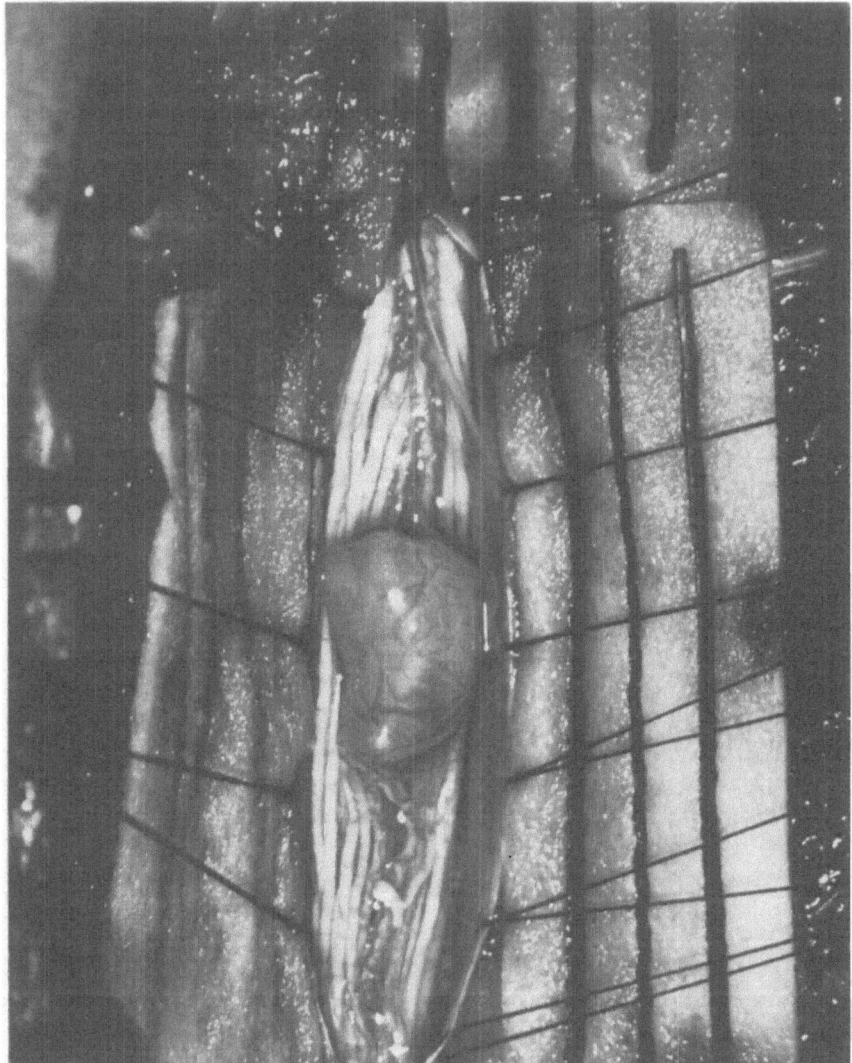

Fig. 7-52. Intraspinal schwannoma arising from a nerve root of the cauda equina. (Courtesy of Hernando Mena, M.D., Washington, D.C.).

Hyalinization of blood vessel walls is common in schwannomas, but other vascular changes may also be observed. Sometimes, especially in the larger tumors, there are large foci of closely packed vascular channels that give the impression of a capillary or cavernous angioma.[88] Kasantikul et al[113] found such angiomas in 14 of 103 acoustic schwannomas. Fibrinoid necrosis of blood vessels or thrombosis may also be present.

Pleomorphism and hyperchromatism of nuclei are common in schwannomas, as are foci of hypercellularity (Fig. 7-56). These features are not indicative of malignancy. Tumors showing such changes are sometimes referred to as "cellular" or "ancient" schwannomas.[50] Mitotic figures, however, are uncommon in schwannomas, and their presence should raise the question of malignancy.

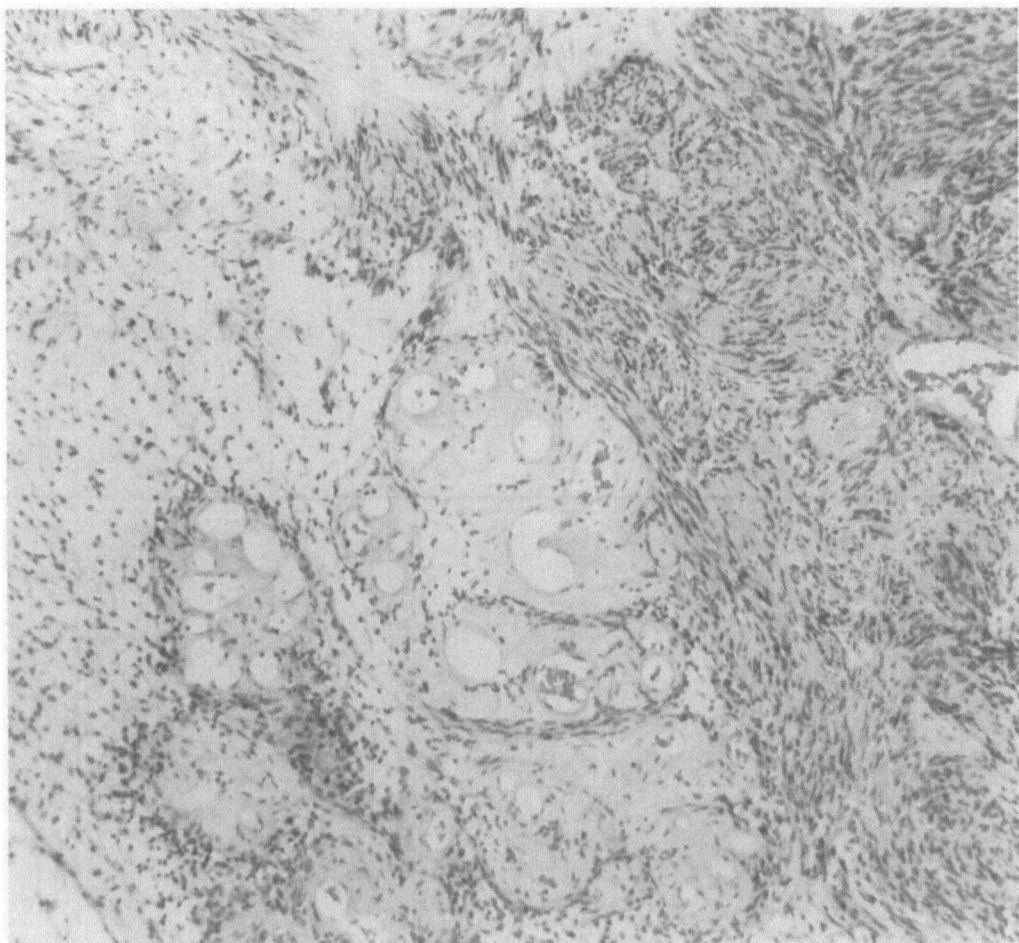

Fig. 7-53. Acoustic schwannoma. There is sharp demarcation between the compact Antoni A tissue in the right half of the field and the loose Antoni B tissue on the left. Clusters of abnormal vascular channels lie near the center of the field (×110).

Specially stained sections from schwannomas show a variable amount of stromal collagen, but reticulin fibers are abundant, separating individual cells and running parallel to the long axis of the cell (Fig. 7-58). Reticulin fibers are most easily found in the Antoni A tissue and only variably in the Antoni B tissue. Axons are rarely found in schwannomas. Immunoreactive S-100 protein, Leu-7 antigen, and vimentin can be demonstrated in most schwannomas.[87,109,115,269] Occasional schwannomas contain cells immunostaining for glial fibrillary acidic protein (GFAP).

By electron microscopy, the neoplastic Schwann cell has a distinct basal lamina, long but thin cell processes, scattered intracytoplasmic filaments, occasional profiles of rough endoplastic reticulum, mitochondria, Golgi complexes, and rare intercellular junctions.[74,213] Intercellular bundles of fibrous long-spacing collagen (Luse bodies) are characteristic, but not specific for schwannoma. In the Antoni A areas, the attenuated Schwann-cell processes interdigitate and occasionally form mesaxon-like structures that wrap around other Schwann-cell processes. In the Antoni B areas, the intercellular

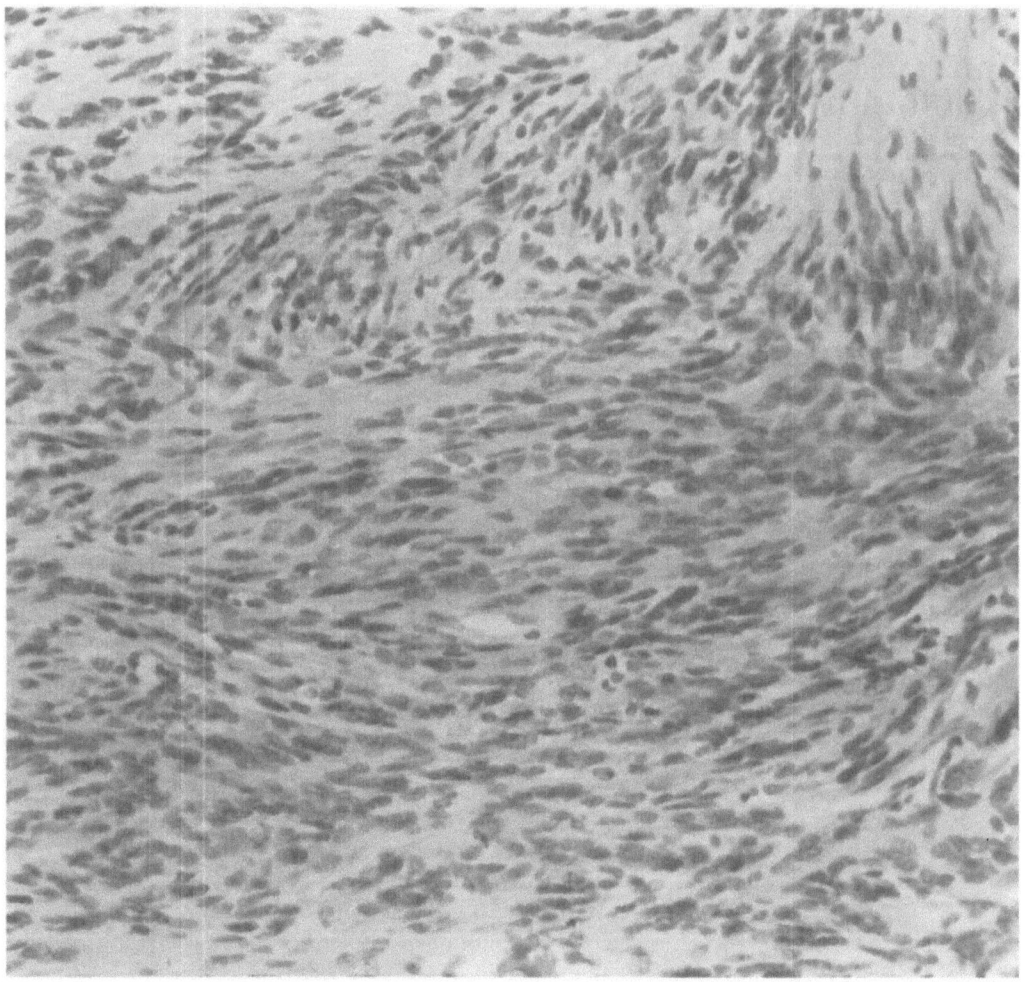

Fig. 7-54. Antoni A pattern within a schwannoma (×290).

space increases; the neoplastic Schwann cells frequently contain cytoplasmic polymorph-ous dense bodies, which have been interpreted as a consequence of degenerative changes.[213]

The differential diagnosis of a cerebellopontine angle tumor includes schwannoma, meningioma, and astrocytoma. A pilocytic astrocytoma from the cerebellum or a fibrillary astrocytoma from the brain stem may grow into the cerebellopontine angle and mimic a schwannoma. A reticulin impregnation adapted for frozen sections quickly differenti-ates between a schwannoma, in which individual cells are outlined by reticulin fibers, and a glioma, with only blood vessels outlined by reticulin fibers.[120] Furthermore, astrocytomas typically immunostain diffusely for GFAP, whereas only occasional schwannomas contain immunoreactive GFAP.[87,109,115]

Fibroblastic meningioma may also be confused with an intracranial or intraspinal schwannoma, but the presence of numerous psammoma bodies, cellular whorls, and interspersed areas of transitional meningioma help to identify the meningioma. Immu-

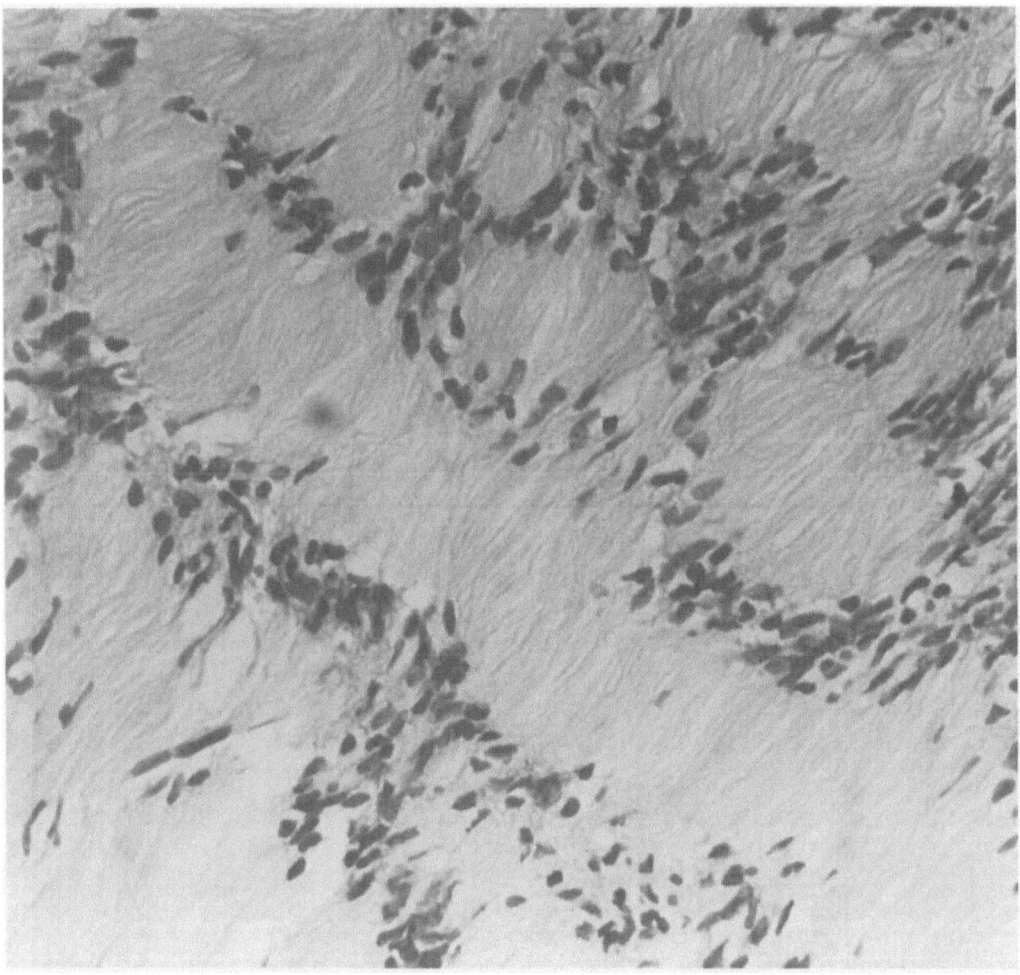

Fig. 7-55. Prominent nuclear palisading in Antoni A tissue of a schwannoma leads to the formation of Verocay bodies (×500).

nostaining for Leu-7 antigen may also be very helpful, since most schwannomas, but only exceptional meningiomas, are positive for Leu-7.[34,182]

Peripheral schwannoma must be distinguished from leiomyoma, well-differentiated leiomyosarcoma and neurofibroma. The smooth muscle tumors are distinguished by PTAH-positive fuchsinophilic intracytoplasmic filaments and no immunoreactivity for S-100 protein or Leu-7 antigen.[182,269] Neurofibroma lacks demarcation into Antoni A and B patterns, is not encapsulated, and contains occasional axons.

Malignant transformation of an intracranial or intraspinal schwannoma has not been documented. Malignant degeneration of a peripheral schwannoma has been reported,[247] but is so rare that several authors have questioned its occurrence.[270,276] The malignant schwannoma (neurofibrosarcoma, malignant peripheral nerve sheath tumor) arises either de novo or from malignant degeneration of a neurofibroma and is discussed later (page 187).

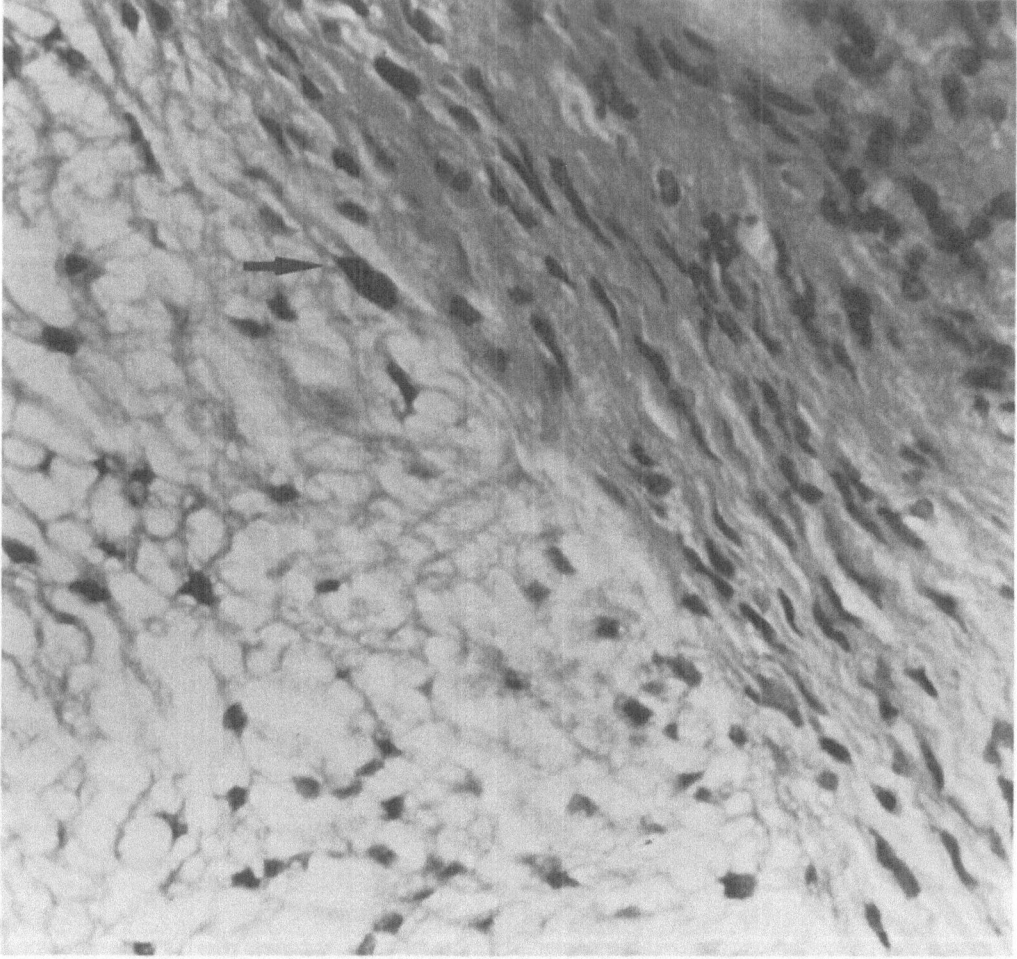

Fig. 7-56. The Antoni B tissue in the left half of the field has a loose edematous stroma. Note the enlarged, hyperchromatic nucleus (arrow) at the border between Antoni A and B areas (×540).

Neurofibroma

Because of some overlap in histologic features and a common cell of origin, some authors have suggested that solitary schwannomas and solitary neurofibromas should be considered as the same clinical entity.[52] Most pathologists think that the close association between neurofibroma and neurofibromatosis, the potential of neurofibroma for malignant degeneration, and distinguishing gross and microscopic features make it both desirable and feasible to distinguish between neurofibroma and schwannoma.[73]

Neurofibromas may be single or multiple and are usually associated with neurofibromatosis. A single, isolated neurofibroma, unaccompanied by other stigmata of neurofibromatosis, however, may occur and is termed a solitary neurofibroma.[95] Neurofibromas may be associated with neurofibromatosis, and perhaps the solitary neurofibroma could be viewed as a forme fruste of the phakomatosis. Such a generalization cannot be

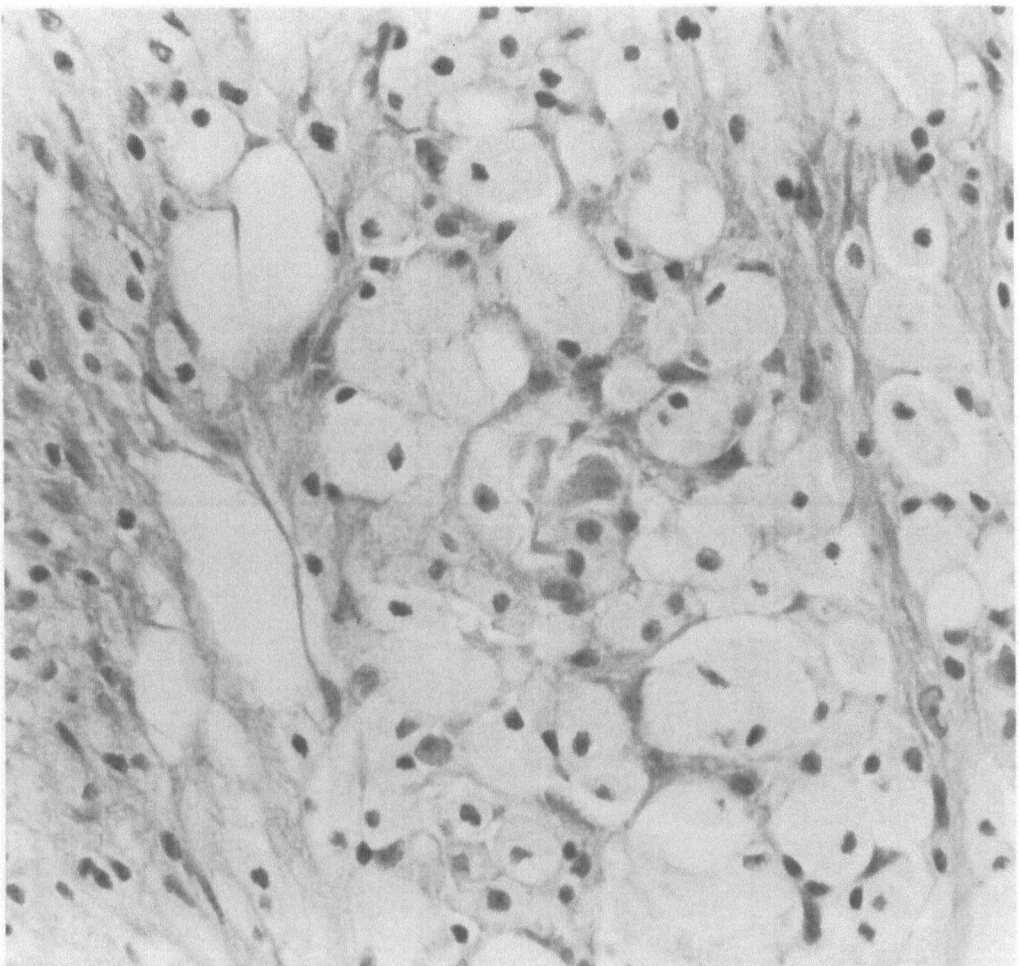

Fig. 7-57. Focal collections of foam cells are one of several degenerative changes frequently found in schwannomas (×500).

made, however, until a sensitive and specific marker for this autosomal-dominant disease is discovered.

Neurofibromas may occur on any peripheral nerve. Deep neurofibromas most commonly arise in the major nerve plexuses, major nerve trunks, retroperitoneum, and gastrointestinal tract.[270] Deep neurofibromas may also involve cranial nerves or spinal nerve roots.[200,270] "Cutaneous" neurofibromas arise from terminal nerve twigs in the dermis.

On larger nerves, the deep neurofibroma forms a fusiform enlargement of the nerve. The tumor is neither encapsulated nor well circumscribed. The fascicular organization of the involved segment of nerve is not only frequently maintained, but the usually small individual fascicles may become so enlarged by the intrafascicular growth of the neoplasm that they appear as the cords of a nerve plexus (plexiform neurofibroma). The cut surfaces of the tumor are soft and light gray, and lack the whorling pattern, cystic degeneration, and hemorrhage so common in large schwannomas.

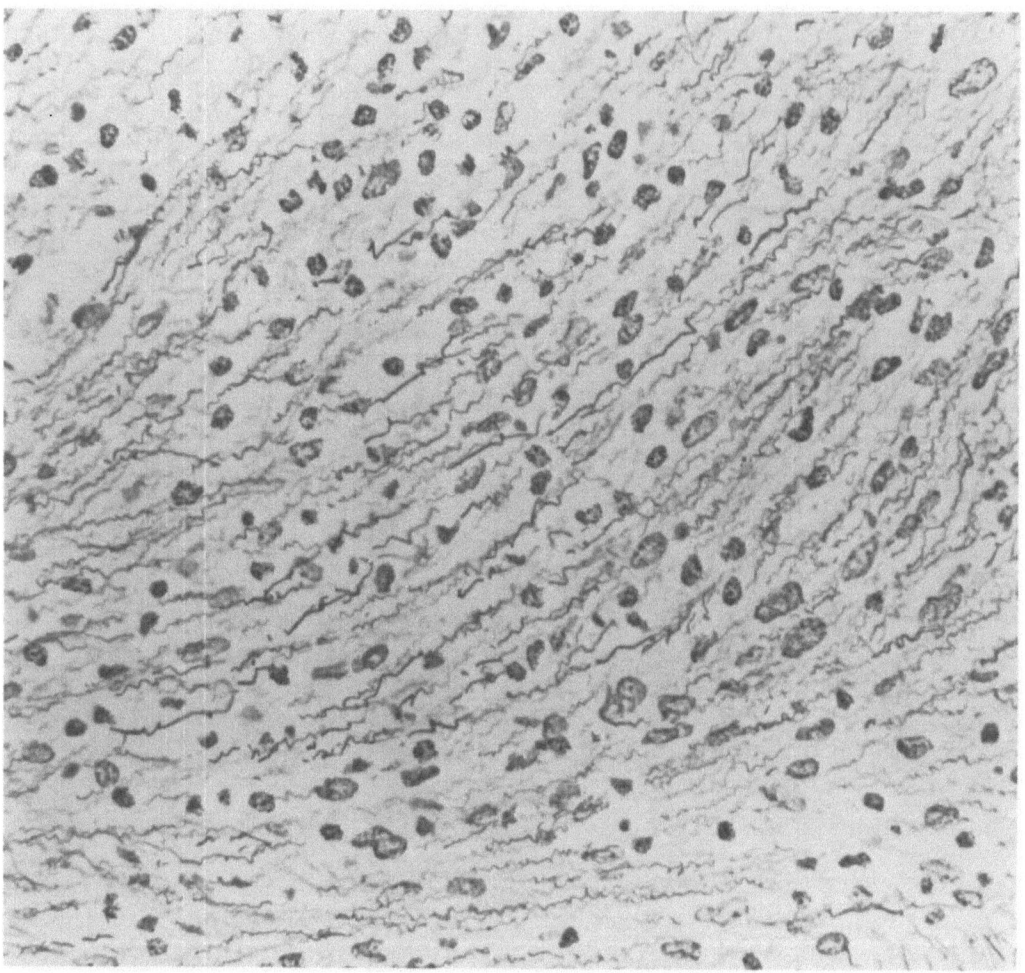

Fig. 7-58. Thick wavy reticulin fibers lie between individual cells in the Antoni A area from a schwannoma (Reticulin impregnation, ×500).

Microscopically, plexiform and other deep neurofibromas are hypocellular to moderately cellular spindle-cell neoplasms (Figs. 7-59, 7-60). The cells have spindle-shaped nuclei and inconspicuous cytoplasm. They are set in an extensive extracellular myxoid matrix, which typically contains numerous mast cells. The spindle-shaped cells frequently associate with bundles of collagen to form long, wavy strands giving the neoplasm a "neural" appearance. Nuclear palisading is uncommon, but structures resembling tactile corpuscles[218,265] or a focus of schwannoma may occasionally be found.[200] If the neurofibroma is of the plexiform type with a prominent intrafascicular pattern of growth, the residual nerve fibers within the involved fascicles are often characteristically grouped near the centers of the grotesquely expanded fascicles (Fig. 7-61).

Plexiform neurofibromas and most deep nonplexiform neurofibromas are a manifestation of neurofibromatosis.[94] The plexiform neurofibroma frequently involves long segments of nerve; the intrafascicular neoplasm may even extend centripetally along the nerve to the spinal cord.[94] There is a small, but real, risk that plexiform and other

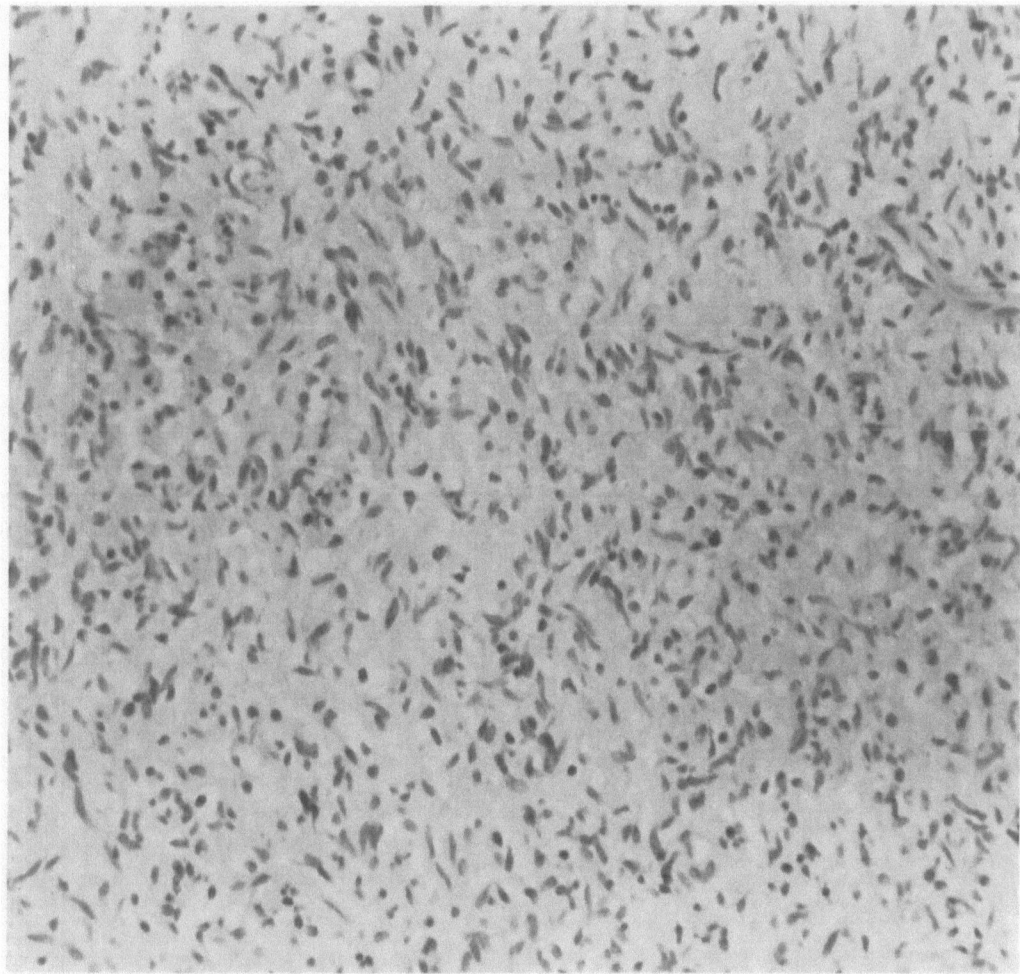

Fig. 7-59. A patternless proliferation of cells with spindle-shaped nuclei characterizes the neurofibroma. In other areas, this tumor had an intrafascicular growth pattern typical of a plexiform neurofibroma (×590).

deep neurofibromas may undergo malignant degeneration to a neurofibrosarcoma (malignant schwannoma).

The cutaneous neurofibroma is typically soft, nodular, and may be pedunculated. The tumor originates from terminal nerve twigs in the dermis. It is well circumscribed, but not encapsulated; the cut surfaces are homogeneous and light gray. Microscopically, the dermal neoplasm is characterized by an extrafascicular (nonplexiform) proliferation of cells with spindle-shaped nuclei in a collagenous stroma (Fig. 7-62). The cells may be arranged haphazardly or in small wavy cords. As in the plexiform neurofibroma, nuclear palisading is uncommon, but structures resembling tactile corpuscles may be found.[218] The stroma focally may have a myxoid appearance and stain positively with Alcian blue. Mast cells are usually scattered throughout the neoplasm. Although the terminal nerve twig from which the dermal neurofibroma originates is usually not identified, special stains frequently reveal occasional axons within the tumor. The overly-

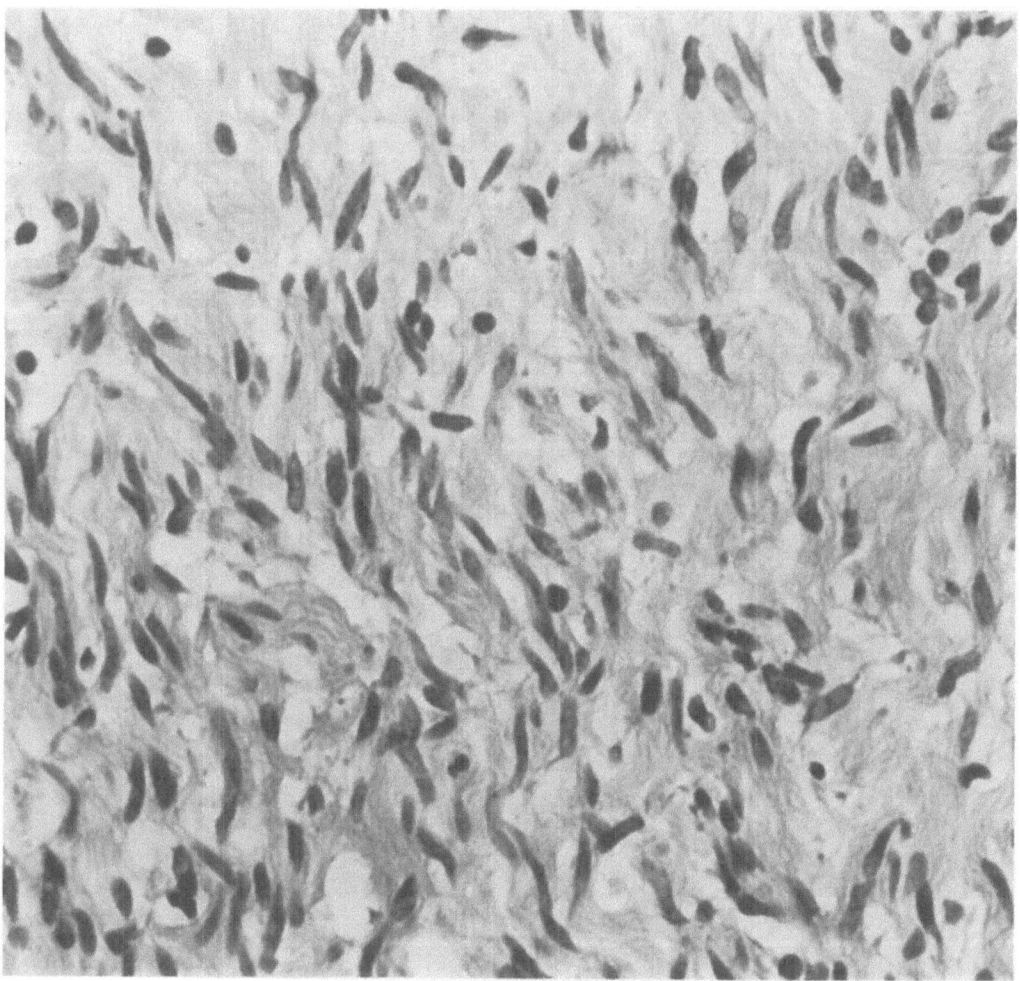

Fig. 7-60. Plexiform neurofibroma. The spindle-shaped nuclei are characteristically wavy and hyperchromatic (×590).

ing epidermis may be thin, but is otherwise unremarkable. The cutaneous neurofibroma must be distinguished from a dermal leiomyoma, a dermatofibroma, and a neural nevus.

Cutaneous neurofibromas may be solitary or multiple. The presence of multiple cutaneous neurofibromas is considered a defining characteristic of peripheral neurofibromatosis.[196] Cutaneous (nonplexiform) neurofibromas, whether solitary or as a manifestation of neurofibromatosis, do not undergo malignant degeneration.[94] Cutaneous neurofibromas should be distinguished from plexiform neurofibromas involving the subcutis and overlying dermis. The latter almost always indicate neurofibromatosis and may undergo malignant degeneration.

Electron microscopy reveals that the major differences between schwannoma and neurofibroma are the greater amount of extracellular collagen and the presence of myelinated and unmyelinated axons in neurofibroma.[213] The neoplastic cells may occasionally form large onion-bulb formations.[9] Most authors consider that the Schwann cell is the principal cell of origin of both schwannoma and neurofibroma; the presence of

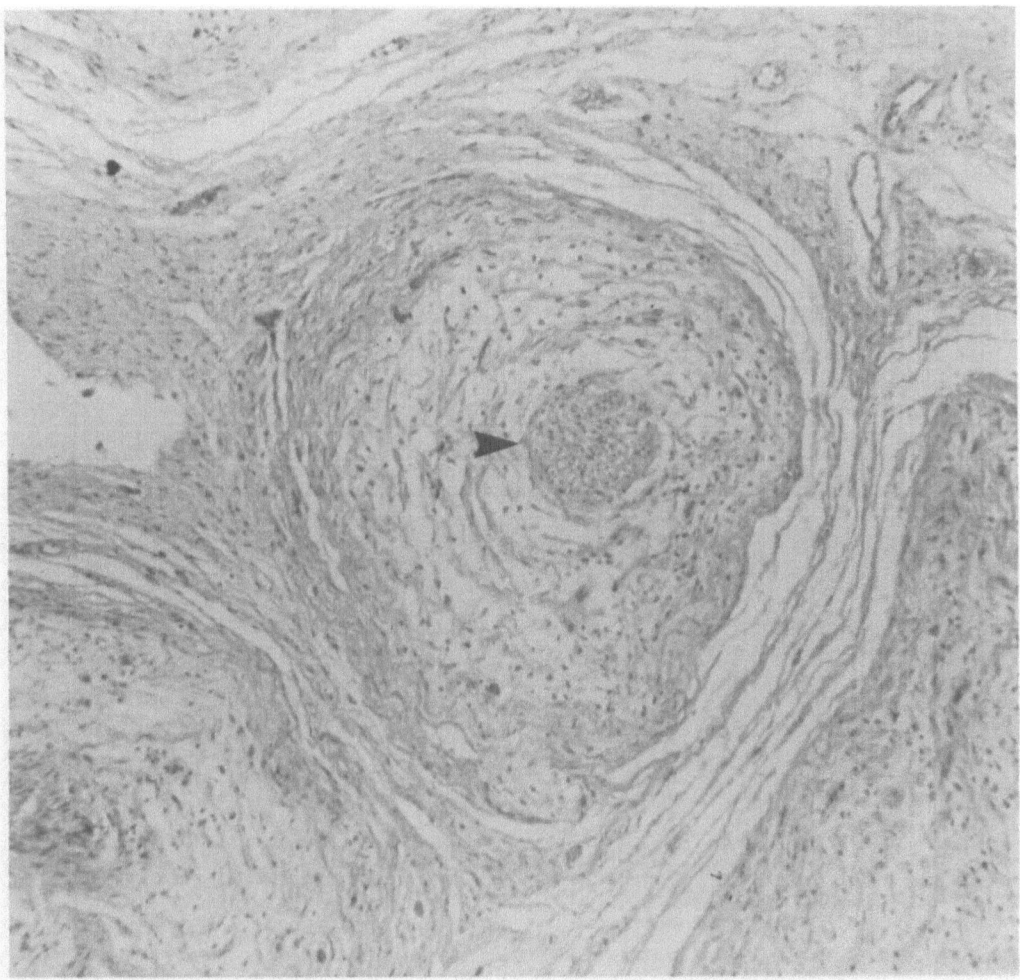

Fig. 7-61. Plexiform neurofibroma. The nerve fascicle in the center of the field is greatly expanded by proliferation of spindle cells in a loose stroma. A group of residual nerve fibers (arrow) is near the center of the distorted fascicle (×115).

immunoreactive S-100 protein in cutaneous and plexiform neurofibromas and schwannomas supports this view.[226] Ultrastructural studies suggest that the perineurial cell and fibroblast also participate in neurofibroma.[74,133]

Malignant Schwannoma

Malignant schwannoma (malignant peripheral nerve sheath tumor, neurofibrosarcoma) is a malignant spindle-cell neoplasm arising in peripheral nerve.[59] The tumor is rare, comprising only 5% of soft tissue sarcomas.[230] The neoplasm may arise de novo or from malignant degeneration of a neurofibroma; it never arises from malignant degeneration of an intracranial schwannoma and only rarely originates from a peripheral schwannoma.[74,247] The tumor occurs in all age groups, but mainly in adults; there is

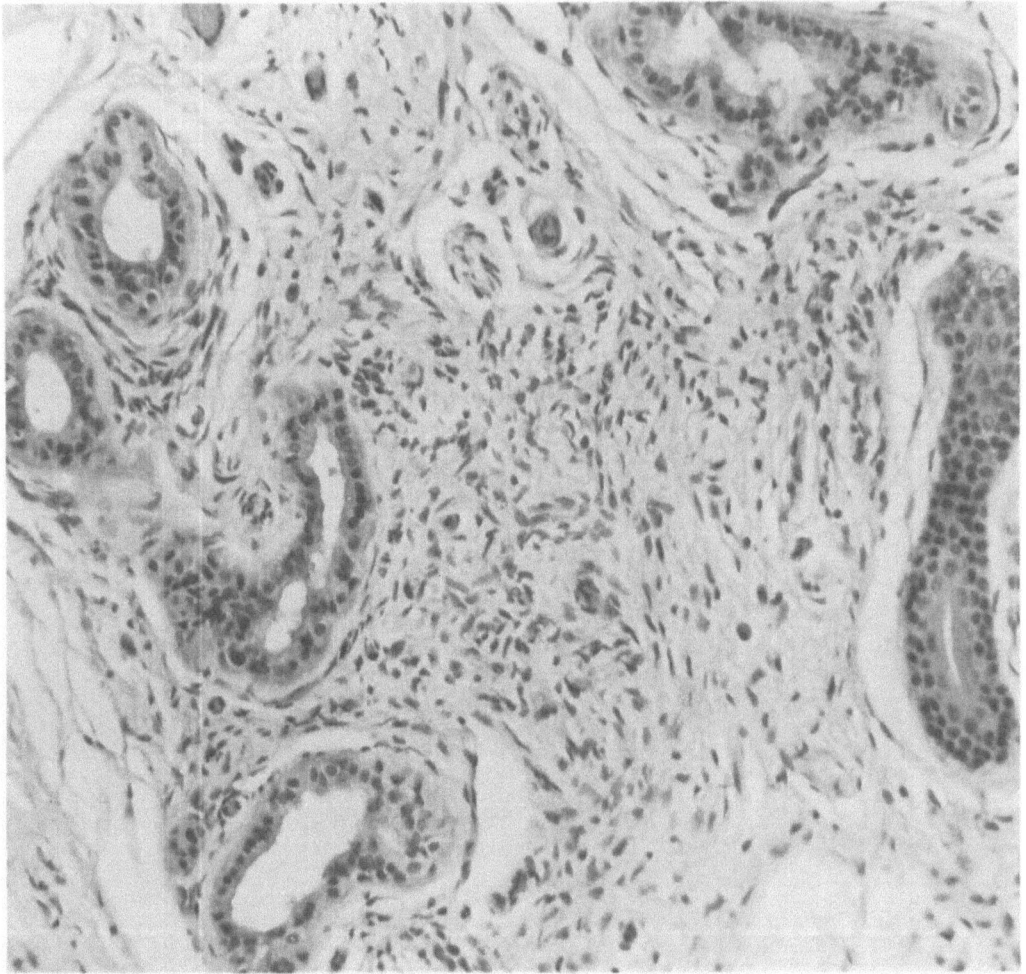

Fig. 7-62. Cutaneous neurofibroma involving sweat gland. Cutaneous neurofibromas are unencapsulated and may infiltrate adjacent tissues (×250).

no sex predilection.[83] Of the 165 cases of malignant schwannoma reviewed by Sordillo et al,[220] 40% of the patients had neurofibromatosis. The five-year survival rate was 23% for malignant schwannomas arising in patients with neurofibromatosis, and 47 percent for malignant schwanommas without neurofibromatosis. The clinical course is generally one of multiple local recurrences and often blood-borne metastases. Malignant schwannoma may arise in an area of previous irradiation, both in patients with or without neurofibromatosis.[58,80,220]

Malignant schwannomas occur in many locations, including the soft tissues of the head and neck, chest wall, retroperitoneum, large nerves of the extremities, cranial nerves, and spinal nerve roots.[48,49,59,89,128,197,220] The neoplasms range from a few centimeters to many centimeters in diameter. If the nerve of origin is seen, the tumor is often a fusiform, but unencapsulated enlargement. Occasionally, the neoplasm may extend for a considerable length within the nerve. The cut surfaces of the neoplasm are soft to firm and white to tan; foci of hemorrhage and necrosis are common.

Microscopically, the malignant schwannoma is a cellular spindle-cell tumor closely resembling a fibrosarcoma (Figs. 7-63 and 7-64). The spindle cells often form tight, interwoven fascicles. However, myxoid, hypocellular areas, rich in hyaluronidase-sensitive acid mucopolysaccharides, are also common and may predominate in some tumors (Fig. 7-65).[89] Other characteristic features are dilated, thin-walled blood vessels and perivascular cuffs of neoplastic cells.[89] Differentiation of the neoplastic cells to malignant osteoid, malignant cartilage, angiosarcoma, rhabdomyosarcoma (malignant triton tumor), mucin-producing glands or squamous epithelium may be observed.[31,59,89,251,275] Structures resembling tactile corpuscles may also be present.[95] Specially stained sections reveal a variable amount of collagen, but usually an abundance of reticulin fibers, which often outline individual neoplastic cells. The tumor is not encapsulated and infiltrates surrounding tissues. Because the neoplasm may infiltrate longitudinally within the nerve of origin, a frozen-section, intraoperative microscopic examination of the proximal end of the resected nerve has been advocated.[48]

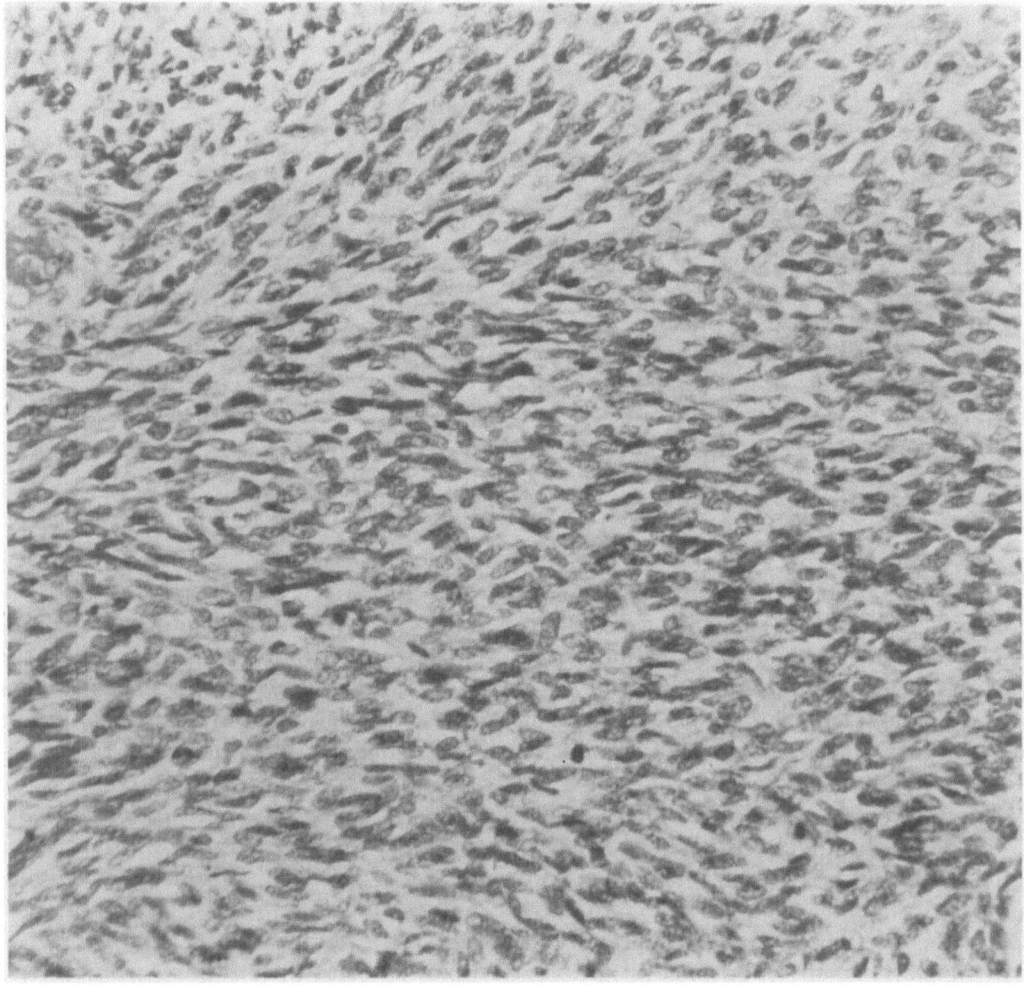

Fig. 7-63. This field from a malignant schwannoma has the nonspecific appearance of a spindle-cell sarcoma (×300).

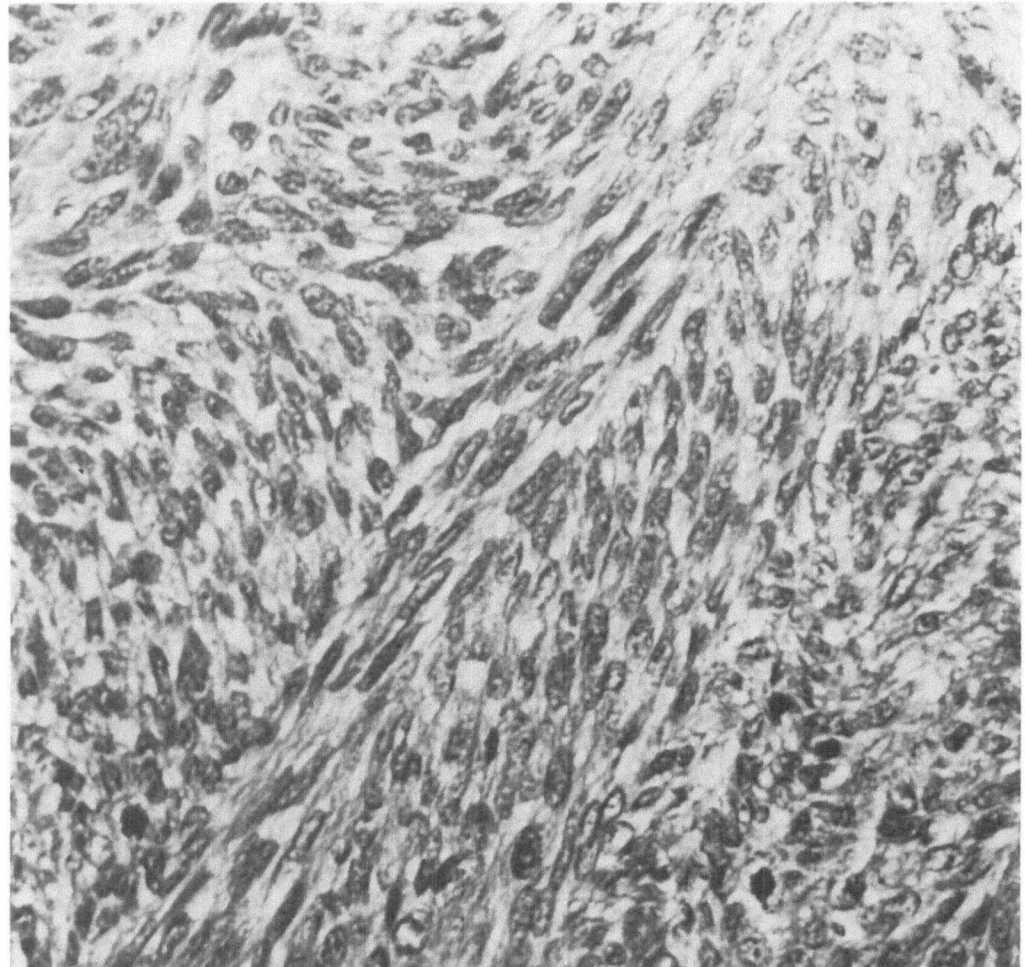

Fig. 7-64. Malignant schwannoma. Intersecting fascicles give the tumor a "herringbone" pattern (×550).

Severe, diffuse cellular polymorphism is uncommon in malignant schwannoma, but foci of highly polymorphic cells or tumor giant cells are occasionally found. Mitotic figures are invariably present. Hemorrhage and necrosis are common, and the neoplastic cells may palisade around the areas of necrosis.[95] If the malignant schwannoma arises from a neurofibroma, there may be areas of increased cellularity within the neurofibroma that suggest a transition from neurofibroma to malignant schwannoma.

As noted, malignant schwannoma may arise from the malignant degeneration of a neurofibroma. Of Guccion and Enzinger's[89] 46 cases of malignant schwannoma arising in patients with neurofibromatosis, 31 cases were associated with a neurofibroma. One must be careful, however, not to misinterpret the occasional presence of enlarged, hyperchromic nuclei, which are frequently found in neurofibromas and schwannomas, as evidence of malignant degeneration. Similarly, the presence of rare mitotic figures, the appearance of hypercellularity due to predominance of the Antoni A component, and bony erosion due to expansion of the encapsulated tumor are not indicators of malignancy in a schwannoma.[276] Reliable criteria for malignancy in peripheral nerve

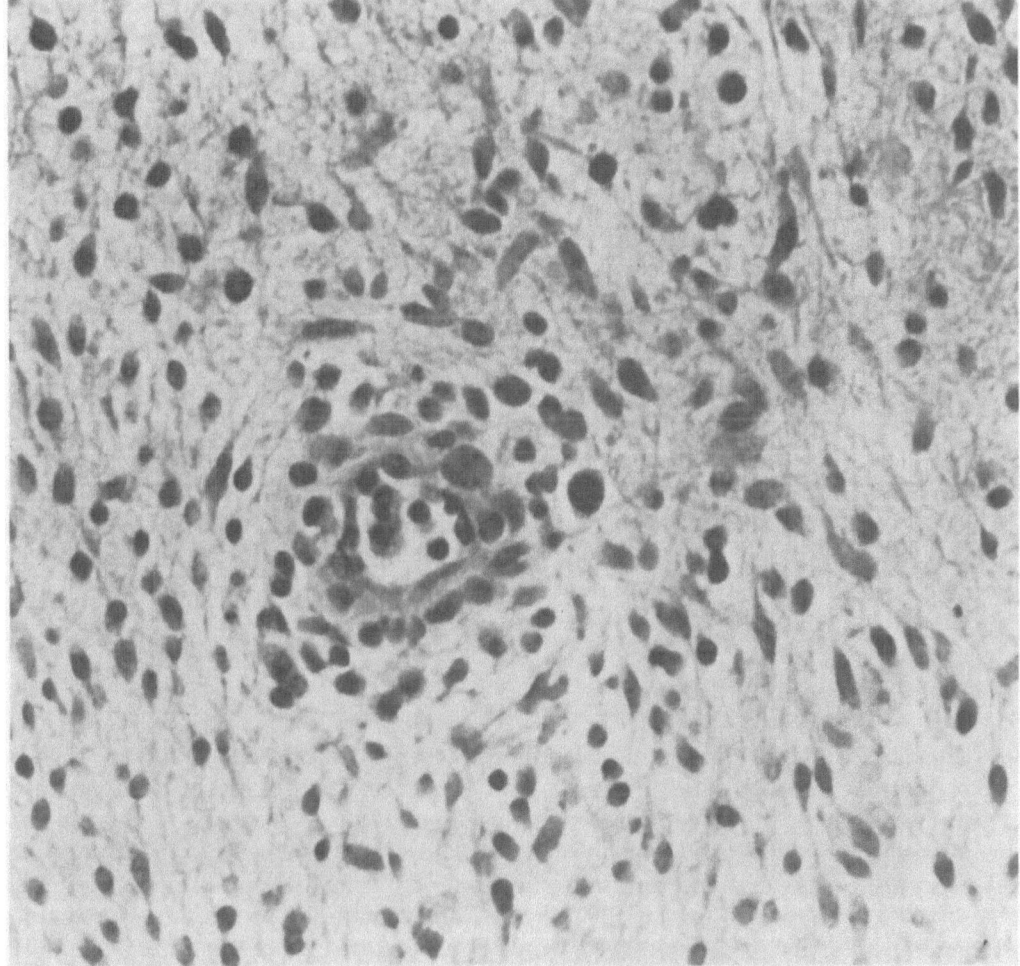

Fig. 7-65. Myxoid area within a malignant schwannoma. Neoplastic cells cluster around a thin-walled blood vessel (×620).

sheath tumors include hypercellularity, nuclear hyperchromatism, the presence of more than occasional mitotic figures, foci of tumor necrosis, and tumor invasion of adjacent tissues.[247,276]

Electron-microscopic and immunocytochemical studies have not resolved the question whether malignant schwannomas arise from Schwann cells, perineurial cells, or nerve sheath fibroblasts.[74,226,235] Of the 10 malignant schwannomas examined by Erlandson and Woodruff,[74] only one contained cells with some ultrastructural features similar to those found in a benign schwannoma. An additional four tumors contained cells with ultrastructural features suggestive of neuroectodermal derivation, (i.e., cells with broad processes covered by discontinuous basal lamina, primitive intercellular junctions, or extracellular long-spacing collagen). The remaining five tumors had only anaplastic cells without distinguishing ultrastructural features. Immunoreactive S-100 is found in only 50% of malignant schwannomas.[269] Immunoreactivity for Leu-7 antigen or myelin basic protein is also found in some tumors.[273]

The lack of distinctive histologic features in malignant schwannoma, both by light and electron microscopy, dictates that certain prerequisites be met before interpreting a malignant spindle-cell tumor as a malignant schwannoma. Criteria for determining nerve sheath origin have been proposed by several investigators.[48,73,74,235,247] For practical purposes, it is reasonable to consider a malignant spindle-cell neoplasm to be of nerve sheath origin if it arises in a nerve, is contiguous with a neurofibroma or schwannoma, or occurs in a patient with neurofibromatosis. Immunohistochemistry and electron microscopy may yield strong supporting evidence for a nerve-sheath origin.[74,269,273]

Rare variants of malignant schwannoma, such as malignant epithelioid schwannoma, are discussed by Harkin and Reed[95] by Enzinger and Weiss.[73]

Ganglion Cyst of Nerve

A mucinous ganglion cyst, identical to those found in the periarticular tissues, may develop in a peripheral nerve and produce nerve compression. The peroneal nerve is most commonly affected.[45] The cyst may be extraneural or intraneural. It contains mucoid material and has no epithelial lining. A ganglion cyst of the nerve must be distinguished from the so-called perineurial cyst of the posterior spinal root ganglion.[234]

Localized Hypertrophic Neuropathy

This rare and poorly understood condition presents clinically as a slowly progressive motor mononeuropathy, and macroscopically as a localized, fusiform enlargement of a peripheral nerve. Microscopically, paraffin-embedded cross-sections of the involved nerve reveal many well-developed onion bulbs. The lesion has been variously interpreted as a localized form of hypertrophic (onion bulb) neuropathy, a chronic entrapment neuropathy, or a neurofibroma.[219,270] Recent ultrastructural and immunocytochemical studies suggest that the onion-bulb lamellae are formed by perineurial cells.[12] The role of perineurial cells in this and other nerve sheath tumors has been reviewed by Weidenheim and Campbell.[267]

Other Tumors of the Nerve Sheath

The nerve sheath myxoma (neurothekeoma) is an uncommon lesion involving the dermis and subcutis.[79,192] The tumor has a characteristic lobulation microscopically and often immunostains for S-100 protein.

Fibrolipomatous hamartoma of the nerve is characterized by a fibrofatty enlargement of the epineurium and fibrosis of the perineurium.[214] The median nerve is typically involved. Macrodactyly may also be present.

References

1. Abarbanel JM, Berginer VJ, Osimani A, et al: Neurologic complications after gastric restriction surgery for morbid obesity. *Neurology* 37:196–200, 1987
2. Adelman LS, Aronson SM: Intramedullary nerve fiber and Schwann cell proliferation within the spinal cord (schwannosis). *Neurology* 22:726–731, 1972

3. Ahonen RE: Peripheral neuropathy in uremic patients and in renal transplant recipients. *Acta Neuropathol* (Berlin) 54:43–53, 1981

4. Anzil P, Dozic S: Peripheral nerve changes in porphyric neuropathy: Findings in a sural nerve biopsy. *Acta Neuropathol* (Berlin) 42:121–126, 1978

5. Arseni C, Cumitrescu L, Constantinescu A: Neurinomas of the trigeminal nerve. *Surg Neurol* 4:497–503, 1975

6. Arts WFM, Busch HFM, Van Der Brand HJ, et al: Hereditary neuralgic amyotrophy. Clinical, genetic, electrophysiological, and histopathologic studies. *J Neurol Sci* 62:261–279, 1983

7. Asbury AK: Proximal diabetic neuropathy. Ann Neurol 2:179–180, 1977

8. Asbury AK: Diagnostic considerations in Guillain-Barré syndrome. *Ann Neurol* 9:1–5, 1981

9. Asbury AK, Johnson PC: *Pathology of Peripheral Nerve.* Philadelphia, W.B. Saunders Company, 1978.

10. Badurska B, Fidzianska A, Jedrezejowska H: A dominant form of neuronal ceroid-lipofuscinosis. An ultrastructural study of sural nerve and peripheral lymphocytes. *J Neurol* 226:205–212, 1981

11. Bailey RO, Baltch AL, Venkatesh R, et al: Sensory motor neuropathy associated with AIDS. *Neurology* 38:886–891, 1988

12. Balboa JM, Khoury NJS, Hudson AR, et al: Perineurioma (localized hypertrophic neuropathy). *Arch Pathol Lab Med* 108:557–560, 1984

13. Behse F, Buchthal F: Peroneal muscular atrophy (PMA) and related disorders. II. Histological findings in sural nerves. *Brain* 100:67–85, 1977

14. Behse F, Buchthal F: Alcoholic neuropathy: Clinical electrophysiological, and biopsy findings. *Ann Neurol* 2:95–110, 1977

15. Behse F, Buchthal F: Sensory action potentials and biopsy of the sural nerve in neuropathy. *Brain* 101:473–493, 1978

16. Behse F, Buchthal F, Carlsen F, et al: Hereditary neuropathy with liability to pressure palsies: Electrophysiological and histopathological aspects. *Brain* 95:777–794, 1972

17. Behse F, Buchthal F, Carlsen F, et al: Endoneurial space and its constituents in the sural nerve of patients with neuropathy. *Brain* 97:773–784, 1974

18. Behse F, Buchthal F, Carlsen F, et al: Unmyelinated fibers and Schwann cells of sural nerve in neuropathy. *Brain* 98:493–510, 1975

19. Behse F, Buchthal F, Carlsen F: Nerve biopsy and conduction studies in diabetic neuropathy. *J Neurol Neurosurg Psychiatry* 40:1072–1082, 1977

20. Benson MD, Cohen AS, Brandt KD, et al: Neuropathy, M Components, and amyloid. *Lancet* 1:10–12, 1975

21. Berciano J, Combarros O, Figlos J, et al: Hereditary motor and sensory neuropathy Type II: Clinicopathological study of a family. *Brain* 109:897–914, 1986

22. Bergouignan FX, Massonnat R, Vital C, et al: Uncompacted lamellae in three patients with POEMS syndrome. *Eur Neurol* 27:173–181, 1987

23. Bergouigan F-X, Vital C: Occurrence of Renaut's bodies in a peripheral nerve. *Arch Pathol Lab Med* 108:330–333, 1984

24. Bird TD, Ott J, Giblett ER, et al: Genetic linkage evidence for heterogeneity in Charcot-Marie-Tooth neuropathy (HMSN Type I). *Ann Neurol* 14:679–684, 1983

25. Bischoff A: Neuropathy in leukodystrophies, in Dyck PJ, Thomas PK, Lambert EH (eds): *Peripheral Neuropathy.* Vol. II, Philadelphia, W.B. Saunders Company, 1975, 891–913

26. Bolton CF: Peripheral neuropathies associated with chronic renal failure. *Can J Neurol Sci* 7:89–95, 1980

27. Bradley WB, Madrid R, Thrush DC, et al: Recurrent brachial plexus neuropathy. *Brain* 98:381–398, 1975

28. Bradley WG, Good P, Rasool CG, et al: Morphometric and biochemical studies of peripheral nerves in amyotrophic lateral sclerosis. *Ann Neurol* 14:267–277, 1983

29. Brechenmacher C, Vital C, Deminiere C, et al: Guillian-Barré syndrome: An ultrastructural study of peripheral nerve in 65 patients. *Clin Neuropathol* 6:19–24, 1987

30. Bridger MW, Farkashidy J: The distribution of neuroglia and schwann cells in the 8th nerve of man. *J Laryngol Otol* 94:1353–1362, 1980

31. Brooks JSJ, Freeman M, Enterline HT: Malignant "triton" tumors: Natural history and immunohistochemistry of nine new cases with literature review. *Cancer* 55:2543–2549, 1985

32. Brown MJ, Martin JR, Asbury AK: Painful diabetic neuropathy. *Arch Neurol* 33:164–171, 1976

33. Byrd JC, Powers JM: Wolman's disease: Ultrastructural evidence of lipid accumulation in central and peripheral nervous systems. *Acta Neuropathol* (Berlin) 45:37–42, 1979

34. Caillaud J-M, Benjelloun S, Bosq J, et al: HNK-1-defined antigen detected in paraffin-embedded neuroectoderm tumors and those derived from cells of the amine precursor uptake and decarboxylation system. *Cancer Res* 44:4432–4439, 1984

35. Calatayud T, Vallejo AR, Dominguez L, et al: Lymphomatoid granulomatosis manifesting as a subacute polyradiculoneuropathy: *A case* report and review of the neurological manifestations. *Eur Neurol* 19:213–223, 1980
36. Carpenter S, Karpati G, Rothman S, et al: Pathological involvement of primary sensory neurons in Werdnig-Hoffman disease. *Acta Neuropath* (Berlin) 42:91–97, 1978
37. Carson FL, Kingsley WB: Nonamyloid green birefringence following Congo red staining. *Arch Pathol Lab Med* 104:333–335, 1980
38. Cavanagh JB: The "dying back" process: A common denominator in many naturally occurring and toxic neuropathies. *Arch Pathol Lab Med* 103:659–664, 1979
39. Chad D, Shoukimas GM, Bradley WG, et al: Peripheral nerve unmyelinated axons following lumbar sympathectomy. *Ann Neurol* 10:486–488, 1981
40. Chad D, Pariser K, Bradley WG, et al: The pathogenesis of cryoglobulinemic neuropathy. *Neurology* 32:725–729, 1982
41. Chari VR, Katiyar BC, Rastogi BL, et al: Neuropathy in hepatic disorders: A clinical, electrophysiological and histopathological appraisal. *J Neurol Sci* 31:93–111, 1977
42. Charnas L, Trapp B, Griffin J: Congenital absence of peripheral myelin: abnormal Schwann cell development causes lethal arthrogryposis multiplex congenita. *Neurology* 38:966–974, 1988
43. Charron L, Peyronnard JM, Marchand L: Sensory neuropathy associated with primary biliary cirrhosis. *Arch Neurol* 37:84–87, 1980
44. Chopra JS, Samanta AK, Murthy JMK, et al: Role of porta-systemic shunt and hepatocellular damage in the genesis of hepatic neuropathy. *Clin Neurol Neurosurg* 82:37–44, 1980
45. Cobb CA, Moiel RH: Ganglion of the peroneal nerve: Report of two cases. *J Neurosurg* 41:255–259, 1974
46. Cornblath DR, McArthur JC, Kennedy PGE, et al: Inflammatory demyelinating peripheral neuropathies associated with human T-cell lymphotrophic virus type III infection. *Ann Neurol* 21:32–40, 1987
47. Croft PB, Urish H, Wilkinson M: Peripheral neuropathy of sensorimotor type associated with malignant disease. *Brain* 90:31–66, 1967
48. D'Agostino AN, Soule EH, Miller RH: Primary malignant neoplasms of nerves (malignant neurilemomas) in patients without manifestations of multiple neurofibromatosis (von Recklinghausen's disease). *Cancer* 16:1003–1014, 1963
49. D'Agostino AN, Soule EH, Miller RH: Sarcomas of the peripheral nerves and somatic soft tissues associated with multiple neurofibromatosis (Von Recklinghausen's disease). *Cancer* 16:1015–1027, 1963
50. Dahl I: Ancient neurilemmoma (schwannoma). *Acta Path Microbiol Scand (Sect A)* 85:812–818, 1977
51. Dalakas MC, Pezeshkpour GH: Neuromuscular diseases associated with human immunodeficiency virus infection. *Ann Neurol* 23:S38–S48, 1988
52. Das Gupta TK, Brasfield RD, Strong EW, et al: Benign solitary schwannomas (neurilemomas). *Cancer* 24:355–366, 1969
53. Dastur DK: Leprosy, in Vinken PJ, Bruyn GW (eds): *Handbook of Clinical Neurology, Vol 33,* Amsterdam, North-Holland Publishing Company, 1978 421–468
54. Davenport J, Farrell DF, Sumi S: Giant axonal neuropathy caused by industrial chemicals: Neuroaxonal masses in man. *Neurology* 26:349, 1976
55. Dinn JJ, Dinn EI: Natural history of acromegalic peripheral neuropathy. *Quarterly J Med* 57(224):833–842, 1985
56. DiTrapani G, David P, LaCara A, et al: Morphological studies of sural nerve biopsies in the pseudopolyneuropathic form of amyotrophic lateral sclerosis. *Clin Neuropathol* 5:134–138, 1986
57. Donaghy M, Hakin RN, Bamford JM, et al: Hereditary sensory neuropathy with neurotrophic keratitis. *Brain* 110:563–583, 1987
58. Ducatman BS, Scheithauer BW: Postirradiation neurofibrosarcoma. *Cancer* 51:1028–1033, 1983
59. Ducatman BS, Scheithauer BW, Piepgras DG, et al: Malignant peripheral nerve sheath tumors: A clinico-pathologic study of 120 cases. *Cancer* 57:2006–2021, 1986
60. Dyck PJ: Neuronal atrophy and degeneration predominantly affecting peripheral sensory and autonomic neurons, in Dyck PJ, Thomas PK, Lambert EH et al (eds): *Peripheral Neuropathy.* 2nd ed. Vol. II, Philadelphia, W.B. Saunders Company, 1984, 791–824
61. Dyck PJ: Inherited neuronal degeneration and atrophy affecting peripheral motor, sensory, and autonomic neurons, in Dyck PJ, Thomas PK, Lambert EH, et al (eds): *Peripheral Neuropathy* 2nd ed. Vol. II, Philadelphia, W.B. Saunders Company, 1984, 1600–1655
62. Dyck PJ, Benstead TJ, Conn DL, et al: Nonsystemic vasculitic neuropathy. *Brain* 110:843–854, 1987
63. Dyck PJ, Conn DL, Okazaki H: Necrotizing angiopathic neuropathy: Three-dimensional morphology of fiber degeneration related to sites of occluded vessels. *Mayo Clin Proc* 47:461–475, 1972

64. Dyck PJ, Johnson WJ, Lambert EH, et al: Segmental demyelination secondary to axonal degeneration in uremic neuropathy. *Mayo Clin Proc* 46:400–431, 1971
65. Dyck PJ, Karnes JL, Daube J, et al: Clinical and neuropathological criteria for the diagnosis and staging of diabetic polyneuropathy. *Brain* 108:861–880, 1985
66. Dyck PJ, Karnes J, Lais A, et al: Pathologic alterations of the peripheral nervous system of humans, in Dyck PJ, Thomas PK, Lambert EH, et al (eds): *Peripheral Neuropathy*. 2nd ed. Vol. I, Philadelphia, W.B. Saunders Co., 1984, 760–870
67. Dyck PJ, Karnes JL, O'Brien P, et al: The spatial distribution of fiber loss in diabetic polyneuropathy suggests ischemia. *Ann Neurol* 19:440–449, 1986
68. Dyck PJ, Karnes LA, Rizza OP, et al: Fiber loss is primary and multifocal in sural nerves in diabetic polyneuropathy. *Ann Neurol* 19:425–439, 1986
69. Dyck PJ, Lais AC, Karnes JL, et al: Permanent axotomy, a model of axonal atrophy and secondary segmental demyelination and remyelination. *Ann Neurol* 9:575–583, 1981
70. Dyck PJ, Lais AC, Ohta M, et al: Chronic inflammatory polyradiculoneuropathy. *Mayo Clin Proc* 50:621–637, 1975
71. Dyck PJ, Oviatt KF, Lambert EH: Intensive evaluation of referred unclassified neuropathies yields improved diagnosis. *Ann Neurol* 10:222–226, 1981
72. Eames RA, Lange LS: Clinical and pathological study of ischaemic neuropathy. *J Neurol Neurosurg Psychiatry* 30:215–226, 1967
73. Enzinger FM, Weiss SW: *Soft Tissue Tumors*. 2nd ed. St. Louis, C.V. Mosby Company, 1988
74. Erlandson RA, Woodruff JM: Peripheral nerve sheath tumors: An electron microscopic study of 43 cases. *Cancer* 49:273–287, 1982
75. Ferriere G, Denef J-F Rodriguez J, et al: Morphometric studies of normal sural nerves in children. *Muscle and Nerve* 8:697–704, 1985
76. Fink LH, Early CB, Bryan RN: Glossopharyngeal schwannomas. *Surg Neurol* 9:239–245, 1978
77. Finkel MF: Lyme disease and its neurologic complications. *Arch Neurol* 45:99–103, 1988
78. Fitting JW, Bischoff A, Regli F, et al: Neuropathy, amyloidosis, and monoclonal gammopathy. *J Neurol Neurosurg Psychiatry* 42:193–202, 1979
79. Fletcher CDM, Chan J K-C, McKee PH: Dermal nerve sheath myxoma: A study of three cases. *Histopathology* 10:135–145, 1986
80. Foley KM, Woodruff JM, Ellis FT, et al: Radiation-induced malignant and atypical peripheral nerve sheath tumors. *Ann Neurol* 7:311–318, 1980
81. Galassi G, Gibertoni M, Mancini A, et al: Sarcoidosis of the peripheral nerve: Clinical, electrophysiological and histological study of two cases. *Eur Neurol* 23:459–465, 1984
82. Ghatak NR, Norwood CW, Davis CH: Intracerebral schwannoma. *Surg Neurol* 3:45–47, 1975
83. Ghosh BC, Ghosh L, Huvos AG, et al: Malignant schwannoma: A clinicopathologic study. *Cancer* 31:184–190, 1973
84. Glenner GG: Amyloid deposits and amyloidosis: The β-fibrilloses. *N Engl J Med* 302:1283–1292, 302:1333–1343, 1980
85. Goebel HH, Lenard HG, Kohlschutter A, et al: The ultrastructure of the sural nerve in Pompe's disease. *Ann Neurol* 2:111–115, 1977
86. Goebel HH, Zeman W, DeMyer W: Peripheral motor and sensory neuropathy of early childhood simulating Werdnig-Hoffmann disease. *Neuropadiatrie* 7:182–195, 1976
87. Gould VE, Moll R, Moll I, et al: The intermediate filament complement of the spectrum of nerve sheath neoplasms. *Lab Invest* 55:463–474, 1986
88. Gruskin P, Carberry JN: Pathology of acoustic tumors, in House WF, Luetje CM (eds): *Acoustic Tumors, Vol 1*, Baltimore, University Park Press, 1979, 85–148
89. Guccion JG, Enzinger F: Malignant schwannoma associated with von Recklinghausen's neurofibromatosis. *Virchows Arch A Path Anat Histol* 383:43–57, 1979
90. Gumbinas M, Larsen M, Liu HM: Peripheral neuropathy in classic Niemann-Pick disease: Ultrastructure of nerves and skeletal muscles. *Neurology* 25:107–113, 1975
91. Gutrecht JA, Dyck PJ: Quantitative teased-fiber and histologic studies of human sural nerve during postnatal development. *J Comp Neurol* 138:117–130, 1970
92. Hall SM: The response of the (myelinating) Schwann cell population to multiple episodes of demyelination. *J Neurocytol* 12:1–12, 1983
93. Harding AE, Thomas PK: The clinical features of hereditary motor and sensory neuropathy types I and II. *Brain* 103:259–280, 1980
94. Harkin JC: Differential diagnosis of peripheral nerve tumors, in Omer GE, Spinner M, (eds): *Management of Peripheral Nerve Problems*. Philadelphia, W.B. Saunders Company, 1980, 657–668

196   *Thomas W. Bouldin*

95. Harkin JC, Reed RJ: Tumors of the Peripheral Nervous System. Bethesda, Armed Forces Institute of Pathology, Inc., 1969
96. Hart RC, Gardner DP, Howieson J: Acoustic tumors: Atypical features and recent diagnostic tests. *Neurology* 33:211–221, 1983
97. Holm TW, Prawe SE, Sahl WJ, et al: Multiple cutaneous neuromas. *Arch Dermatol* 107:608–610, 1973
98. Horwich MS, Cho L, Porro RS, et al: Subacute sensory neuropathy: A remote effect of carcinoma. *Ann Neurol* 2:7–19, 1977
99. Hudson AR, Kline DG: Progression of partial experimental injury to peripheral nerve. Part 2: Light and electron microscopic studies. *J Neurosurg* 42:15–22, 1975
100. Hughes RAC, Cameron JS, Hall SM, et al: Multiple mononeuropathy as the initial presentation of systemic lupus erythematosus—nerve biopsy and response to plasma exchange. *J Neurol* 228:239–247, 1983
101. Ikeda S-I, Hanyu N, Hongo M, et al: Hereditary generalized amyloidosis with polyneuropathy: clinico-pathological study of 65 Japanese patients. *Brain* 110:315–337, 1987
102. Ilyas AA, Quarles RH, MacIntosh TD, et al: IgM in a human neuropathy related to paraproteinemia binds to a carbohydrate determinant in the myelin-associated glycoprotein and to a ganglioside. *Proc Natl Acad Sci* 81:1225–1229, 1984
103. Iwashita T, Enjoji M: Plexiform neurilemoma: A clinicopathological and immunohistochemical analysis of 23 tumours from 20 patients. *Virchows Archiv A* 411:305–309, 1987
104. Jacobs JM, Love S: Qualitative and quantitative morphology of human sural nerve at different ages. *Brain* 108:897–924, 1985
105. Jacobs JM, Shetty VP, Antia NH: Teased fibre studies in leprous neuropathy. *J Neurol Sci* 79:301–313, 1987
106. Jefferson D, Eames RA: Renaut body distribution at sites of human peripheral nerve entrapment. *J Neurol Sci* 49:19–29, 1981
107. Johnson PC, Brendel K, Meezan E: Human diabetic perineurial cell basement membrane thickening. *Lab Invest* 44:265–270, 1981
108. Johnson PC, Doll SC, Cromey DW: Pathogenesis of diabetic neuropathy. *Ann Neurol* 19:450–457, 1986
109. Johnson MD, Glick AD, Davis BW: Immunohistochemical evaluation of Leu-7, myelin basic-protein, S100-protein, glial-fibrillary acidic-protein, and LN3 immunoreactivity in nerve sheath tumors and sarcomas. *Arch Pathol Lab Med* 112:155–160, 1988
110. Jonsson V, Jensen TS, Friis ML, et al: Immunoglobulin deposits in peripheral nerve endings detected by skin biopsy in patients with IgM M proteins and neuropathy. *Neurology* 37:303–306, 1987
111. Johnson PC, Rolak LA, Hamilton RH, et al: Paraneoplastic vasculitis of nerve: A remote effect of cancer. *Ann Neurol* 5:437–44, 1979
112. Julien J, Vital C, Vallet J-M, et al: Polyneuropathy in Waldenström's macroglobulinemia. *Arch Neurol* 35:423–525, 1978
113. Kasantikul V, Netsky MG, Glasscock ME, et al: Acoustic neurilemmoma. Clinicoanatomical study of 103 patients. *J Neurosurg* 52:28–35, 1980
114. Katrak SM, Pollock M, O'Brien CP, et al: Clinical and morphological features of gold neuropathy. *Brain* 103:671–693, 1980
115. Kawahara E, Oda Y, Ooi A, et al: Expression of glial fibrillary acidic protein (GFAP) in peripheral nerve sheath tumors: A comparative study of immunoreactivity of GFAP, vimentin, S-100 protein, and neurofilament in 38 schwannomas and 18 neurofibromas. *Am J Surg Path* 12:115–120, 1988
116. Kelly JJ: Peripheral neuropathies associated with monoclonal proteins: a clinical review. *Muscle & Nerve* 8:138–150, 1985
117. Kelly JJ, Kyle RA, Miles JM, et al: The spectrum of peripheral neuropathy in myeloma. *Neurology* 31:24–31, 1981
118. Kelly JJ, Kyle RA, Miles JM, et al: Osteosclerotic myeloma and peripheral neuropathy. *Neurology* 33:202–210, 1983
119. Kennedy WR, Sung JH, Berry JF: A case of congenital hypomyelination neuropathy. *Arch Neurol* 34:337–345, 1977
120. Kepes JJ, Morantz RA, England AM: Reticulin stain in differentiating astrocytomas from neurilemmomas on frozen sections. *J Neurosurg* 51:124–125, 1979
121. King RHM, Thomas PK: Electron microscope observations on aberrant regeneration of unmyelinated axons in the vagus nerve of the rabbit. *Acta Neurpathol* (Berlin) 18:150–159, 1971
122. King RHM, Thomas PK: The occurrence and significance of myelin with unusually large periodicity. *Acta Neuropathol* (Berlin) 63:319–329, 1984
123. Kissel JT, Slivka AP, Warmolts JR, et al: The clinical spectrum of necrotizing angiopathy of the peripheral nervous system. *Ann Neurol* 18:251–257, 1985

124. Kocen RS, King RH, Thomas PK, et al: Nerve biopsy findings in two cases of Tangier disease. *Acta Neuropathol* (Berlin) 26:317–327, 1973
125. Koch T, Schultz P, Williams R, et al: Giant axonal neuropathy: A childhood disorder of microfilaments. *Ann Neurol* 1:438–451, 1977
126. Konishi T, Saida K, Ohnishi A, et al: Perineuritis in mononeuritis multiplex with cryoglobulinemia. *Muscle Nerve* 5:173–177, 1982
127. Kosik KS, Mullins TF, Bradley WG, et al: Coma and axonal degeneration in vitamin B_{12} deficiency. *Arch Neurol* 27:590–592, 1980
128. Kudo M, Matsumoto M, Terao H: Malignant nerve sheath tumor of acoustic nerve. *Arch Pathol Lab Med* 107:293–297, 1983
129. Landrieu P, Said G: Peripheral neuropathy in type A Niemann-Pick disease: A morphological study. *Acta Neuropathol* (Berlin) 63:66–71, 1984
130. Lascelles RG, Thomas PK: Changes due to age in internodal length in the sural nerve in man. *J Neurol Neurosurg Psychiatry* 29:40–44, 1966
131. Lassmann G: Morton's toe. Clinical, light and electron microscopic investigations in 133 cases. *Clin Orthopaedics* 142:73–84, 1979
132. Low PA, Dyck PJ, Lambert EH, et al: Acute panautonomic neuropathy. *Ann Neurol* 13:412–417, 1983
133. Lazarus SS, Trombetta LD: Ultrastructural identification of a benign perineurial cell tumor. *Cancer* 41:1823–1829, 1978
134. Lewis RA, Sumner AJ, Brown MJ, et al: Multifocal demyelinating neuropathy with persistent conduction block. *Neurology* 32:958–964, 1982
135. Lippa CF, Chad DA, Smith TW, et al: Neuropathy associated with cryoglobulinemia.. *Muscle and Nerve* 9:626–631, 1986.
136. Low, FN: The perineurium and connective tissue of peripheral nerve, in Landon DN (ed): *The Peripheral Nerve.* London, Chapman and Hall, 1976, pp 159–187
137. Low PA, Burke WJ, McLeod JG: Congenital sensory neuropathy with selective loss of small myelinated fibers. *Ann Neurol* 3:179–182, 1978
138. Low PA, McLeod JG, Prineas JW: Hypertrophic Charcot-Marie-Tooth disease. *J Neurol Sci* 35:93–115, 1978
139. Lowman RM, Livolsi VA: Pigmented (melanotic) schwannomas of the spinal cord. *Cancer* 46:391–397, 1980
140. Ludwig J, Dyck PJ, LaRusso NF: Xanthomatous neuropathy of liver. *Hum Pathol* 13:1049–1051, 1982
141. Madrid R, Bradley WG: The pathology of neuropathies with focal thickening of the myelin sheath (tomaculous neuropathy): Studies on the formation of the abnormal myelin sheath. *J Neurol Sci* 25:415–448, 1975
142. Madrid R, Bradley WG, David CJ: The peroneal muscular atrophy syndrome: Clinical, genetic, electrophysiological and nerve biopsy studies. Part 2. Observations on pathological changes in sural nerve biopsies. *J Neurol Sci* 32:91–122, 1977
143. Martin JJ, Leroy JG, Farriaux JP, et al: I-cell disease (mucolipidosis II): A report on its pathology. *Acta Neuropathol* (Berlin) 33:185–305, 1975
144. Martin JJ, Lowenthal A, Ceuterick C, et al: Adrenomyeloneuropathy: A report on two families. *J Neurol* 226:221–232, 1982
145. Martinez AJ, Taylor JR, Dyck PJ, et al: Chlordecone intoxication in man. II. Ultrastructure of peripheral nerves and skeletal muscle. *Neurology* 28:631–635, 1978
146. Martuza RL, Eldridge R: Neurofibromatosis 2 (bilateral acoustic neurofibromatosis). *N Engl J Med* 318:684–688, 1988
147. Maury CPJ, Teppo A-M, Karinemi A-L, et al: Amyloid fibril protein in familial amyloidosis with cranial neuropathy and corneal lattice dystrophy (FAP Type IV) is related to transthyretin. *Am J Clin Pathol* 89:359–364, 1988
148. McCombe PA, McLeod JG: The peripheral neuropathy of vitamin B_{12} deficiency. *J Neurol Sci* 66:117–126, 1984
149. McCombe PA, Pollard JD, McLeod, JG: Chronic inflammatory demyelinating polyradiculoneuropathy: A clinical and electrophysiological study of 92 cases. *Brain* 110:1617–1630, 1987
150. McCombe PA, McLeod JG, Pollard JD, et al: Peripheral sensorimotor and autonomic neuropathy associated with systemic lupus erythematosus. *Brain* 110:533–549, 1987
151. McLeod JG: An electrophysiological and pathological study of peripheral nerves in Friedreich's ataxia. *J Neurol Sci* 12:333–349, 1971
152. McLeod JG, Evans WA: Peripheral neuropathy in spinocerebellar degenerations. *Muscle Nerve* 4:51–61, 1981

153. McLeod JG, Low PA: Peroneal muscular atrophy with autosomal dominant inheritance. *Clin Exp Neurol* 14:142–153, 1977
154. Meachim G, Abberton MJ: Histological findings in Morton's metatarsalgia. *J Pathol* 103:209–217, 1971
155. Meier C: Survey of progress: Polyneuropathy in paraproteinaemia. *J Neurol* 232:204–214, 1985
156. Meier C, Bischoff A: Polyneuropathy in hypothyroidism: Clinical and nerve biopsy study of 4 cases. *J Neurol* 215:103–114, 1977
157. Meier C, Kauer B, Muller U, et al: Neuromyopathy during chronic amiodarone treatment: A case report. *J Neurol* 220:231–239, 1979
158. McLeod JG, Tuck RR, Pollard JD, et al: Chronic polyneuropathy of undetermined cause. *J Neurol Neurosurg Psychiatry* 47:530–535, 1984
159. Miller RG, Davis CJ, Illingworth DR, et al: The neuropathy of abetalipoproteinemia. *Neurology* 30:1286–1291, 1980
160. Nakanishi T, Sobue I, Toyokura Y, et al: The Crow-Fukase syndrome: a study of 102 cases in Japan. *Neurology* 34:712–720, 1984
161. Neary D, Eames RA: The pathology of ulnar nerve compression in man. *Neuropathol Appl Neurobiol* 1:69–88, 1975
162. Nemni R, Bottacchi E, Fazio R, et al: Polyneuropathy in hypothyroidism: Clinical, electrophysiological and morphological findings in four cases. *J Neurol Neurosurg Psychiatry* 50:1454–1460, 1987
163. Nemni R, Corbo M, Fazio R, et al: Cryoglobulinaemic neuropathy: A clinical, morphological and immuno-cytochemical study of 8 cases. *Brain* 3:541–552, 1988
164. Neuen E, Seitz RJ, Langenbach M, et al: The leakage of serum proteins across the blood-nerve barrier in hereditary and inflammatory neuropathies. An immunohistochemical and morphometric study. *Acta Neuropathol* (Berlin) 73:53–61, 1987
165. Nobile-Orazio E, Marmiroli P, Baldini L, et al: Peripheral neuropathy in macroglobulinemia: Incidence and antigen-specificity of M proteins. *Neurology* 37:1506–1514, 1987
166. Nukada H, Dyck PJ: Decreased axon caliber and neurofilaments in hereditary motor and sensory neuropathy, Type I. *Ann Neurol* 16238–16241, 1984
167. Ochoa J: The sural nerve of the human foetus: Electron microscope observations and counts of axons. *J Anat* 18:231–245, 1971
168. Ochoa J: The primary nerve fiber pathology of plantar neuromas. A model of chronic entrapment. *J Neuropathol Exp Neurol* 35:370, 1976
169. Ochoa J: Recognition of unmyelinated fiber disease: Morphologic criteria. *Muscle Nerve* 1:375–387, 1978
170. Ochoa J, Mair WG: The normal sural nerve in man. I. Ultrastructure and numbers of fibres and cells. *Acta Neuropathol* (Berlin) 13:197–216, 1969
171. Ochoa J, Mair WG: The normal sural nerve in man. II. Changes in the axons and Schwann cells due to ageing. *Acta Neuropathol* (Berlin) 13:217–239, 1969
172. Ohi T, Kyle RA, Dyck PJ: Axonal attenuation and secondary segmental demyelination in myeloma neuropathies. *Ann Neurol* 17:255–261, 1985
173. Ohnishi A, Dyck PJ: Loss of small peripheral sensory neurons in Fabry disease. *Arch Neurol* 31:120–127, 1974.
174. Ohnishi A, Hirano A: Uncompacted myelin lamellae in dysglobulinemic neuropathy. *J Neurol Sci* 51:131–140, 1981
175. Ohnishi A, Peterson CM, Dyck PJ: Axonal degeneration in sodium cyanate-induced neuropathy. *Arch Neurol* 32:530–534, 1975
176. Ohnishi A, Tsuji S, Igisu H, et al: Beriberi neuropathy. *J Neurol Sci* 45:177–190, 1980
177. O'Neill BP, Marmion LC, Feringa ER: The adrenoleukomyeloneuropathy complex: Expression in four generations. *Neurology* 31:151–156, 1981
178. Ongerboer de Visser BW, Feltkamp-Vroom TM, Feltkamp CA: Sural nerve immune deposits in polyneuropathy as a remote effect of malignancy. *Ann Neurol* 14:261–266, 1983
179. Ono J, Senba E, Okada S, et al: A case report of congenital hypomyelination. *Eur J Pediatr* 138:265–270, 1982
180. Ouvrier RA, McLeod JG, Conchin TE: The hypertrophic forms of hereditary motor and sensory neuropathy. A study of hypertrophic Charcot Marie-Tooth disease (HMSN Type I) and Dejerine-Sottas disease (HMSN Type III) in childhood. *Brain* 110:121–148, 1987
181. Parry GJ: Peripheral neuropathies associated with human immunodeficiency virus infection. *Ann Neurol* 23:S49–S53, 1988
182. Perentes E, Rubinstein LJ: Immunohistochemical recognition of human nerve sheath tumors by anti-leu 7 (HNK-1) monoclonal antibody. *Acta Neuropathol* (Berlin) 68:319–324, 1985

183. Peyronnard JM, Charron L, Beaudet F, et al: Vasculitic neuropathy in rheumatoid disease and Sjögren syndrome. *Neurology* 32:839–845, 1982

184. Pezeshkpour G, Krarup C, Buchthal F, et al: Peripheral neuropathy in mitochondrial disease. *J Neurol Sci* 77:285–304, 1987

185. Pollock M, Nukada N, Taylor P, et al: Comparison between fascicular and whole sural nerve biopsy. *Ann Neurol* 13:65–68, 1983

186. Powell HC: Pathology of diabetic neuropathy: New observations, new hypotheses. *Lab Invest* 49:515–518, 1983

187. Powell HC, Haas, R, Hall CL, et al: Peripheral nerve in type III glycogenosis: Selective involvement of unmyelinated fiber Schwann cells. *Muscle & Nerve* 8:667–671, 1985

188. Powers JM, Schaumburg HH: Adrenoleukodystrophy: Similar ultrastructural changes in adrenal cortical and Schwann cells. *Arch Neurol* 30:406–408, 1974

189. Prineas JW: Acute idiopathic polyneuritis: An electron microscope study. *Lab Invest* 26:133–147, 1972

190. Prineas JW: Pathology of the Guillain-Barré syndrome. *Ann Neurol* 9:6–19, 1981

191. Prineas JW, McLeod JG: Chronic relapsing polyneuritis. *J Neurol Sci* 27:427–458, 1976

192. Pultizer DR, Reed RJ: Nerve-sheath myxoma (perineurial myxoma). *Am J Dermatopathol* 7:409–421, 1985

193. Raine CS: Schwann cell responses during recurrent demyelination and their relevance to onion-bulb formation. *Neuropathol Appl Neurobiol* 3:453–470, 1977

194. Reed RJ, Bliss BO: Morton's neuroma. *Arch Pathol* 95:123–129, 1973

195. Reed RJ, Fine RM, Meltzer HD: Palisaded, encapsulated neuromas of the skin. *Arch Dermatol* 106:865–870, 1972

196. Riccardi VM: Von Recklinghausen neurofibromatosis. *N Engl J Med* 305:1617–1626, 1981

197. Robertson I, Cook MG, Wilson DF, et al: Malignant schwannoma of cranial nerves. *Pathology* 15:421–429, 1983

198. Robitaille Y, Carpenter S, Karpati G, et al: A distinct form of adult polyglucosan body disease with massive involvement of central and peripheral neuronal processes and astrocytes. *Brain* 103:315–336, 1980

199. Rosenblum JL, Keating JP, Prensky AL, et al: A progressive neurologic syndrome in children with chronic liver disease. *N Engl J Med* 304:503–508, 1981

200. Russell DS, Rubinstein LJ: Pathology of Tumors of the Nervous System. 4th ed. Edward Arnold (Publishers) Ltd, Great Britain, 1977

201. Sabin TD, Swift TR: Leprosy, in Dyck PJ, Thomas PK, Lambert EH (eds): *Peripheral Neuropathy* 2nd ed. Vol II, Philadelphia, W.B. Saunders Company, 1984, 1955–1987

202. Said G: Perhexiline neuropathy: A clinicopathological study. *Ann Neurol* 3:259–266, 1978

203. Said G: A clinicopathologic study of acrodystrophic neuropathies. *Muscle Nerve* 3:491–501, 1980

204. Said G, Marion M-H, Selva J, et al: Hypotrophic and dying-back nerve fibers in Friedreich's ataxia. *Neurology* 36:1292–1299, 1986

205. Said G, Slama G, Selva J: Progressive centripetal degeneration of axons in small fiber diabetic polyneuropathy. *Brain* 106:791–807, 1983

206. Schaumburg H, Kaplan J, Windebank A, et al: Sensory neuropathy from pyridoxine abuse. A new megavitamin syndrome. *N Engl J Med* 309:445–448, 1983

207. Schochet SS, McCormick WF, Powell GF: Krabbe's disease: a light and electron microscopic study. *Acta Neuropathol* (Berlin) 36:153–160, 1976

208. Schold SC, Cho ES, Somasundaram M, et al: Subacute motor neuropathy: A remote effect of lymphoma. *Ann Neurol* 5:271–289, 1979

209. Schroder JM: Proliferation of epineurial capillaries and smooth muscle cells in angiopathic peripheral neuropathy. *Acta Neuropathol* (Berlin), 72:29–37, 1986

210. Schroder JM, Bohl J, Brodda K: Changes of the ratio between myelin thickness and axon diameter in the human developing sural nerve. *Acta Neuropathol* (Berlin) 43:169–178, 1978

211. Shetty VP, Mehta LN, Antia NH, et al: Teased fiber study of early nerve lesions in leprosy and in contacts, with electrophysiological correlates. *J Neurol Neurosurg Psychiatry* 40:708–711, 1977

212. Shield LK, King RHM, Thomas PK: A morphometric study of human fetal sural nerve. *Acta Neuropathol* (Berlin) 70:60–70, 1986

213. Sian CS, Ryan SF: The ultrastructure of neurilemoma with emphasis on Antoni B tissue. *Hum Pathol* 12:145–160, 1981

214. Silverman TA, Enzinger FM: Fibrolipomatous hamartoma of nerve: A clinicopathologic analysis of 26 cases. *Am J Surg Pathol* 9:7–14, 1985

215. Sima AAF, Lattimer SA, Yagihashi S, et al: Axoglial dysjunction: a novel structural lesion the accounts

for poorly reversible slowing of nerve conduction in the spontaneously diabetic bio-breeding rat. *J Clin Invest* 77:474–484, 1986

216. Sluga E, Poewe W: Chronic idiopathic polyneuritis. *Clin Neuropathol* 2:31–41, 1983
217. Smith IS, Kahn SN, Lacey BW, et al: Chronic demyelinating neuropathy associated with benign IgM paraproteinaemia. *Brain* 106:169–195, 1983
218. Smith TW, Bhawan J: Tactile-like structures in neurifibromas: An ultrastructural study. *Acta Neuropathol* (Berlin) 50:233–236, 1980
219. Snyder M, Cancilla PA, Batzdorf U: Hypertrophic neuropathy simulating a neoplasm of the brachial plexus. *Surg Neurol* 7:131–134, 1977
220. Sordillo PP, Helson L, Hajdu SI, et al: Malignant schwannoma: clinical characteristics, survival, and response to therapy. *Cancer* 47:2503–2509, 1981
221. Spencer PS: The traumatic neuroma and proximal stump. *Bull Hosp Joint Diseases* 35:85–102, 1974
222. Spencer PS, Schaumburg HH: Experimental and Clinical Neurotoxicology. Baltimore, Williams and Wilkins, 1980
223. Stafford CR, Bogdanoff BM, Green L, et al: Mononeuropathy multiplex as a complication of amphetamine angiitis. *Neurology* 25:570–572, 1975
224. Staunton H, Dervan P, Kale R, et al: Hereditary amyloid polyneuropathy in North West Ireland. *Brain* 110:1231–1245, 1987
225. Steck AJ, Murray N, Dellagi K, et al: Peripheral neuropathy associated with monoclonal IgM autoantibody. *Ann Neurol* 22:764–767, 1987
226. Stefansson K, Wollmann R, Jerkovic M: S-100 protein in soft-tissue tumors derived from Schwann cells and melanocytes. *Amer J Pathol* 106:261–268, 1982
227. Steiman GS, Rorke LB, Brown MJ: Infantile neuronal degeneration masquerading as Werdnig-Hoffmann disease. *Ann Neurol* 8:317–324, 1980
228. Steinman L, Tharp BR, Dorfman LJ, et al: Peripheral neuropathy in the cherry-red spot-myoclonus syndrome (Sialidosis type I). *Ann Neurol* 7:450–456, 1980
229. Stewart TJ, Liland J, Schuknecht HG: Occult schwannomas of the vestibular nerve. *Arch Otolaryngol* 101:91–95, 1975
230. Storm FK, Eilber FR, Mirra J, et al: Neurofibrosarcoma. *Cancer* 45:126–129, 1980
231. Sunderland S: Nerves and Nerve Injuries. 2nd ed. Edinburgh, Churchill Livingstone, 1978
232. Sung JH, Mastri AR, Chen KTK: Aberrant peripheral nerves and neuromas in normal and injured spinal cords. *J Neuropathol Exp Neurol* 40:551–565, 1981
233. Takatsu M, Hays AP, Latov N, et al: Immunofluorescence study of patients with neuropathy and IgM M proteins. *Ann Neurol* 18:173–183, 1985
234. Tarlov IM: Spinal perineurial and meningeal cysts. *J Neurol Neurosurg Psychiat* 33:833–843, 1970
235. Taxy JB, Battifora H, Trujillo Y, et al: Electron microscopy in the diagnosis of malignant schwannoma. *Cancer* 48:1381–1391, 1981
236. Thomas PK, Eliasson SG: Diabetic neuropathy, in Dyck PJ, Thomas PK, Lambert EH. et al (eds): *Peripheral Neuropathy*. 2nd ed. Vol. I, Philadelphia, W.B. Saunders Company, 1984, 1773–1810
237. Thomas PK, Hollinrake K, Lascelles RG, et al: The polyneuropathy of chronic renal failure. *Brain* 94:761–780, 1971
238. Thomas PK, King RH: Peripheral nerve changes in amyloid neuropathy. *Brain* 97:395–406, 1974
239. Thomas PK, King RH: The degeneration of unmyelinated axons following nerve section: An ultrastructural study. *J Neurocytol* 3:497–512, 1974
240. Thomas PK, Lascelles RG: The pathology of diabetic neuropathy. *Q J Med* 35:489–509, 1966
241. Thomas PK, Walker JG: Xanthomatous neuropathy in primary biliary cirrhosis. *Brain* 88:1079–1088, 1965
242. Thomas PK, Walker RWH, Rudge P, et al: Chronic demyelinating peripheral neuropathy associated with multifocal central nervous system demyelination. *Brain* 110:53–76, 1987
243. Tohgi H, Tsukagoshi H, Toyokura Y: Quantitative changes with age in normal sural nerves. *Acta Neuropathol* (Berlin) 38:213–220, 1977
244. Trapani GD, Tulli A, La Cara A, et al: Peripheral neuropathy in course of progressive systemic sclerosis. *Acta Neuropathol* (Berlin) 72:103–110, 1986
245. Tredici G, Minoli G: Peripheral nerve involvement in familial spastic paraplegia. *Arch Neurol* 36:236–239, 1979
246. Trockel U, Schroder JM, Reiners KH, et al: Multiple exercise-related mononeuropathy with abdominal colic. *J Neurol Sci* 60:431–442, 1983

247. Trojanowski JQ, Kleinman GM, Proppe KH: Malignant tumors of nerve sheath origin. *Cancer* 46:1202–1212, 1980

248. Trotter JL, Engel WK, Ignaezak TF: Amyloidosis with plasma cell dyscrasia: An overlooked cause of adult onset sensorimotor neuropathy. *Arch Neurol* 34:209–214, 1977

249. Tsukada N, Koh CS, Owa M, et al: Chronic neuropathy associated with immune complexes of hepatitis B virus. *J Neurol Sci* 61:193–221, 1983

250. Ulrich J, Hirt HR, Kleihues P, et al: Connatal polyneuropathy: A case with proliferated microfilaments in Schwann cells. *Acta Neuropathol* (Berlin) 55:39–46, 1981

251. Uri AK, Witzleben CL, Raney RB: Electron microscopy of glandular schwannoma. *Cancer* 53:493–497, 1984

252. Vainio K: Morton's metatarsalgia in rheumatoid arthritis. *Clin Orthopaedics* 142:85–89, 1979

253. Vallat JM, Desproges-Gotteron R, Leboutet MJ, et al: Cryoglobulinemic neuropathy: A pathological study. *Ann Neurol* 8:179–185, 1980

254. Vallat JM, Gil R, Leboutet MJ, et al: Case reports: Congenital hypo- and hypermyelination neuropathy. Two cases. *Acta Neuropathol* (Berlin) 74:97–201, 1987

255. Verghese JP, Bradley WG, Nemni R, et al: Amyloid neuropathy in multiple myeloma and other plasma cell dyscrasias. *J Neurol Sci* 59:237–246, 1983

256. Vital A, Vital C: Polyarteritis nodosa and peripheral neuropathy: ultrastructural study of 13 cases. *Acta Neuropathol* (Berlin) 67:136–141, 1985

257. Vital A, Vital C, Riviere JP: Variability of morphological features in early infantile polyneuropathy with defective myelination. *Acta Neuropathol* (Berlin) 73:295–300, 1987

258. Vital C, Aubertin J, Ragnault JM, et al: Sarcoidosis of the peripheral nerve: A histological and ultrastructural study of two cases. *Acta Neuropathol* (Berlin) 58:111–114, 1982

259. Vital C, Brechenmacher C, Reiffers J, et al: Uncompacted myelin lamellae in two cases of peripheral neuropathy. *Acta Neuropathol* (Berlin) 60:252–256, 1983

260. Vital C, Brachenmacher C, Serise JM, et al: Ultrastructural study of peripheral nerve in arteritic diabetic patients. *Acta Neuropathol* (Berlin) 61:225–231, 1983

261. Vital C, Vallat JM: *Ultrastructural Study of the Human Diseased Peripheral Nerve. 2nd edition.* New York, Elsevier, 1987

262. Voiculescu V, Alexianu M, Popescu-Trismana G, et al: Polyneuropathy with lipid deposits in Schwann cells and axonal degeneration in cerebrotendinous xanthomatosis. *J Neurol Sci* 82:89–99, 1987

263. Vos A, Gabreels-Festen A, Joosten E, et al: The neuropathy of Cockayne syndrome. *Acta Neuropathol* (Berlin) 61:153–156, 1983

264. Vos AJM, Joosten EMG, Gabreels-Festen AAWM: Adult polyglucosan body disease: Clinical and nerve biopsy findings in two cases. *Ann Neurol* 13:440–444, 1983

265. Watabe K, Kumanishi F, Ikuta F, et al: Tactile-like corpuscles in neurofibromas: Immunohistochemical demonstration of S-100 protein. *Acta Neuropathol* 61:173–177, 1983

266. Watanabe S, Ohnishi A: Subperineurial space of the sural nerve in various peripheral nerve diseases. *Acta Neuropathol* 46:227–230, 1979

267. Weidenheim KM, Campbell WG: Perineurial cell tumor. *Virchows Arch [Pathol Anat]* 408:375–383, 1986

268. Weinstein EM, Chui H, Lane S, et al: Churg-Strauss syndrome (allergic granulomatous angiitis): Neuro-ophthalmologic manifestations. *Arch Ophthalmol* 101:1217–1220, 1983

269. Weiss SW, Langloss JM, Enzinger FM: Value of S-100 protein in the diagnosis of soft tissue tumors with particular reference to benign and malignant Schwann cell tumors. *Lab Invest* 49:299–308, 1983

270. Weller RO, Cervós-Navarro J: *Pathology of Peripheral Nerves.* London, Butterworths, 1977

271. Weller RO, Das Gupta TK: Experimental hypertrophic neuropathy: An electron microscope study. *J Neurol Neurosurg Psychiatry* 31:34–42, 1968

272. Wichman A, Buchthal F, Pezeshkpour GH, et al: Peripheral neuropathy in abetalipoproteinemia. *Neurology* 35:1279–1289, 1985

273. Wick MR, Swanson PE, Scheithauer BW, et al: Malignant peripheral nerve sheath tumor: An immunohistochemical study of 62 cases. *Am J Clin Pathol* 87:425–433, 1987

274. Wisniewski H, Terry RD, Whitaker JN, et al: Landy-Guillain-Barré syndrome: A primary demyelinating disease. *Arch Neurol* 21:269–276, 1969

275. Woodruff JM: Peripheral nerve tumors showing glandular differentiation (glandular schwannomas). *Cancer* 37:2399–2413, 1976

276. Woodruff JM, Susin M, Godwin TA, et al: Cellular schwannoma: A variety of schwannoma sometimes mistaken for a malignant tumor. *Am J Surg Pathol* 5:733–7444, 1981

277. Yasuda H, Dyck PJ: Abnormalities of endoneurial microvessels and sural nerve pathology in diabetic neuropathy. *Neurology* 37:20–28, 1987
278. Yiannikas C, McLeod JG, Pollard JD, et al: Peripheral neuropathy in mitochondrial disease. *J Neurol Sci* 77:285–304, 1987
279. Zochodne DW, Bolton CF, Wells GA, et al: Critical illness polyneuropathy: A complication of sepsis and multiple organ failure. *Brain* 110:819–842, 1987

8

Muscle Biopsy

Hans H. Goebel

Introduction

A muscle biopsy is expected to be diagnostic of the structural abnormalities of the musculature, which comprises about 40% of the body volume. Clinical examination, including family history, electrophysiologic studies by electromyography and electroneurography, serologic tests, especially creatine kinase (CK) levels, and muscle biopsy are the preferred methods to establish the diagnosis of a neuromuscular disease. The pathologist may receive the tissue specimens without any pertinent clinical information, or only a brief note such as "amyotrophic lateral sclerosis suspected" or "rule out polymyositis." Frequently, both the clinical information and the method of supplying the tissue to the pathologist are inadequate.

The 1988 World Federation of Neurology classification of neuromuscular diseases[209] lists more than 600 disorders affecting skeletal muscle. Many are conditions that clinically involve skeletal muscles foremost; these are the neuromuscular disorders in a restricted sense. Other diseases affect skeletal muscle secondarily or concomitantly with other organs bearing the brunt of these disease processes as in many metabolic, endocrine, and collagen disorders. A double classification based on that of the World Federation of Neurology and a second purely morphologic one may confuse the clinician and prevent the pathologist from appropriately diagnosing the morphologic findings. To avoid such frustration, a minimum of clinical and ancillary data on the patient should accompany the request for a morphologic evaluation of the muscle biopsy specimen.

The Muscle Biopsy

The introduction of enzyme histochemistry, immunohistology, and electron microscopy has greatly enlarged the morphologic interpretation of muscle lesions. Pathologists

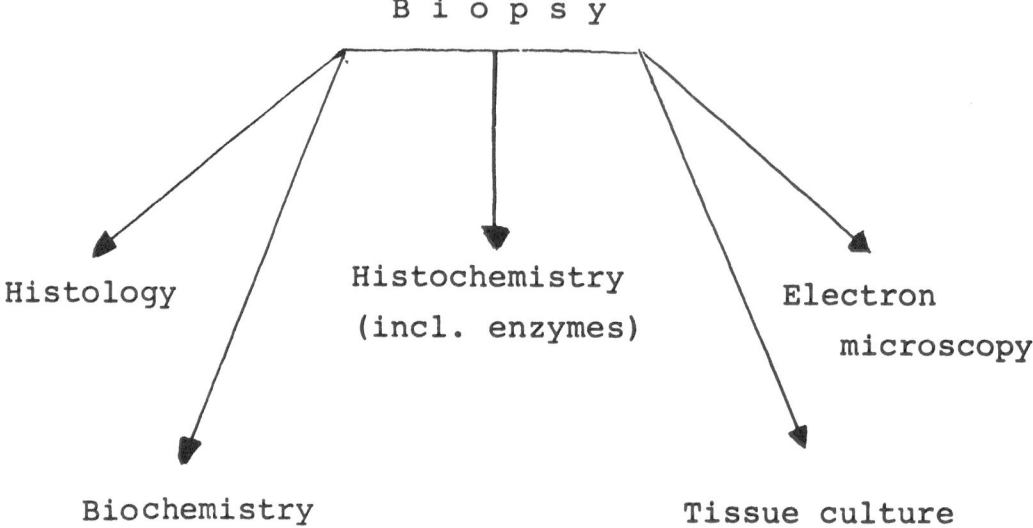

Fig. 8-1. Investigative procedures employed in muscle biopsy tissues.

should be consulted about how to process the muscle biopsy specimen before it is taken. Comprehensive workup of a muscle biopsy tissue cannot be done with formalin-fixed material. Primary fixation in formaldehyde or similar fixatives has largely been abandoned since the introduction of enzyme histochemistry. For enzyme and immuno-histologic studies, the muscle should be kept unfixed in a moist chamber before being frozen in liquid nitrogen, isopentane in liquid nitrogen, or Freon.[68]

The muscle biopsy is then subjected to light microscopy (Fig. 8-1), which entails freezing the muscle (Fig. 8-2) so that cross-sections of the muscle fibers become available

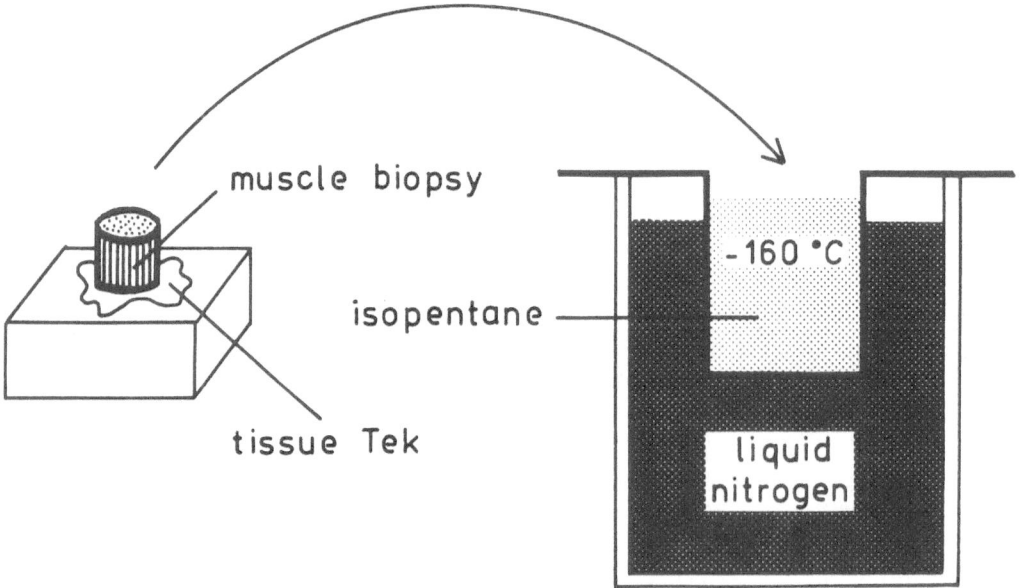

Fig. 8-2. Handling of the unfixed muscle tissue for cryostat sections. (Courtesy of S. Schwarting, D.D.S.)

in histologic preparations. These sections are important for enzyme and immunohisto-chemical studies and histographic analysis.

Histographic analysis may be completed either by using the "smaller diameter" technique[31] or by measuring the entire area of the cross-sectioned muscle fiber. Sections of paraffin-embedded muscle fibers may be helpful in diagnosing inflammatory processes, necrosis, and regeneration of muscle fibers as well as vascular diseases. They are useless for evaluating muscle tissue showing selective fiber type involvement, fiber type grouping, or certain metabolic abnormalities.

For electron microscopy, the tissue should be fixed in buffered glutaraldehyde at the time of removal. A sterile clamp may be applied in situ to the muscle, and the clamped specimen then immersed in glutaraldehyde. If the muscle fibers are extended at the time of clamping, they will remain so during fixation and will render the I- and A-bands of the sarcomeres more conspicuous. In special cases, such as myasthenia gravis or myasthenic syndromes, neuromuscular junctions or motor endplates should be studied. Various techniques to obtain the muscle biopsy at the motor point have been described.[50,113,207] Short muscles (i.e., the external intercostal or peroneal brevis) do not require preoperative identification of the motor point; excision of the entire length of the muscle will provide motor endplates.

The application of enzyme histochemistry (Table 8.1), immunohistology and electron microscopy to the study of muscle tissue requires close proximity between operating room and laboratory. Transport from one room to the other should be completed within two hours after removal of the muscle specimen. This time interval is compatible with adequate morphologic study of referred muscle tissue. If long distances are involved, the muscle specimen must be mounted and frozen in the operating room and transported

Table 8-1.
Histologic and Enzyme Histochemical and
Immunohistologic Stains

Hematoxylin–eosin	Acid phosphatase
Modified trichrome	Amylophosphorylase
Oil red O	Nonspecific esterase
PAS (+ digestion)	Acetylcholinesterase
Elastic van Gieson	Myoadenylate deaminase
Unstained (autofluorescence)	Phosphofructokinase
	Desmin
Alizarin red	Vimentin
Azur B	Immunoglobulins, especially IgG
Iron	
NADH-tetrazolium reductase	Complement factors
	Immune complexes
Menadione-linked alpha-glycerophosphatedehydrogenase (and other oxidative enzymes, e.g., SDH, COX, LDH, mitochondrial ATPase)	Labeling of B and T-lymphocytes
	T subsets
	monocytes
	macrophages
	acetylcholine receptors
ATPase after alkaline (pH 9.4/10.4) and acid (pH 4.5/4.6 and 4.2/4.3; 3/9) preincubations	
Alkaline phosphatase	

to the laboratory, wrapped in parafilm, and placed on dry ice. After the muscle has been properly frozen on wooden or cork chucks, it may be stored in a deep freezer until it is ready for distant transportation. The author has found this type of long distance two-step preparation to be satisfactory, provided a skilled and careful technician handles the muscle specimen immediately after its surgical removal.

The growing awareness of metabolic myopathies in children and adults frequently requires the separate availability of unfixed, muscle tissue immediately deep frozen for subsequent biochemical diagnostic studies.

Normal Morphologic Appearances

A muscle fascicle consists of densely packed polygonal muscle fibers measuring, on cross-section, between 40 and 80 μm in adult men and 30–70 μm in adult women.[68] Data on normal adult myofiber diameters are limited to certain muscles, i.e., the biceps and quadriceps muscles; data on myofiber diameters in children are incomplete but available[33] (Table 8-2).

There is usually a checkerboard pattern of type I, type IIA, and type IIB muscle fibers (Table 8-3), based on the adenosin triphosphatase (ATPase) technique after acid preincubation (pH 4.5).[68] In the biceps and quadriceps muscles, these three fiber types usually comprise one-third each of the muscle fiber population.[68] Other muscles may have different patterns of distribution and size of type I and type II fibers.[127,170] Type IIC fibers are regarded as immature fibers and as those that are in the process of regeneration or reinnervation. They give an intermediate reaction at pH 4.3 and their

Table 8-2.
Approximate Mean Diameters of Type I and Type II Myofibers[a]

Age (Years)	Mean Diameter (μm)		Range (± 2 Standard Deviation) (μm)	
	Type I	Type II	Type I	Type II
1	16	14	8–24	7–21
2	18	16	9–27	8–24
3	20	18	10–30	9–27
4	22	20	11–33	10–30
5	24	23	12–36	12.5–35.5
6	27	26	13.5–40.5	13–39
7	30	29	15–45	14.5–43.5
8	33	32	16.5–49.5	16–48
9	36	35	18–54	17.5–52.5
10	40	38	20–60	19–57
11	44	42	22–66	21–63
12	48	46	24–72	23–69
13	52	50	26–78	25–75
14	56	55	28–84	27.5–82.5
15	60	58	30–90	29–87

[a] Obtained largely from Quadriceps and Gastrocnemius in children aged 1–15 years; ATPase preparations.

Table 8-3.
Fiber Types

Type I Myofibers	Type II Myofibers
Low in alkaline ATPase	High in alkaline ATPase
High in acid ATPase	Low in acid ATPase
Low in phosphorylase	High in phosphorylase
Low in MAG	High in MAG
High in NADH	Low in NADH
High oxidative capacity	High glycolytic capacity
Abundant triglyceride stores	Scanty triglyceride stores
	Sparse capillary bed
Rich capillary bed	Fast twitch
Slow twitch	

evaluation may be particularly helpful in the muscle tissue of young children afflicted with congenital muscular dystrophy, with certain congenital myopathies, and with aspects of immaturity or maturational arrest. Alkaline (pH 9.4) and acid (pH 4.3) ATPase preparations, and oil red O and PAS stains also identify type I and type II fibers.[68] The amylophosphorylase preparation shows a lack of enzyme activity in type V glycogenosis (McArdle's disease), and denervated fibers are also frequently found without phosphorylase activity. The two-step technique that demonstrates phosphofructokinase (PFK)[23] identifies type VII glycogenosis (Tarui's disease) on grounds of an absent PFK histochemical reaction. The acid phosphatase preparation indicates lysosomal activity. Degenerating and denervated fibers show considerable activity of this enzyme, as do macrophages invading necrotic muscle fibers.

Alkaline phosphatase is normally confined to endothelial cells; regenerating muscle fibers may also show some activity of this enzyme. Such regenerating fibers also have a basophilic hue in the hematoxylin–eosin (H&E) preparation, and they are faintly blue in the Azur B stain. Nonspecific esterase activity is demonstrable at sites having increased lipofuscin content and at motor endplates. An acetylcholine esterase preparation may outline further the size and shape of individual normal and abnormal motor endplates. The NADH–tetrazolium reductase (NADH) and menadione-linked alpha-glycerophosphate dehydrogenase (MAG) preparations exhibit reciprocity of enzyme activity in the individual muscle fiber: a strong reaction in type I fibers in the NADH preparation corresponds to a weak reaction in the MAG preparation. Type II fibers have the opposite features. The NADH preparation also shows a regular fine sarcoplasmic network, indicating that this enzyme activity is not confined to mitochondria.

Distortion of this sarcoplasmic reticular network is emphasized in moth-eaten fibers, whorled fibers, minicores and central cores, as well as in target fibers. Tubular aggregates, usually located in the subsarcolemmal regions, give a strong NADH reaction but no MAG reaction; however, aggregates of abnormal mitochondria have a strong reaction in both oxidative enzyme preparations. Such mitochondrial aggregates are usually seen as "ragged red fibers" in modified trichrome preparations. Other mitochondrial enzymes might be successfully employed when suspecting mitochondrial myopathies such as SDH (succinic dehydrogenase) or COX (cytochrome c oxidase), two exclusively mitochondrial enzymes that are more strongly reacting in type I than in type II myofibers and that accentuate "ragged red fibers." They and mitochondrial ATPase with and without

DNP (a decoupler of oxidative phosphorylation) also identify enzyme-deficient myofibers as an expression of their respective partial enzyme deficiency. The amount of fat within muscle fibers varies considerably, but is usually higher in type I than in type II fibers. If excessive, as in lipid myopathies, lipid droplets may occur as vacuoles and should not be confused with the effects of ice crystal formation. Glycogen is usually shown in the PAS preparation and is more abundant in type II than in type I fibers.

Connective tissue in the normal muscle is recognized as perimysium and epimysium. Intramuscular vessels may be seen in the elastic van Gieson stain and in alkaline phosphatase and ATPase preparations (especially after preincubation at pH 3.9). The normal vascular network has an even distribution among and within the fascicles.

Muscle enzyme activity is preserved for a few hours after death. Phosphorylase activity is lost first, then alkaline ATPase. NADH and ATPase activities, after acid preincubation, are preserved the longest time.

Light-microscopic studies are generally conducted on cross-sectioned myofibers, but electron microscopy is usually done on longitudinally embedded muscle fibers. If the muscle is extended prior to in situ clamping and fixed in a clamp, sarcomeres will be well extended, showing distinct Z-disks and I- and A-bands. The sarcoplasmic reticulum and particularly the triads are usually discernible at the junction of the I- and A-bands, and they may be further visualized by lanthanum, which is applied to the muscle specimen together with osmium tetroxide before embedding. Mitochondria are usually small and show a regular and uniform pattern of cristae. Clusters of mitochondria may be located in the subsarcolemmal region, particularly close to nuclei. Lipid droplets may also be seen beneath the sarcolemmal membrane as well as deeper within muscle fibers. With increasing age of the patient, lipofuscin granules accumulate next to the nucleus. The basal lamina closely follows the plasma membrane of the muscle fiber.

Among muscle fibers, capillaries with a thin basement membrane may be seen along with some collagen fibrils. The motor endplate is a region in the periphery of the muscle fiber, where the sarcolemma, (i.e., the plasmalemma and the basal lamina), is conspicuously folded. Subsarcolemmal electron densities on the crests of the subneural apparatus are the site of acetylcholine receptors. The subneural area of the motor endplate also contains many mitochondria. The axon terminal, covered on either side by Schwann cell processes, may contain clear vesicles. A basal lamina covers both the muscle fiber, the Schwann cell, and axon terminal at the motor endplate, and courses across the entire cleft between the axon terminal and the subneural apparatus of the muscle fiber.

Sectioning and examining all biopsied muscle tissues ultrastructurally is time-consuming, and in most instances, unnecessary for diagnosis. Selective electron microscopy is therefore recommended. Visualizing acetylcholine receptors at and beyond motor endplates and anti-acetylcholine receptor antibodies, in patients with myasthenia gravis remains a future goal. Recently developed and introduced techniques of immunohistology concern three aspects of myopathology:

1. identification of immunoglobulins and complement factors as well as immunocomplexes, most often by immunofluorescence, by applying respective antisera to unfixed muscle tissue sections;
2. classification of cells within inflammatory infiltrates as to B and T-lymphocytes as well as T subsets, monocytes and macrophages by applying respective antibodies to unfixed tissue sections[2,5,78];
3. Immunohistochemical identification of filament-related proteins as actin, desmin or myosin by applying antibodies to either unfixed or fixed tissue sections

using immunofluorescence or immunoenzyme (peroxidase, alkaline phosphatase) methods or to ascertain the presence or absence of the recently discovered protein dystrophin,[120] which may become of diagnostic importance in establishing or eliminating the diagnoses of Duchenne and Becker's muscular dystrophies or other muscular dystrophies, respectively.

Nonspecific Structural Changes

Compared to the many clinical entities affecting skeletal muscles, either primarily or secondarily, the morphologic expression of neuromuscular diseases is narrow. As a result, structural abnormalities among different neuromuscular diseases overlap widely and the changes are often nonspecific.

The application of histochemistry and electron microscopy has widened the range of possible morphologic changes. Muscle fibers contain organelles similar to those in other cells—i.e., mitochondria, endoplasmic reticulum, lysosomes, and glycogen, and also some that are specific for muscle fibers, (e.g., myofilaments, the T-tubular system, multiple nuclei, and satellite cells). This dual population of specific and nonspecific cellular constituents is responsible for many useful diagnostic features.

The muscle fiber is more dependent on innervation than other extraneural cells; impairment of this innervation adds another expression to neuromuscular diseases.

Atrophy

Decrease in volume of muscle fibers (Fig. 8-3), particularly in diameter, is one of the most conspicuous abnormal features of skeletal muscle. Simple atrophy probably reflects the loss of myofilaments and some organelles; nuclei persist, later forming pyknotic clumps (Fig. 8-3). Attenuation of myofilaments and shrivelling of the basal lamina around a shrunken muscle fiber indicates atrophy. Denervation is the most frequent cause of small muscle fibers. Chronic ischemia may cause perifascicular atrophy in patients with dermatomyositis. The small muscle fibers characteristic of primary myopathies, especially muscular dystrophy, are a primary change of the myofiber. Atrophy of muscle fibers may be reversible, but the exact "point of no return" is unknown. Selective fiber atrophy is a frequent feature of muscle tissue. Generally, type I fiber atrophy occurs in congenital or hereditary diseases (Table 8-4), and type II fiber atrophy may develop, sometimes as a reversible phenomenon, in acquired neuromuscular diseases (Table 8-4). Hypotrophy of muscle fibers indicates lack of muscle fiber growth.

Hypertrophy

Enlargement of muscle fibers frequently coexists with atrophic fibers. Such enlargement is ascribed to compensatory mechanisms activated by the atrophy of adjacent myofibers. In certain instances, hypertrophy of muscle fibers may be unassociated with muscle fiber atrophy, as in the case of female carriers of Duchenne muscular dystrophy, primary myopathies and muscular dystrophies, and in circumscribed denervation caused by radiculopathy.[17] Excessive hypertrophy of muscle fibers is thought

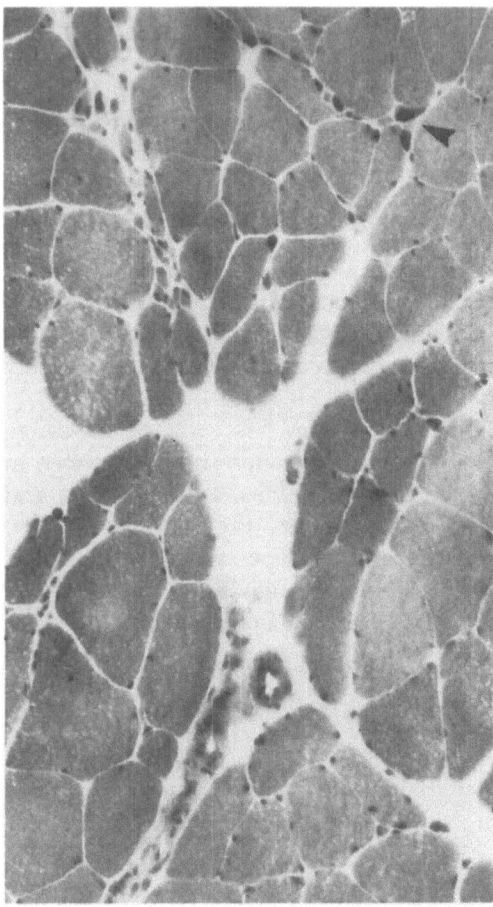

Fig. 8-3. Several small, angular, atrophic muscle fibers and a few pyknotic nuclear clumps (arrow): 38-year-old woman, myopathia distalis juvenilis Biemond; gastrocnemius (Modified trichrome; ×184).

to result in fiber splitting. This concept has recently been criticized, based on experimental studies attributing "splitting" to a fusion of regenerating myofibers.[184] Selective hypertrophy of one fiber type (often type II) is rare and diagnostically it is less useful than selective fiber type atrophy.

Necrosis

Muscle fibers may undergo coagulation necrosis. This change occurs segmentally, leaving other parts of the fiber intact. An early stage preceding necrosis may be represented by plasma membrane loss that needs repair to prevent muscle fiber necrosis.[40] Such breaks or holes in the plasma membrane have been demonstrated in cases of Duchenne muscular dystrophy.[28,160] Necrosis of muscle fibers is reflected in coagulation of sarcomeres (Fig. 8-4), organelles, and nuclei. In cases of contraction bands or in hyaline (opaque) fibers, the sarcomeres are enormously contracted and the individual myofilaments are indistinct; organelles, such as mitochondria, are intact or even swollen. Autophagocytosis, morphologically marked by "rimmed vacuoles" is another form of necrosis that results in cell death rather than regeneration.

Table 8-4.
Type I and Type II Fiber Atrophies

Mainly Type I Fiber Atrophy	Mainly Type II Fiber Atrophy
Dystrophic myotonia (adult and juvenile)	Disuse or cachexia
Congenital myotonia	Supranuclear lesions
Congenital myopathies	pyramidal disorders
Congenital fiber type disproportion	mental retardation
Rigid spine syndrome	hemiparesis
Distal myopathy	Parkinson's syndrome
Periodic paralysis	Collagen vascular diseases
Myositis	polymyalgia rheumatica
Rheumatoid arthritis (stages III and IV)	rheumatoid arthritis (stages I and II)
Tenotomy	Myasthenia gravis
	Steroid therapy, Cushing's syndrome
	Carcinoid myopathy
	Renal insufficiency (uremia)
	Early, severe denervation predominantly affecting type II fibers
	Guillain–Barré syndrome
	polyneuropathy
	experimental denervation

Coagulation necrosis is followed by macrophage invasion (Fig. 8-4) and phagocytosis of the necrotic debris reflected in strong acid phosphatase activity (Fig. 8-5).

Regeneration seems to start by activation of dormant satellite cells that form myoblasts and later fuse to form myotubes. The latter may be recognized by abundant ribosomes, polysomes, and rough endoplasmic reticulum (Figs. 8-6 and 8-7).[48] Regenerating muscle fibers often show activity of alkaline phosphatase, an enzyme not demonstrable in either adult or fetal normal muscle fibers.

Inclusion Bodies

Many inclusions (Table 8-5) have been observed in muscle fibers. Defining the precise nature of each inclusion usually requires electron microscopy. Histochemical preparations may help identify some inclusions. Nemaline bodies or rods (Fig. 8-8) are characteristic of nemaline myopathy; they also are a nonspecific feature of other neuromuscular diseases, often in atrophic fibers and recently also seen in the acquired immunodeficiency syndrome (AIDS),[55,109] and consist of large, wedge-shaped structures, showing the typical lattice of Z-disks (Fig. 8-9). Nemaline bodies often form subsarcolemmal clusters. The cytoplasmic body (Fig. 8-10) is a core of electron-dense, amorphous

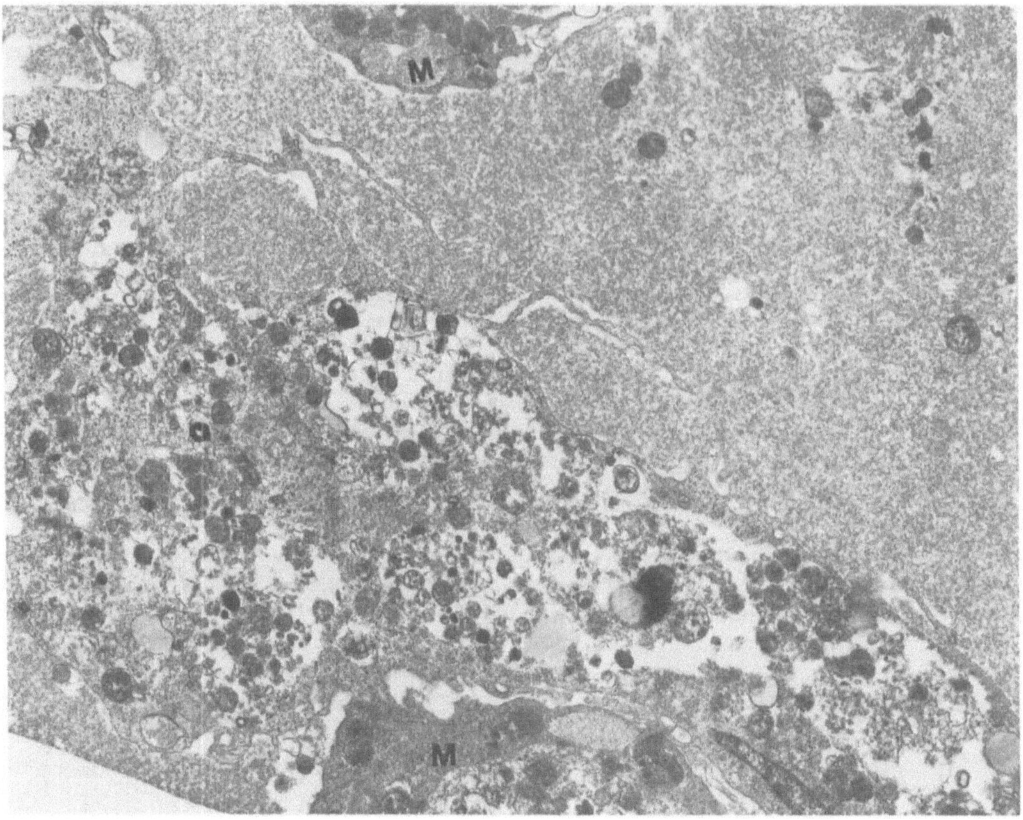

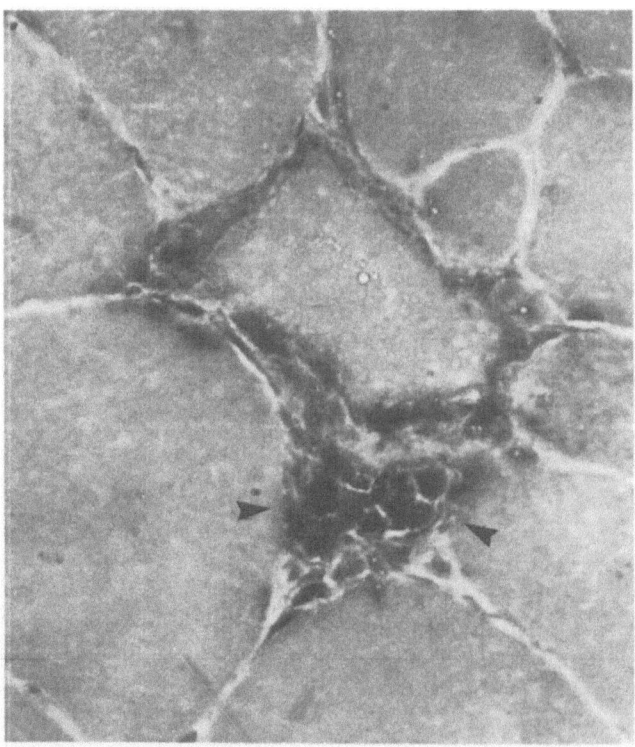

Fig. 8-4. Coagulation necrosis of a muscle fiber and invasion by macrophages (M): 21-year-old woman, necrotizing myositis; biceps (×8,288).

Fig. 8-5. A small necrotic muscle fiber (arrows) is filled with macrophages rich in acid phosphatase: 23-year-old woman, clinically affected carrier of Duchenne's muscular dystrophy; biceps (×575).

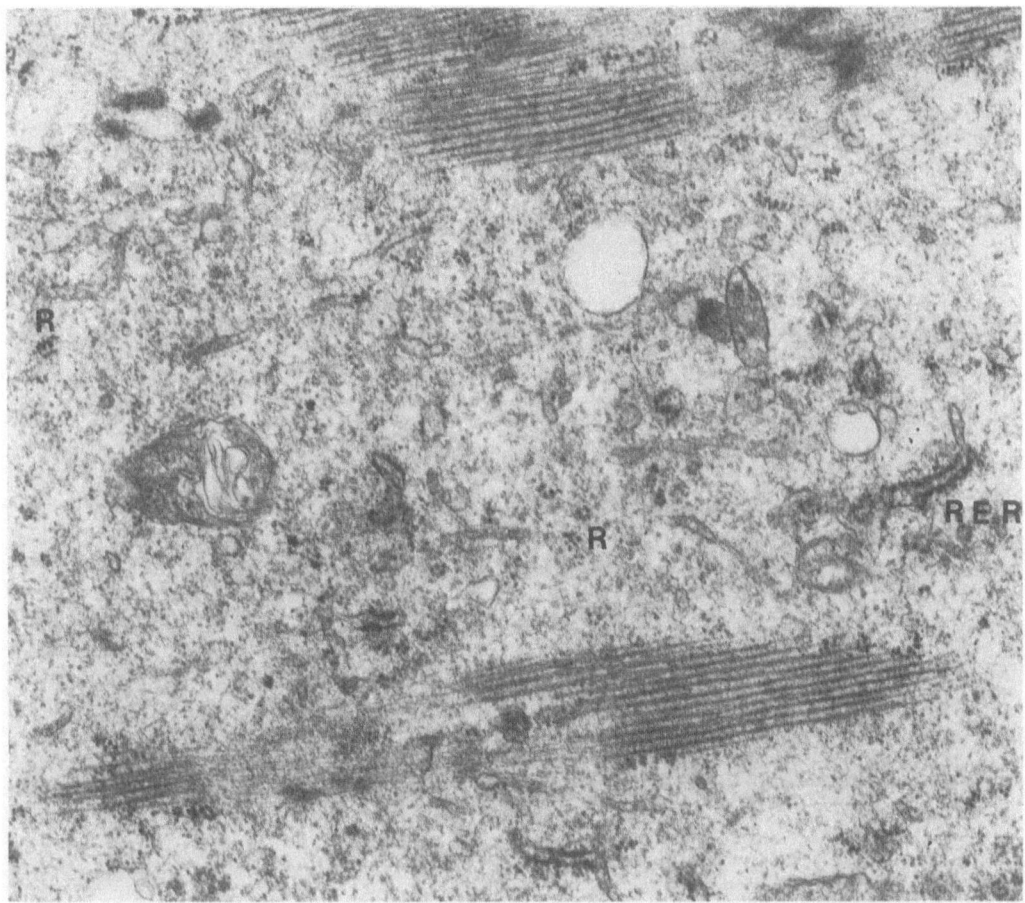

Fig. 8-6. Ribosomes (R) and rough endoplasmic reticulum (RER) are present in a regenerating fiber: 21-year-old woman, necrotizing myositis; biceps. Same biopsy as in Fig. 8-4 (×34,100).

material surrounded by a halo of fine filaments (Fig. 8-11), representing intermediate desmin filaments of 8–10 nm (Table 8-6) as demonstrated by immunofluorescent studies. They are often nonspecific and seen in congenital myopathy.[106] The filamentous body is a subsarcolemmal, usually single, inclusion consisting of fine, densely packed filaments (Table 8-6; Fig. 8-12). Transitional stages between filamentous and cytoplasmic bodies may exist.[106] The zebra body (Fig. 8-13) or leptomere is a small subsarcolemmal inclusion, in which dense areas alternate with fine filaments arranged in parallel. Zebra bodies are prominent in zebra body myopathy and in extraocular muscle fibers.[145]

Concentrically arranged lamellae in *concentric laminated bodies* occur in clusters at the periphery of muscle fibers (Fig. 8-14). They are a nonspecific feature of various neuromuscular disorders, including Marfan's syndrome[102] among other conditions.[95] Concentric laminated bodies resemble mitochondria, from which they were thought to derive; instead, they seem to be peculiar membranes (Table 8-6) of unkown origin.

Strong reactions in both NADH and MAG preparations, as well as other oxidative enzyme preparations, are typical of aggregates of abnormal mitochondria. Such clusters of mitochondria give the light-microscopic feature of "ragged red fibers" (Fig. 8-15),

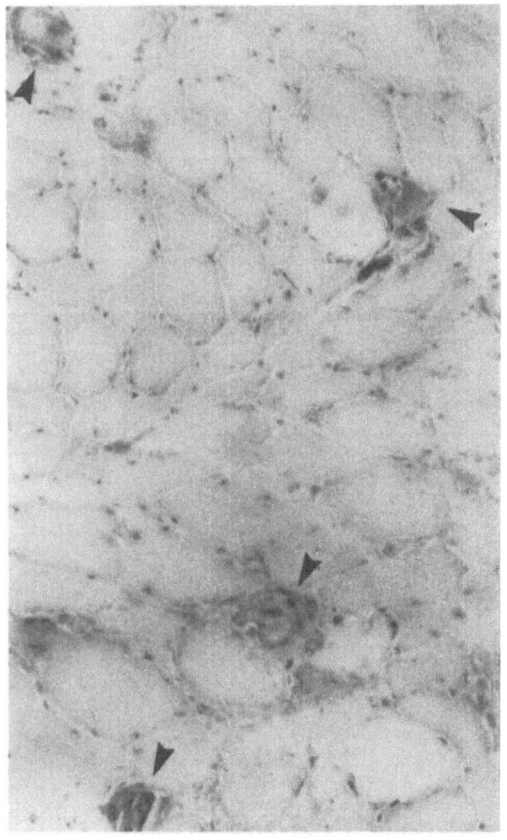

Fig. 8-7. A few small muscle fibers stain intensely with Azure-B (arrows) indicating regeneration. 66-year-old woman, necrotizing myopathy; biceps (×164).

which are clearly seen in myoadenylate deaminase preparations (Fig. 8-16). Skeletal muscle mitochondria are uniform compared to hepatic and cardiac mitochondria. Abnormal mitochondria may occur rarely and nonspecifically in various neuromuscular diseases, occasionally in polymyalgia rheumatica, oculopharyngeal muscular dystrophy, and regularly in the mitochondrial myopathies. Mitochondrial abnormalities involve increases in the number and size of mitochondria as well as in structural changes. Increased formation of cristae may result in densely packed cristae frequently arranged

Table 8-5.
Inclusion Bodies in Muscle Fibers

Nemaline bodies	Filamentous bodies
Zebra bodies	Tubular aggregates
Fingerprint bodies	Abnormally structured
Spheroid bodies	mitochondria
Cytoplasmic bodies	Concentric laminated
Reducing bodies	bodies
Sarcoplasmic bodies	Cylindrical spiral bodies
	Mallory body-like inclusions

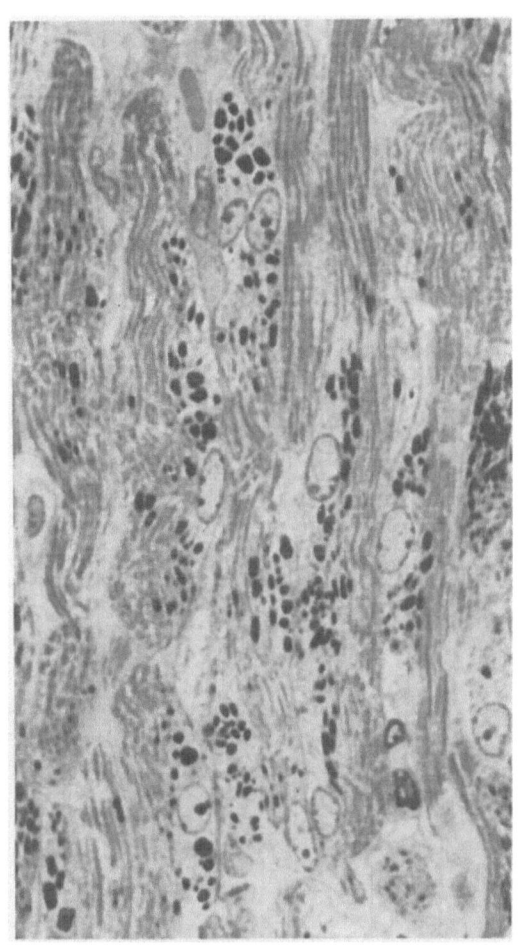

Fig. 8-8. Numerous muscle fibers are filled with small, dark, round or spindle-shaped rods or nemaline bodies: 18-month-old girl, nemaline myopathy; quadriceps. (Toluidine-blue-stained, 1-μm-thick, resin-embedded section; ×864).

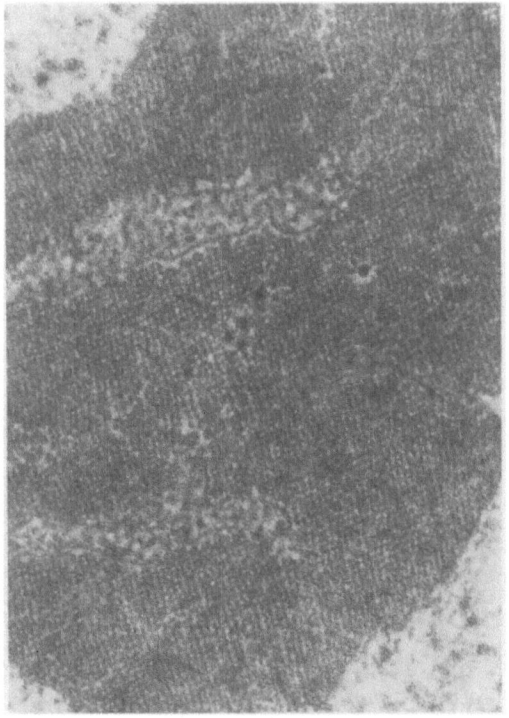

Fig. 8-9. A rod shows the typical lattice pattern of the Z-disk. Same biopsy as in Fig. 8-8. (×106,-750).

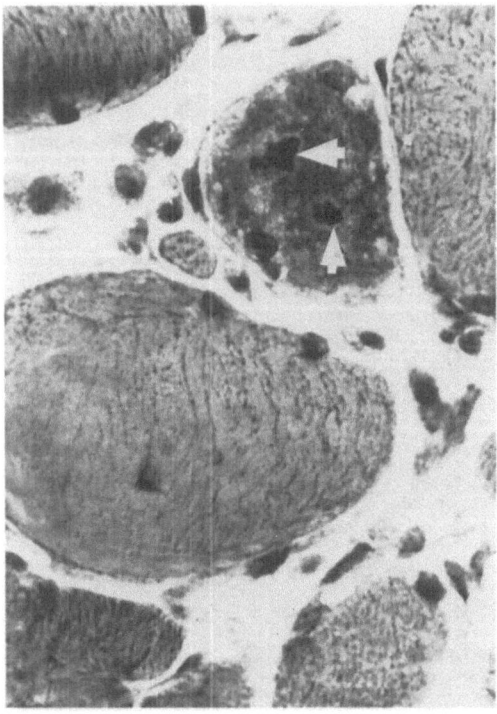

Fig. 8-10. A muscle fiber contains two cytoplasmic bodies (arrows): 38-year-old man, adult-type acid-maltase deficiency; quadriceps. (Modified trichrome; ×600).

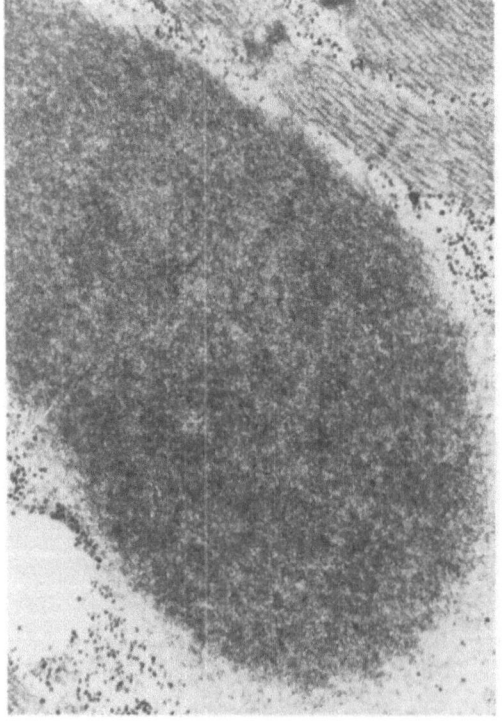

Fig. 8-11. A cytoplasmic body consists of an electron-dense core and a light halo: 15-year-old girl, cytoplasmic body myopathy; quadriceps (×25,600).

Table 8-6.
"Filaments" in Muscle Fibers

Thin myofilaments	6 nm	Sarcomeres
Thick myofilaments	16 nm	Sarcomeres
Intermediate/desmin (skeletin) filaments	8–10 nm	Cytoplasmic bodies (halo), Mallory body-like inclusions Sarcoplasmic bodies
Serrated filaments	14–16.5 nm	Mallory body-like inclusions
Marginal fine filaments	6–8 nm	Mallory body-like inclusions
Cytoplasmic and intranuclear tubular filaments	15–18 nm	Inclusion body myositis
Intranuclear filaments	8.5 nm	Oculopharyngeal muscular dystrophy
Filaments	8–15 nm	Filamentous bodies
Filaments	12–15 nm 15–20 nm	Spheroid bodies
Lamellae	6.5–16 nm	Fingerprint bodies
Lamellae	8 nm	Concentric laminated bodies

circularly or semicircularly (Fig. 8-17A), or intrinsic cristae may be largely absent. Spheroid inclusions of different electron densities, and crystal inclusions thought to derive from excessive crista formation,[199] are characteristic features (Fig. 8-17B). Crystalline inclusions have now been classed as types I and II, the former appearing in type I fibers and located within the intracristal space, the latter in type II myofibers and located between the internal and external mitochondrial membranes.[87]

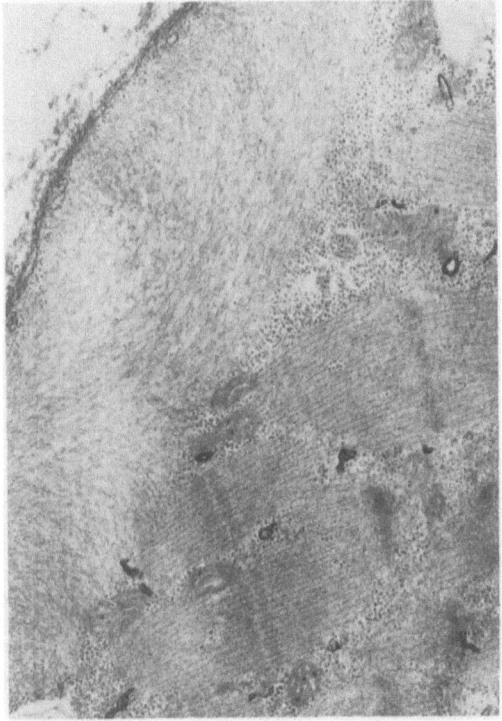

Fig. 8-12. A filamentous body, located beneath the sarcolemma, consists of fine filaments only: 6-month-old boy, generalized hypotonia; quadriceps (×22,178).

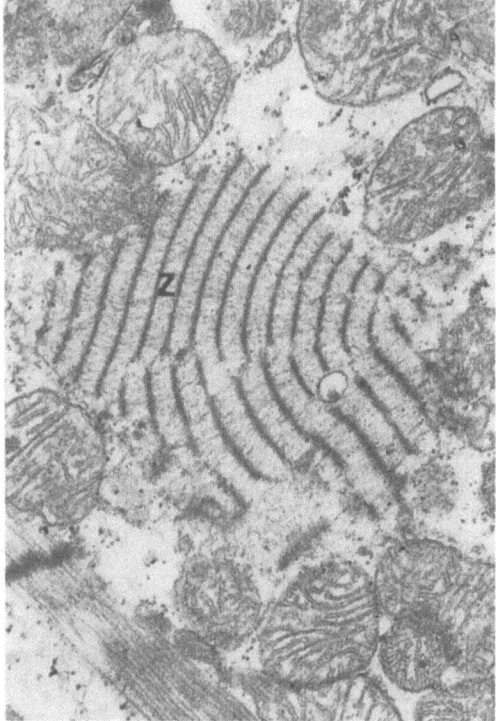

Fig. 8-13. A zebra body (Z) is located among numerous mitochondria in an extraocular muscle fiber. Neuronal ceroid-lipofuscinosis (×23,030).

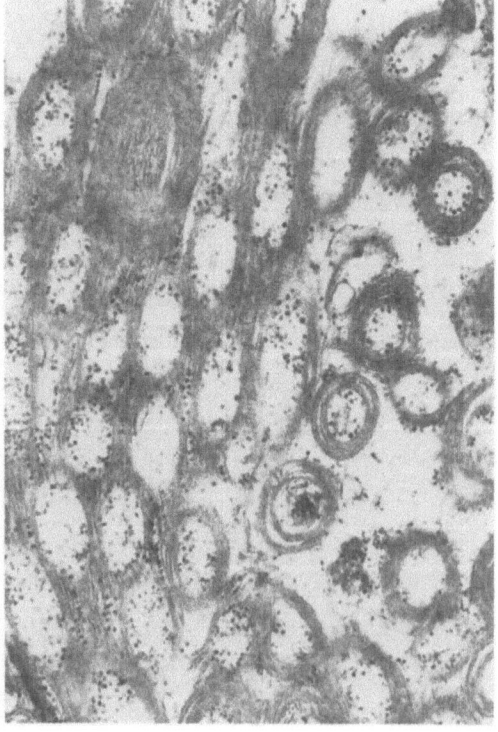

Fig. 8-14. Numerous concentric laminated bodies are cut in cross section or obliquely and consist of serrated lamellae: 20-year-old man, mitochondrial myopathy; gastrocnemius. These concentric laminated bodies are not the equivalent of abnormal mitochondria (×19,200).

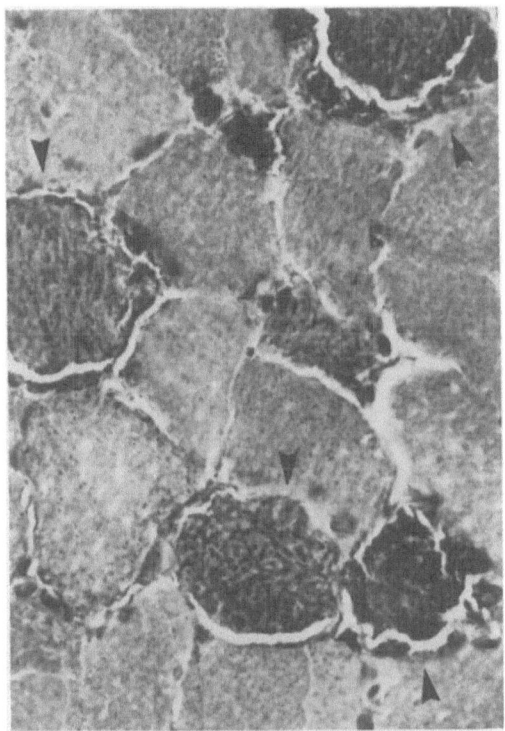

Fig. 8-15. There are several "ragged red fibers" (arrows) in this muscle: 35-year-old woman, oculocraniosomatic syndrome; quadriceps, postmortem. A daughter had the same disease. (Modified trichrome; ×275).

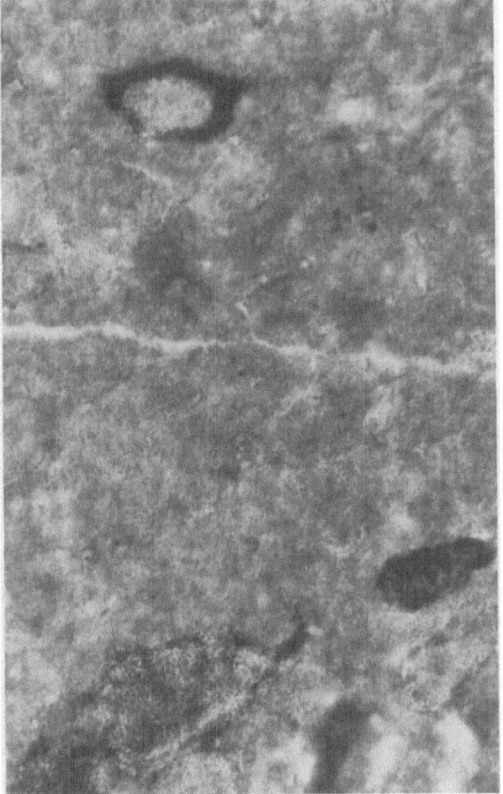

Fig. 8-16. "Ragged red fibers" are prominent in the myoadenylate deaminase preparation. Same muscle as in Fig. 8-15 (×275).

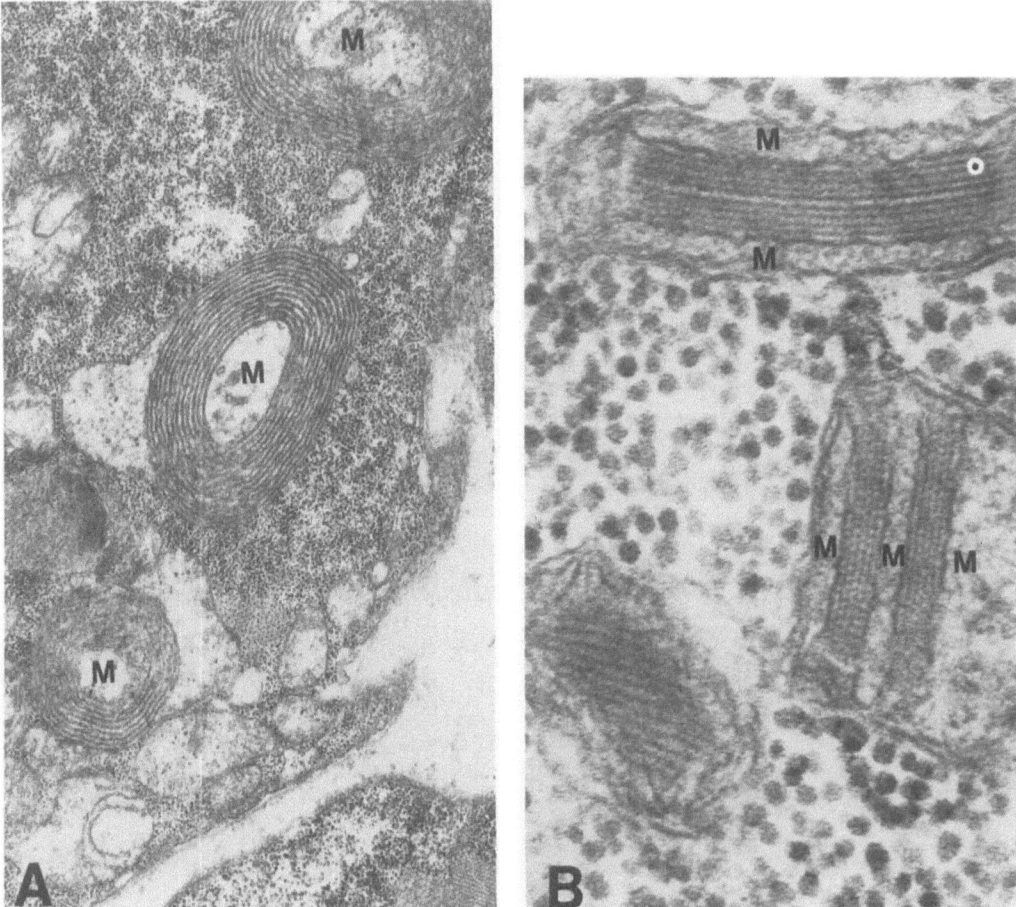

Fig. 8-17. (A) Abnormal mitochondria (M) show circular cristae: 2-month-old boy, mitochondrial myopathy and lactic acidosis; quadriceps (×17,682). (B) Several mitochondria contain crystal inclusions located in the intracristal space outside the mitochondrial matrix (M): 61-year-old man, mitochondrial myopathy; quadriceps (×140,700).

Tubular aggregates (Fig. 8-18) are densely packed, long hollow tubes frequently occurring in cases of periodic paralysis, in congenital myotonia,[188] and in a congenital myopathy associated with tubular aggregates.[161] These tubular aggregates (Fig. 8-19A) are marked by a strong reaction in the NADH preparation (Fig. 8-19B), but a negative reaction in the MAG preparation (Fig. 8-19C). They probably derive from the sarcoplasmic reticulum.

Proliferation of T-tubules may result in honeycomb structures more clearly visualized by using lanthanum, an electron-dense marker that enters the muscle fiber through the T-tubules (Fig. 8-20).

Abnormalities of sarcoplasmic reticulum–T-tubule junctions, normally appearing as triads, may be encountered as dyads, pentads, or heptads. They may be a reliable marker of highly atrophic or immature muscle fibers lacking myofilaments arranged in sarcomeres.

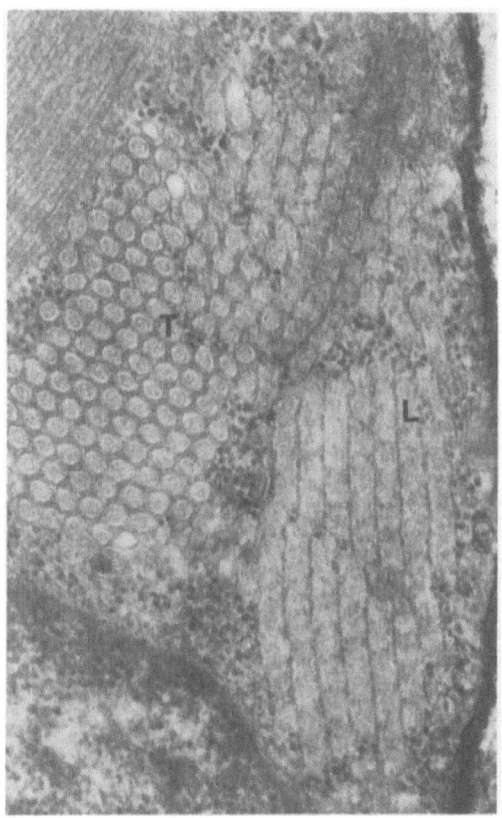

Fig. 8-18. Aggregates of tubules cut longitudinally (L) and transversely (T) beneath the sarcolemma: 8-year-old boy, congenital myotonia; quadriceps (×49,680).

Some inclusions, seen by light microscopy but better defined by electron microscopy, are features of specific "structured" congenital myopathies, such as cylindrical spirals,[26] granulofilamentous material,[86] or reducing bodies.[35]

Vacuoles

Vacuolation is a nondescript feature of several neuromuscular disorders. Such vacuoles may be derived from lysosomes exhibiting activity of acid phosphatase (Fig. 8-21) or from severely enlarged terminal sacs of the sarcoplasmic reticulum (Fig. 8-22) often seen in periodic paralysis. Circumscribed fiber splitting may also surround a vacuolar space. The precise origin of vacuoles in polymyositis has not been determined. Lipid droplets, when extracted by the embedding procedure, may appear as vacuoles although a fat-specific stain (e.g., oil red O) reveals their lipid nature. Ice crystal artifacts and severely swollen mitochondria may mimic vacuoles. The "rimmed vacuole" (Fig. 8-23A) is another nonspecific feature particularly seen in cases of inclusion body myositis,[42] oculopharyngeal muscular dystrophy,[68] distal myopathy,[165] and other neuromuscular disorders. These "rimmed" vacuoles have only scant acid phosphatase activity; they may represent autophagocytotic vacuoles. Electron microscopically (Fig. 8-23B), rimmed vacuoles show characteristic whorls of membranes, debris, and sometimes remnants of cell constituents. As glycogen accumulates within lysosomes in type II glycogenosis,

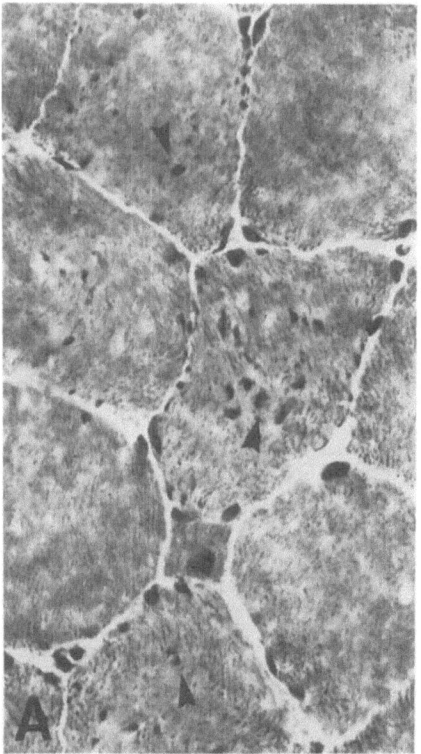

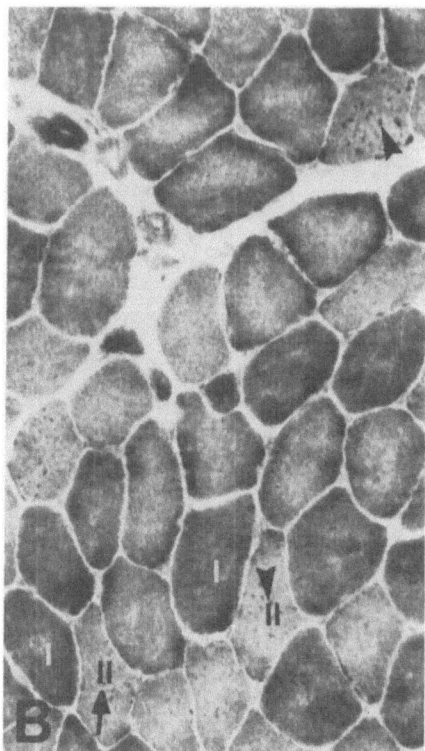

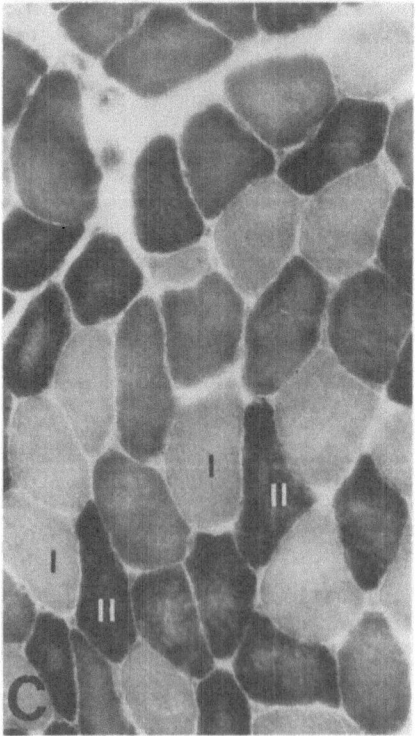

Fig. 8-19. (A) Numerous dots within muscle fibers (arrows) represent tubular aggregates: 8-year-old boy, congenital myotonia; quadriceps. (Modified trichrome; ×470). (B) The tubular aggregates are present in type II (light) fibers and give a positive reaction (arrows). Same biopsy as in Fig. 8-18A. (NADH reaction. ×160). (C) Serial sections to Fig. 8-19B do not show reaction of tubular aggregates in the respective type II fibers. (MAG preparation; ×160).

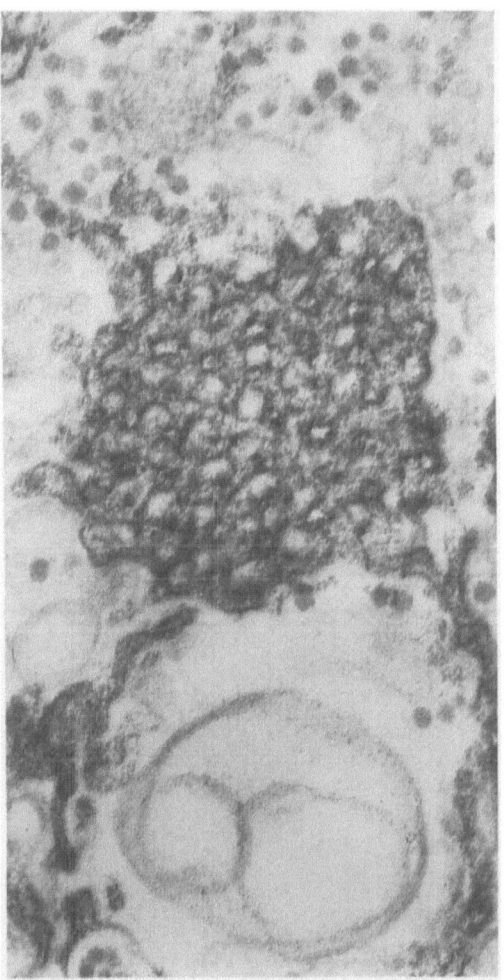

Fig. 8-20. A honeycomb structure representing proliferated T-tubules is in greater contrast when using
lanthanum: 6-month-old boy, generalized hypotonia; quadriceps (×128,100).

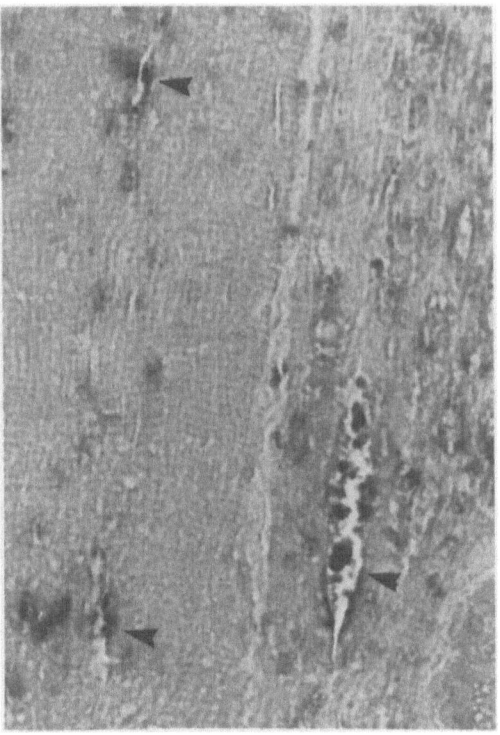

Fig. 8-21. Small vacuoles (arrows) within myofibers
exhibit acid phosphatase activity: 37-year-old
man, adult acid maltase deficiency; quadriceps
(×720).

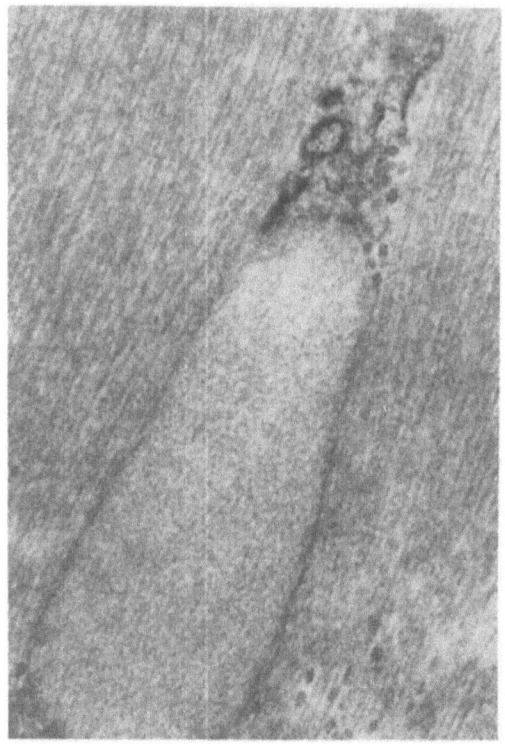

Fig. 8-22. Enlarged terminal sac of the sarcoplasmic reticulum, a vacuole by light microscopy: 18-year-old woman, hypokalemic periodic paralysis; gastrocnemius (×81,200).

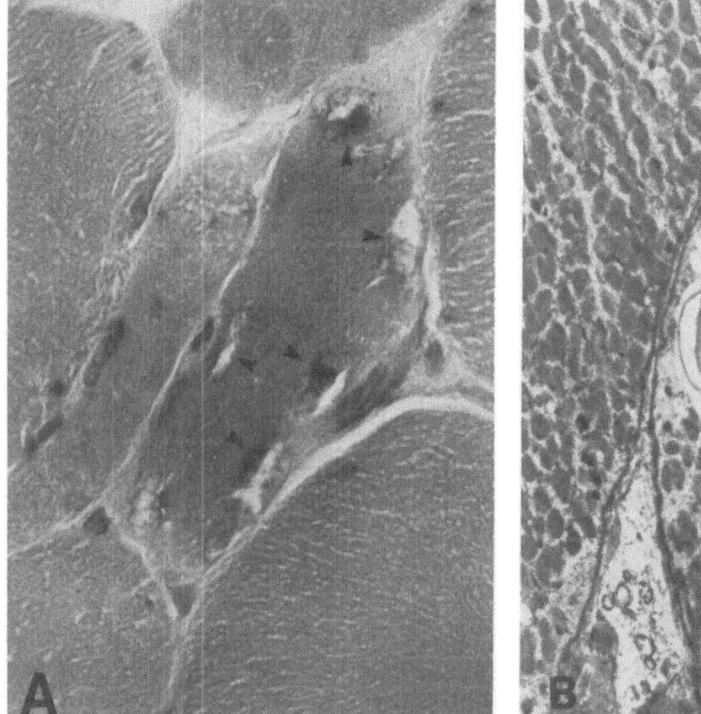

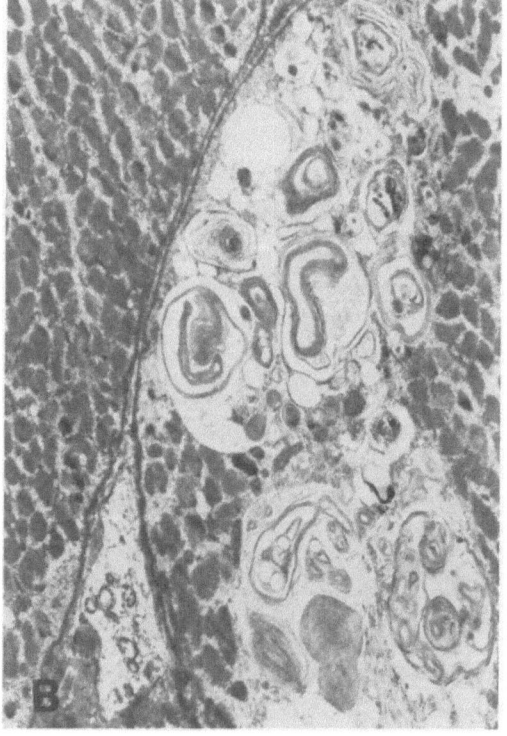

Fig. 8-23. (A) A centrally located muscle fiber contains several "rimmed vacuoles" exhibiting minimal marginal acid phosphatase activity: 47-year-old woman; biceps (×600). (B) A "rimmed" vacuole consists of many membranous whorls and a vacuolar space, sharply separated from surrounding sarcomeres. Same biopsy as Fig. 8-23A (×5,630).

vacuolation of myofibers may be present in muscle specimens, partly related to the lysosomal compartment (Fig. 8-24), partly due to autophagocytosis as seen in "rimmed" vacuoles, or occurring after preparative removal of excessive cytoplasmic glycogen, particularly in the glycogenoses.

Abnormal Myofilaments and Sarcomeres

Using light microscopy, abnormalities of the sarcomeres may be encountered as "target" fibers, "cores" or "core-targetoid" features, as well as a loss of cross-striation; the changes occur largely in type I fibers and are best seen in NADH preparations. Target fibers have single, central substrate defects in the NADH preparation, surrounded by a round margin of increased substrate and peripherally by regular features of the muscle fiber (Figs. 8-25A–C). In core-targetoid fibers (Fig. 8-25B), only the central zone of deficient substrate is present. Cores and targets may be present in many successive sarcomeres, although probably not through the entire length of the fiber. Target fibers are thought to indicate denervation or reinnervation. They may occur together with targetoid fibers (Fig. 8-25B).

Electron microscopically, substrate-deficient central areas of core myofibers lack mitochondria and sarcoplasmic reticulum. Sarcomeres are in considerable disarray, the so-called unstructured cores. Multi- or mini-cores or focal loss of cross-striation have a similar appearance, though many occur within a muscle fiber. More subtle changes of the sarcomeres may be seen, such as "streaming" or "smearing" of the Z-disk (Fig. 8-26), a nonspecific feature frequently located close to adjacent capillaries. In addition,

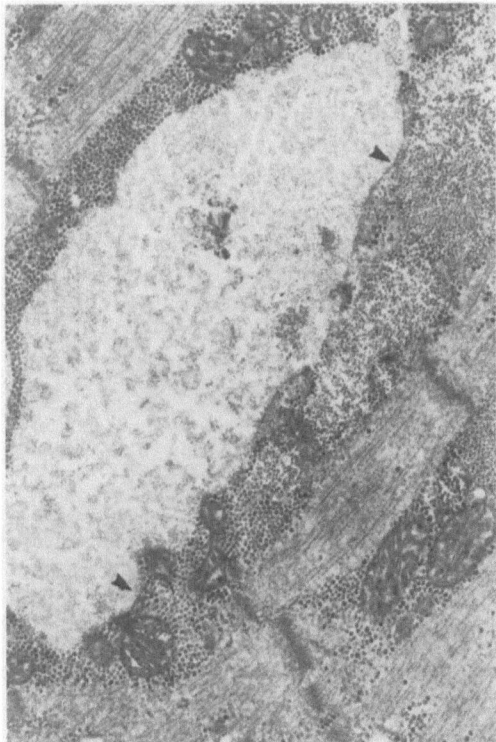

Fig. 8-24. A membrane bound (arrows) lysosomal vacuole filled with glycogen, 1-month-old boy, infantile acid maltase deficiency (Pompe's disease); quadriceps (×18,400).

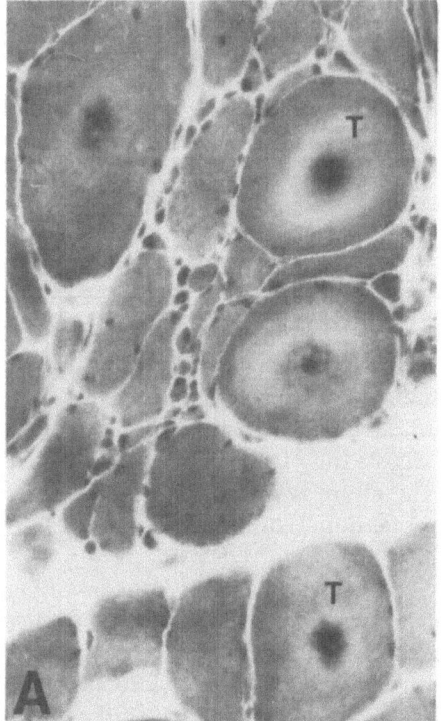

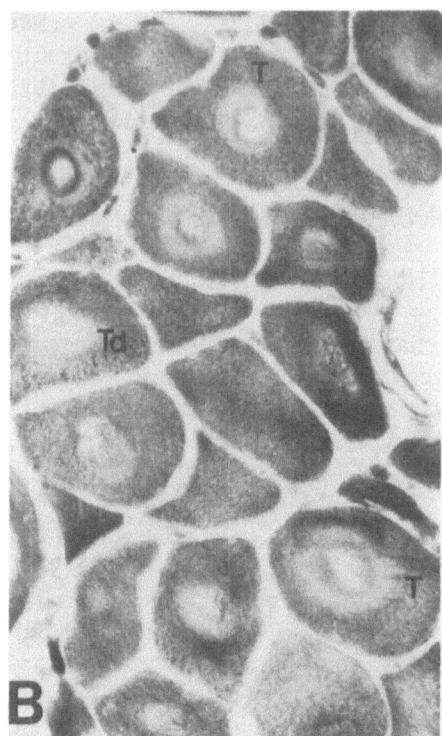

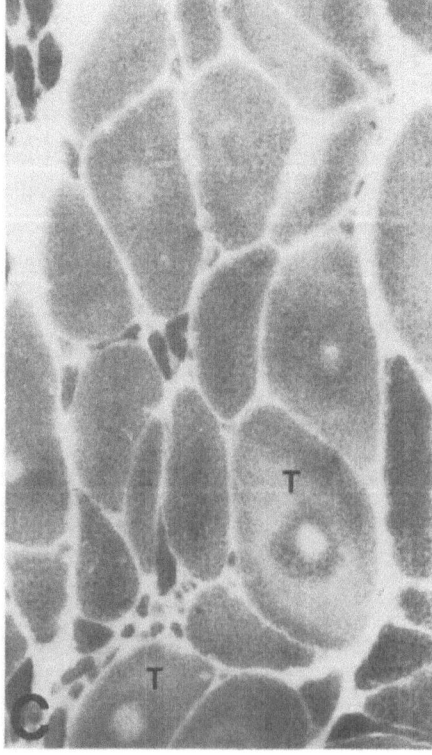

Fig. 8-25. Target (T) fibers are of type I and consist of three zones in the NADH preparation; targetoids (Td) are substrate-free areas: 21-year old man, neurogenic atrophy; gastrocnemius. [(A) modified trichrome, ×250; (B) NADH preparation, ×200; (C) ATPase preparation (pH 10.4), ×228.]

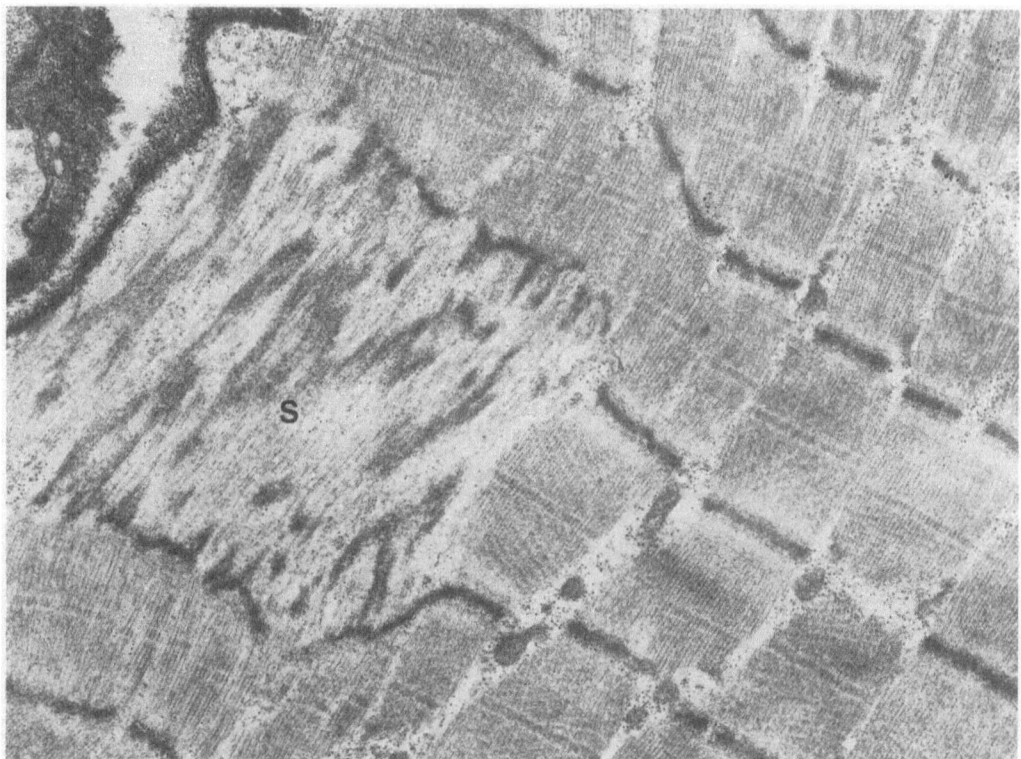

Fig. 8-26. A sarcomere (S) shows "streaming" or "smearing" of the Z-disk: 72-year-old woman, polymyalgia rheumatica; deltoid (×16,768).

zigzag appearance of Z-disks or circumscribed enlargement of Z-disks may be an early stage of rod body formation. Selective loss of myosin has been observed in a case of congenital myopathy[212] and in infantile neurogenic atrophy.[101] Ringbinden are myofibrils running perpendicular to the long axis of the muscle fiber, chiefly beneath the sarcolemma. Sarcoplasmic masses are subsarcolemmal zones largely devoid of any fibrils, but replete with sarcoplasm, organelles, and glycogen. Both features are typical of late dystrophic myotonia.

Cellular constituents fueling the energy process, glycogen and fat, may be increased within myofibers. Glycogen may accrue either in the cytoplasm or within lysosomes in several glycogenoses. Cytoplasmic glycogen may also accumulate in atrophic muscle fibers. Lipid droplets may increase in lipid myopathies but also as a nonspecific, probably reversible phenomenon. A decrease of glycogen and lipid droplets may be difficult to ascertain and is of little diagnostic significance.

Nuclei

Nuclei are located in the periphery of the mature muscle fiber and are small. Internal nuclei in as many as 3% of myofibers are regarded as normal.[57,68] The number of nuclei per unit of muscle fiber volume may increase in muscle atrophy, but these nuclei are still in the periphery. Increase in the number of internal nuclei occurs in various muscular disorders, especially dystrophic myotonia, and is usually regarded as a myopathic feature, though it may also occur in chronic peripheral neuropathy of Charcot–Marie–Tooth.[68] Muscle fibers may be large and vesicular, as in regenerating muscle fibers, or large as in centronuclear myopathy. Intranuclear inclusions are rare. They may, by electron microscopy, represent cytoplasmic invaginations or genuine inclusions, usually filaments. Filaments of 15–18 nm in diameter occur in inclusion body myositis; 8.5 nm filaments are typical of oculopharyngeal muscular dystrophy (Table 8-6).

Interstitial Lesions

Interstitial changes among muscle fibers include endomysial fibrosis, aggregates of inflammatory cells, intramuscular nerve twigs depleted of myelinated axons, and abnormal vessels. The endomysium is usually thicker in endplate regions. Otherwise, endomysial fibrosis is indicative of chronic myopathy. Inflammatory cells may surround degenerating or necrotic muscle fibers in muscular dystrophies and necrotizing myopathies, such as rhabdomyolysis, and then they may be nonspecific, or a primary lesion as in various forms of myositis. Such inflammatory aggregates may be rare or they may abound. In myositis, they are often found in the perimysium, around vessels, or even within walls of larger veins and arteries. Lymphocytes, histiocytes, mononuclear cells, and macrophages (the latter confirmed by their acid phosphatase activity) may compose inflammatory aggregates, and are classifiable as immunohistochemical by respective antibodies.[2,5,78] Granulomas also contain epitheloid cells and multinucleated giant cells, some also rich in acid phosphatase.

Apart from inflammation, changes in intramuscular capillaries are subtle. Necrosis and regeneration of capillary endothelium are characteristic of dermatomyositis. Loops of thickened capillary basement membranes may indicate necrosis, removal, and regeneration of the capillary. Undulating tubules within membrane-bound compartments are also seen in endothelial cells of dermatomyositis. Thick basement membranes may be a nonspecific feature encountered in many neuromuscular diseases as well as in metabolic disorders, but they are especially prominent in cases of diabetes mellitus (Table 8-7). A peculiar feature of interstitial lesions is when one or two capillaries inside a usually hypertrophic muscle fiber are found, which most frequently occurs in the gastrocnemius muscle and is associated with considerable variation in muscle fiber diameters and other nonspecific myopathic features. It is seen especially in Becker's muscular dystrophy

Table 8-7.
Increased Thickness of Capillary Basement Membrane

Aging	Sclerodema
Diabetes mellitus	Chronic alcoholism
Myxedema	Cardiomyopathy and
Familial hypercholester-	congestive heart failure
inemia	Polymyositis
Gout	Obstructive angiopathy
Lupus erythematosus	

and is frequently associated with myalgia. Internalized capillaries conceivably were formed during the process of myofibers splitting and/or fusion.

Intramuscular nerve twigs are normally densely packed with myelinated axons, except in the distant segments close to motor endplates. Loss of myelinated axons and subsequent endoneurial fibrosis may be recognized in neurogenic neuromuscular diseases, but the presence of fairly normal intramuscular nerve twigs does not exclude a neurogenic process.

The muscle spindle undergoes few and nonspecific changes in human neuromuscular disorders. Thickening of capsules has been seen in myositis. An increased number of intrafusal fibers, probably related to splitting, has sometimes occurred in dystrophic myotonia. The scarcity and small size of both the intrafusal fiber and the entire spindle make the systematic evaluation of these structures difficult. Neurogenic atrophy of extrafusal fibers is not associated with atrophy of intrafusal fibers, but precise data are lacking on the state of innervation of intrafusal fibers in denervated human muscle.

Artifacts

Ice crystal holes may form either because of prolonged and slow freezing of the muscle biopsy or because of refreezing. The crystals may distort the contours of muscle fibers preventing accurate morphometry and some enzyme-histochemical reactions, but usually they do not disturb fiber typing. Ice crystal clefts are not reversible.

Hyaline or opaque muscle fibers, a frequent finding in Duchenne muscular dystrophy, have been regarded as artificial but diagnostic changes. They may also occur, albeit less often, in other neuromuscular diseases.

Depletion of glycogen and decreased activity of amylophosphorylase may be related to delayed time processing and early autolysis. Phosphorylase activity is usually absent from autopsy specimens. Drying of muscle fibers may result in the appearance of large areas that stain red in modified trichrome preparations. Transporting muscle specimens in either watery or saline fluids may result in a swelling and separation of muscle fibers that sometimes resembles liquefaction.

For diagnostic purposes, the numerous features of muscle diseases have been patterned in bar graphs[68] for individual neuromuscular disorders. These bar graphs outline the characteristic (though not pathognomonic) patterns of various neuromuscular disorders, such as individual muscular dystrophies, and various forms of neurogenic atrophy. They may represent the pathologic patterns among several patients with the same neuromuscular disorder. They do not always provide the morphologic abnormalities required to diagnose an individual's condition.

Classification of Neuromuscular Disorders

Classification of neuromuscular disorders on purely morphologic grounds is not reliable. Necrotizing myopathy, vacuolar myopathy, or mitochondrial myopathy would be typical morphologic diagnoses, but these are nonspecific and would not consistently help the clinician to integrate the biopsy findings with the clinical problem. Muscle fiber necrosis may occur in metabolic myopathies, myositis, muscular dystrophies, and ischemia. Vacuoles within muscle fibers may occur in glycogenoses, periodic paralyses, chloroquine myopathy, and polymyositis. Formulating a morphologic diagnosis of a muscle specimen according to the World Federation of Neurology classification, however, is impractical. Neuromuscular diseases and the lesions should therefore be tabulated into simple categories.

The diagnostic structural changes of these eight classes of neuromuscular disorders will now be considered.

Muscular Dystrophies

The morphologic range of the muscular dystrophies (MD) is nonspecific. The various forms are classified according to clinical and genetic criteria. Generally, necrosis and regeneration are associated with chronic myopathy as well as atrophy and hypertrophy of muscle fibers, rounding of the contour of individual muscle fibers, an increase in internally located nuclei, endomysial fibrosis, and often, abnormalities in enzyme-histochemical preparations. The structural alterations are not pathognomonic for either the group of MD or any particular clinical form. Some instances, however, have characteristic features. The morphologic diagnosis should always be made in correlation with the clinical data.

Duchenne's Muscular Dystrophy (DMD)

This x-linked, recessively inherited, progressive, and fatal muscular dystrophy is accompanied by morphologic muscle abnormalities even in a preclinical state[169] (Fig. 8-27A). The characteristic lesions include groups of necrotic, phagocytosed, or regenerating muscle fibers. Necrosis of muscle fibers is segmental. Regeneration probably occurs from satellite cells of muscle fibers.

Opaque or hyaline muscle fibers may also abound (Fig. 8-27B). Calcium may be present in abnormally high concentrations within myofibers as demonstrated by calcium-specific stains, such as alizarin red or other dyes.[21] Small regenerating fibers often display increased activity of alkaline phosphatase (Fig. 8-27C), an enzyme that is histochemically inactive in normal, fetal, and nonregenerating diseased muscle fibers. Type I fibers may predominate and type IIB fibers may be absent.

Fiber typing may be difficult in alkaline ATPase preparations but it is more easily made in acid ATPase preparations. Single or small regenerating fibers or groups are often of type IIC.[166] Inflammatory cells are scant and usually confined to necrotic and phagocytosed muscle fibers. Morphometric evaluation of the intramuscular vascular network does not support the concept of quantitative deficiencies in the microcirculation.[126] Electron microscopy does not contribute to the diagnosis of DMD, but it has provided data on changes of plasma membranes, necrosis, and regeneration, as well as on methods of phagocytosis and nonspecific structural abnormalities.

Later in the course of the disease, muscle fibers disappear, endomysial fibrosis and intrafascicular fat cells increase, finally resulting in "end-stage myopathy." Replacement of muscle fibers by connective tissue and adipose cells may be so extensive that recognizing the remaining muscle fibers may be difficult. Small muscle fibers preserve ATPase activity for a long time, aiding in their identification as myofibers.

The association of chronic myopathy with repetitive necrosis and regeneration of muscle fibers, often in small groups, is the typical and most widely observed morphologic expression of DMD. These abnormalities are not found in muscle biopsies from DMD

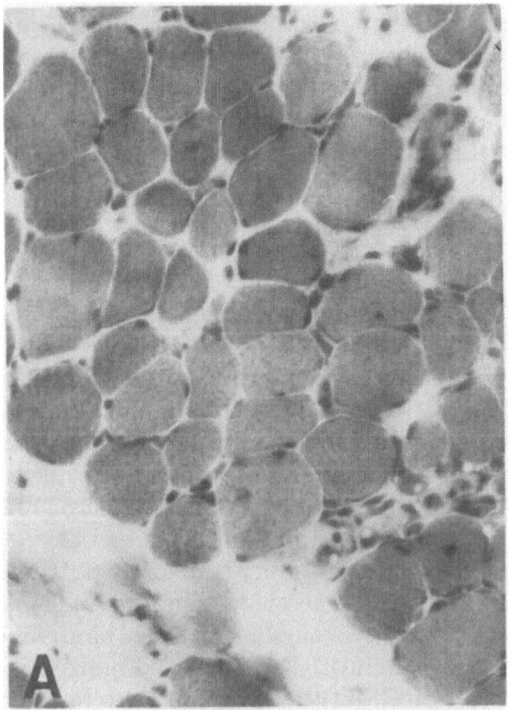
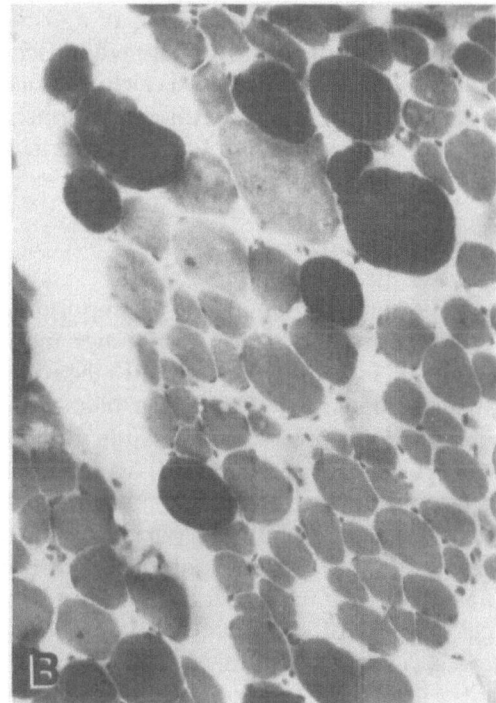
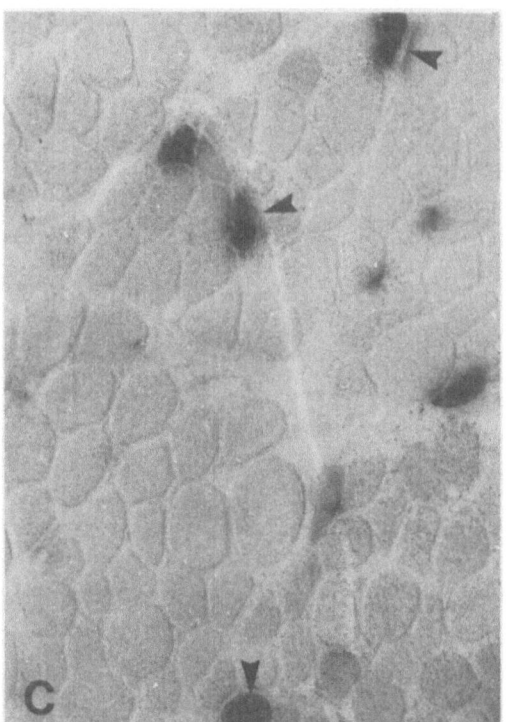

Fig. 8-27. Duchenne's muscular dystrophy in a 3-year-old boy, CK 6760 U/l; quadriceps. (A) Chronic myopathy with rounding of muscle fibers, numerical increase of internal nuclei. (Modified trichrome; ×230). (B) Numerous opaque fibers (Modified trichrome; ×172). (C) Disseminated small muscle fibers positive of alkaline phosphatase activity (arrows) (×184).

patients at or before 2 months of age.[29] The prenatal morphologic diagnosis of DMD is therefore difficult, especially when ischemic (autolytic) changes in muscles of aborted fetuses are added. Increased calcium concentration,[72] enlarged myofiber diameters,[202,211] and subtle myofiber alterations demonstrable by electron microscopy[204] have been described in instances of presumed (at risk) fetal DMD muscle specimens.

Carriers of DMD

Carrier detection in DMD is important for genetic counseling. Though CK determination remains the crucial test, other methods to identify DMD carriers have been attempted, including clinical and electromyographic examinations and muscle biopsies. In most instances the muscle biopsy in DMD carriers is normal; the abnormalities described in a few patients include individual necrotic muscle fibers, nonspecific myopathy (Fig. 8-28), focal lesions, variation in fiber diameter, increase in internal nuclei, and endomysial fibrosis,[154] as well as subtle histochemical and ultrastructural abnormalities.[157,162,182] Hypertrophy of muscle fibers and numerical increase of type I fibers may also be encountered in carriers. Systematic light-microscopic quantitation, including enzyme histochemistry, has been strongly recommended when studying muscle biopsies of presumed or definite DMD carriers.[151] Evaluation of such borderline cases, however, requires adequate control biopsies. Similarly, the reported nonspecific ultrastructural alterations of muscle specimens from DMD carriers should also be interpreted with caution and not be used alone to identify a DMD carrier.[52] There are rare instances of women afflicted with a DMD-like neuromuscular disorder.[63,156] They are

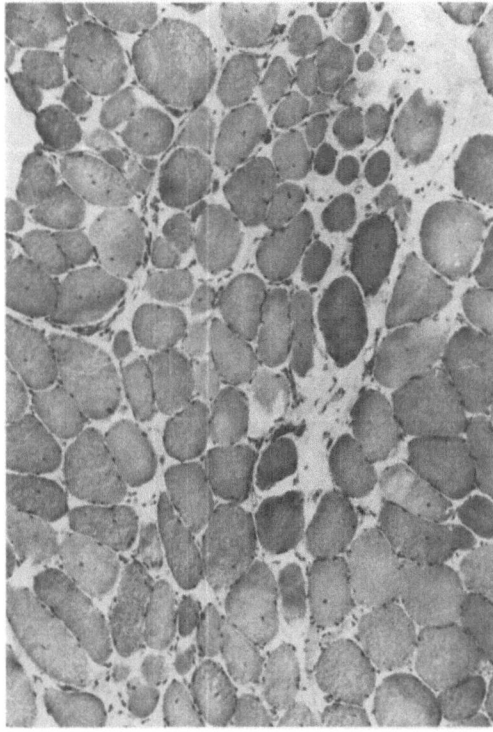

Fig. 8-28. Nonspecific myopathy, marked by a rounding of muscle fibers, and numerical increase of internal nuclei: 27-year-old carrier of Duchenne muscular dystrophy; quadriceps. (PAS; ×69).

either female carriers of DMD with clinical and morphologic expression of the DMD trait, possibly related to extensive inactivation of the paternal normal X-chromosome,[156] or patients afflicted with a severe form of autosomal-recessive limb-girdle dystrophy.

Becker's Muscular Dystrophy (BMD)

This form of muscular dystrophy[12] also has an X-linked recessive mode of inheritance, but the clinical course is protracted and the clinical expression is late. Muscle abnormalities in young boys may be similar to those of DMD;[68,176] muscle tissues obtained later in life show a chronic myopathy[105] in which type IIB fibers are present[105] and myofibers are split.[30,176] Pyknotic nuclear clumps[30,105] and small angulated fibers[105] are features of BMD. Some findings have been interpreted as being neurogenic.[30] Ultrastructural alterations are nonspecific. The differential diagnosis includes DMD, juvenile spinal muscular atrophy, and limb-girdle dystrophy. These entities may be difficult to separate from one another on morphologic grounds alone.

The recent dramatic molecular genetic results concerning the localization of the DMD (and BMD) gene and dystrophin (Fig. 8-29), which is absent in DMD and altered or reduced in BMD, may revolutionize the diagnostic regimen, including muscle biopsy and muscle morphology in these two types of muscular dystrophy and in DMD and BMD prenatal and carrier detection.

From DMD and BMD, an autosomal recessive form of muscular dystrophy has been separated[16,96] that is not as severe as DMD but may be marked by highly elevated CK and groups of necrotic and/or regenerating myofibers within an otherwise little myopathic background.

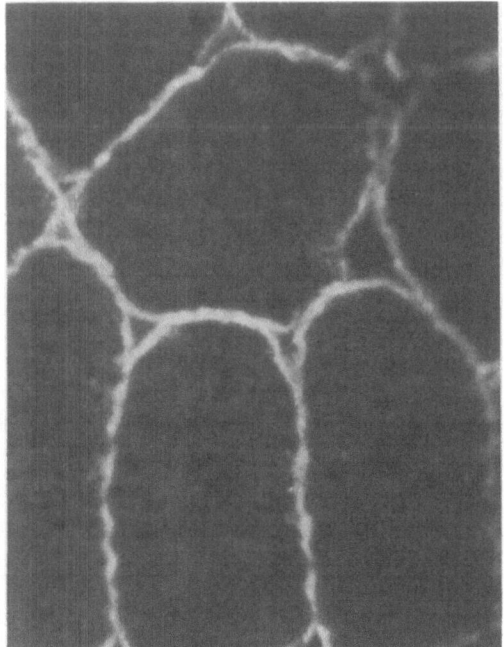

Fig. 8-29. Enlarged fiber diameter spectrum and multiple internal nuclei indicate myopathic features: 22-year-old man, Becker's muscular dystrophy; biceps. (Modified trichrome; ×164).

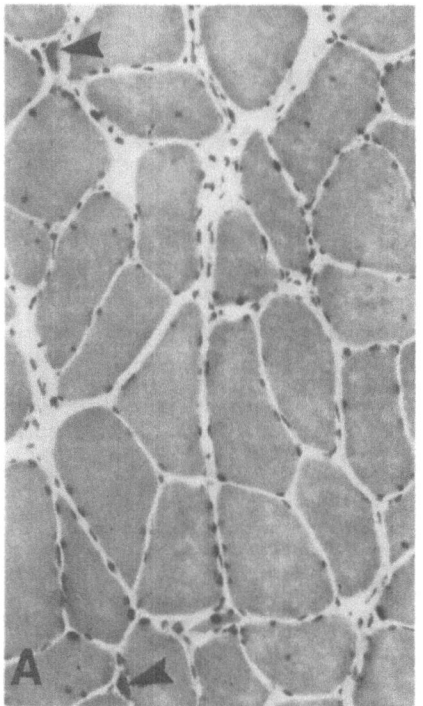

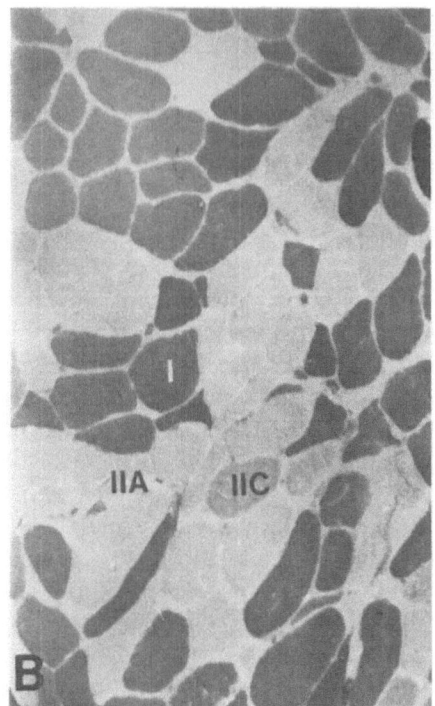

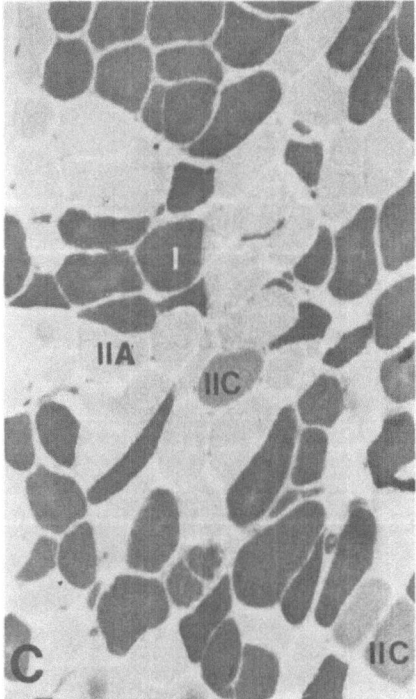

Fig. 8-30. Emery–Dreifuss muscular dystrophy: 40-year-old man; quadriceps. (A) Atrophic and hypertrophic myofibers and pyknotic nuclear clumps (arrows) (Hematoxylin–eosin; ×144). (B) ATPase preparation (pH 4.5). (C) ATPase preparation (pH 4.3). Deficiency of type IIB fibers; only type I, type IIA, and a few type IIC fibers are encountered (×82).

Emery–Dreifuss Type (EDMD)

The Emery–Dreifuss type[73] of X-linked recessive muscular dystrophy is associated with cardiomyopathy.[181] The abnormalities include: nonspecific myopathic features (Fig. 8-30A), fiber type disproportion and type I fiber predominance, and atrophy and type IIB fiber deficiency (Figs. 8-30B,C),[181] or type I fiber atrophy alone.[122]

The clinical features of rigid spine and contracted elbow joints and morphologic changes of type I fiber atrophy, type II fiber hypertrophy, and type IIB fiber deficiency resemble those of the rigid spine syndrome.[103] These two entities may be variants of the same disease.[206]

Limb Girdle Dystrophy (LGD)

Patients afflicted with LGD probably represent a group of heterogenous neuromuscular disorders called "limb-girdle syndromes"[27]; distinctive entities have not been unequivocally separated. The muscle pathology (Fig. 8-31) ascribed to LGD[68] may not occur in all patients. Atrophy and hypertrophy of muscle fibers are random, muscle fiber splitting may be prominent, and moth-eaten fibers may abound. Type I fiber predominance and type IIB fiber deficiency may occur as well as necrosis, phagocytosis, and regeneration of muscle fibers.

The differential diagnosis includes DMD, BMD, EDMD, and juvenile spinal muscular atrophy (JSMA). Differentiation of these clinical entities is usually done only in conjunction with clinical and electromyographic data.

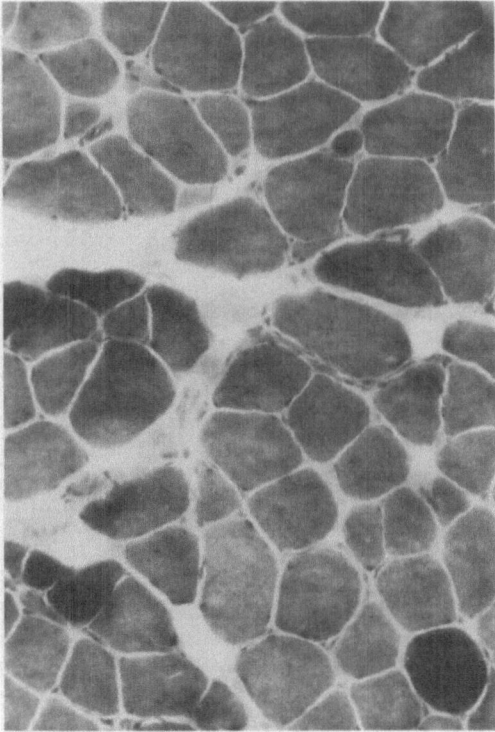

Fig. 8-31. Variation in fiber size and internal nuclei are apparent: 11-year-old boy, one of three affected siblings, limb girdle dystrophy; quadriceps. (Modified trichrome; ×180).

Facioscapulohumeral Dystrophy (FSHD)

This autosomal, dominantly inherited disorder may have a protracted course, but rarely progresses rapidly. Infantile and late clinical forms have been identified.[6] Muscle changes are usually mild (Fig. 8-32A) and may be absent in some patients. When present, they are largely nonspecific and myopathic. Angulated fibers may be scattered throughout. Inflammatory aggregates may be seen within or among the muscle fascicles[68] (Fig. 8-32B) and may be conspicuous. The presence of these aggregates in a biopsy specimen also showing nonspecific myopathic abnormalities poses a difficult diagnostic dilemma of polymyositis versus FSHD. Patients with either disease have similar complaints: sporadic weakness of shoulder girdle and facial muscles. Hypertrophic muscle fibers, particularly of type II, are more common among FSHD patients.[68] Sometimes, even prolonged observation of the patient and extensive family studies may leave the problem unresolved.

Scapuloperoneal muscular dystrophy may be separated from FSHD only on clinical grounds and may be a variant of FSHD. Differentiation of FSHD from the facioscapulohumeral syndrome with abnormally structured mitochondria[129] must be based on ultrastructural analyses.

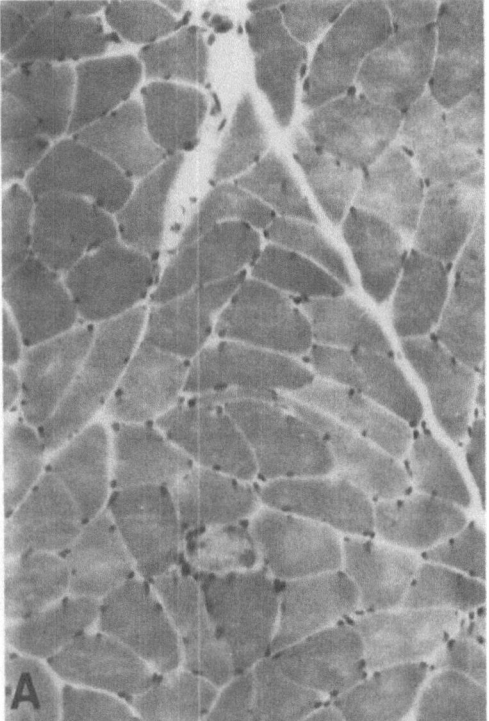 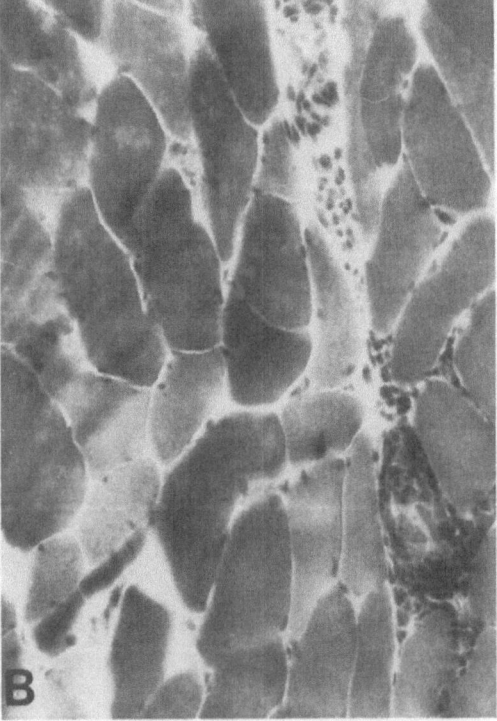

Fig. 8-32. Facioscapulohumeral dystrophy (FSHD) in a 59-year-old woman; deltoid. (A) Only minimal lesions may be present in this form of muscular dystrophy (hematoxylin–eosin; ×180). (B) Inflammatory infiltrates are sometimes encountered in FSHD. (Modified trichrome; ×228).

Oculopharyngeal Muscular Dystrophy (OPMD)

This autosomal dominantly inherited muscular dystrophy usually begins in late adulthood. The muscle biopsy discloses nonspecific features, of which "rimmed" vacuoles have been emphasized as being a frequent morphologic feature in OPMD.[68] Rimmed or autophagic vacuoles contain cellular constituents and large whorls of densely packed membranes. Recently,[201] peculiar 8.5 nm filaments have been found in the myonuclei of these patients. These intranuclear filaments, however, may occur in less than 10% of muscle nuclei and are not related to the rimmed vacuoles and their filaments. Abnormally shaped mitochondria also occur in OPMD.[128]

Distal Myopathy

These heterogenous neuromuscular disorders include several clinical forms of sporadic and autosomal-dominant or autosomal-recessive modes of inheritance. They may occur as congenital, infantile, juvenile, or adult forms. This heterogenous group is largely defined on the basis of clinical and genetic criteria; muscle abnormalities are either inconspicuous or nonspecific. Type I fiber atrophy[11,70] and type I fiber predominance[146] occur in a few patients,[205] but nonspecific myopathic features prevail. A special form has been separated on the basis of the consistent occurrence of rimmed vacuoles,[138,165] similar to those of inclusion body myositis. Another form of distal myopathy had sarcoplasmic bodies and skeletin (intermediate) filaments.[71] Distal myopathy is the same as distal muscular dystrophy.[158] The Welander or Swedish type has been suggested to be of neurogenic origin.[24]

Juvenile distal myopathy of Biemond is a neurogenic disease[119] (Fig. 8-3).

Congenital Muscular Dystrophy (CMD)

Congenital muscular dystrophy differs from other forms of dystrophy because clinical symptoms are noted at birth or shortly thereafter, often with contractures. According to available reports,[164] several forms of CMD may be distinguished, either as clinically benign, malignant forms,[215,216] or associated with special clinical symptoms. The latter includes the atonic-sclerotic type of Ulrich,[94] the Fukuyama type of CMD in Japanese children who have CMD associated with cerebral lesions,[93] and non-Japanese children who had CMD and cerebral lesions.[137] Histopathologic changes may differ in severity. A specific pattern of morphologic lesions has not been delineated to separate clinical forms of CMD. Myopathic features are often associated with fat cell aggregates (Fig. 8-33) inside the muscle fascicles. Endomysial fibrosis may abound, and even end-stage myopathy may be encountered in muscles of young children. CMD may occasionally result in arthrogryposis multiplex congenita. Necrosis and regeneration (Fig. 8-34) of muscle fibers may also occur and be a regular feature in young children afflicted with the Fukuyama type of CMD.[167] A striking discrepancy between severity of muscle lesions and mild clinical disability has been emphasized by Dubowitz.[66] Type I fiber atrophy and immature type IIC fibers may be numerous.[167]

The association of cerebral lesions and CMD has also been found in non-Japanese children.[99] A separate group of patients has, in addition to cerebral morphology and CMD, ocular lesions, also known as oculo-cerebro-muscular dystrophy, which exists

238   Hans H. Goebel

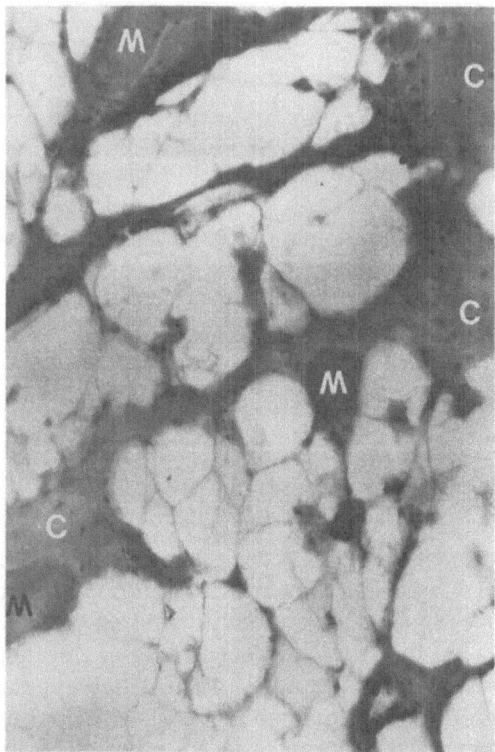

Fig. 8-33. Only a few muscle fibers (M) are left as an "end-stage myopathy," surrounded by connective (C) tissue and aggregates of fat cells: 8-year-old girl, congenital muscular dystrophy; quadriceps. (hematoxylin–eosin; ×156).

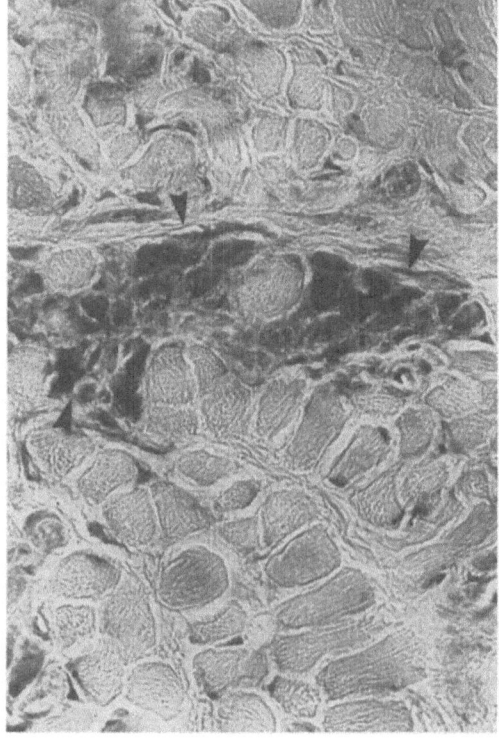

Fig. 8-34. Several small, dark myofibers in clusters indicate regeneration in a specific Azure B stain (arrows): 7-month-old girl, congenital muscular dystrophy; quadriceps (×430).

in at least two types[203] among them the "muscle-eye-brain-syndrome."[173] Occasional patients afflicted with the Fukuyama type of CMD may also have ocular lesions.[44]

VI. Neurogenic Atrophies

The denervated muscle fiber loses volume and becomes atrophic in diameter but not in length. In neuromuscular disorders marked by denervation, the muscle only shows indirect evidence of denervation based on a characteristic pattern of atrophy. Damage to the lower motor neuron may occur at different levels: the anterior horn; the anterior spinal root (radiculopathy); proximally or distally along the peripheral nerve; and at the motor endplate. Theoretically, therefore, neurogenic myofiber atrophy ranges from single fiber atrophy to large group or even fascicular atrophy. Denervation processes requiring muscle biopsy for diagnostic purposes in humans are usually chronic processes. By contrast, a single complete trans-section of the peripheral nerve is induced either by trauma or experimentally.

Chronic denervation is accompanied by sprouting of axons from surviving peripheral nerve fibers. Such sprouts may reinnervate denervated muscle fibers. Innervation determines the typing of muscle fibers. Individual muscle fibers of the same motor unit (i.e., supplied by the same neuron) are scattered, rather than grouped, within a single muscle fascicle. Fiber types normally have a checker-board distribution. Reinnervation of muscle fibers may result in a change of the original fiber type and pattern of fiber grouping (Fig. 8-35). Such change can best be appreciated in enzyme-histochemical

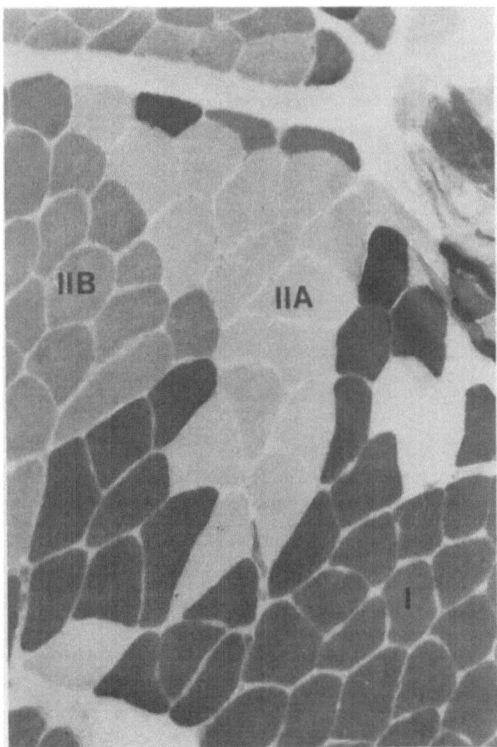

Fig. 8-35. Grouping of fiber types I, IIA, and IIB indicates reinnervation: 46-year-old man; peroneal muscular atrophy. (ATPase preparation pH 4.5; ×122.5).

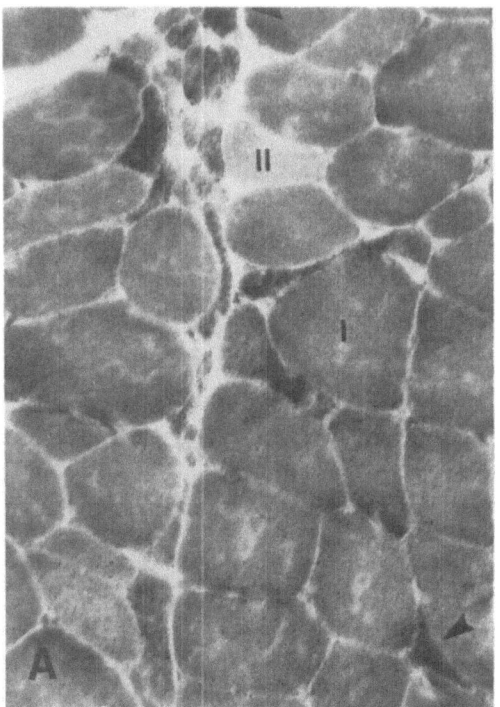

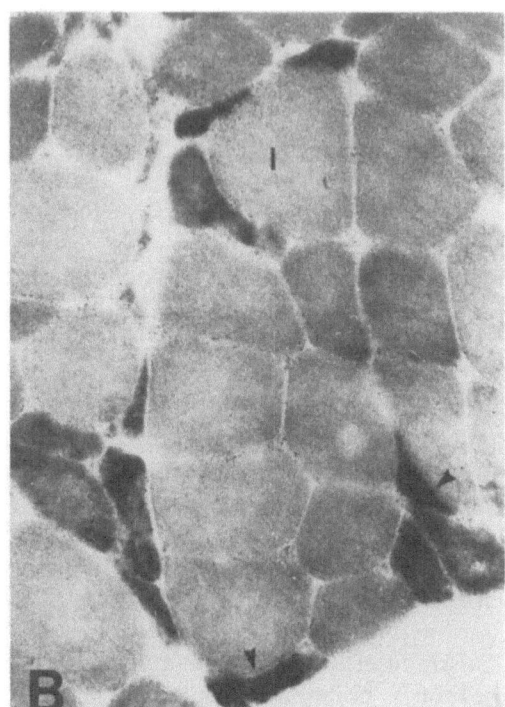

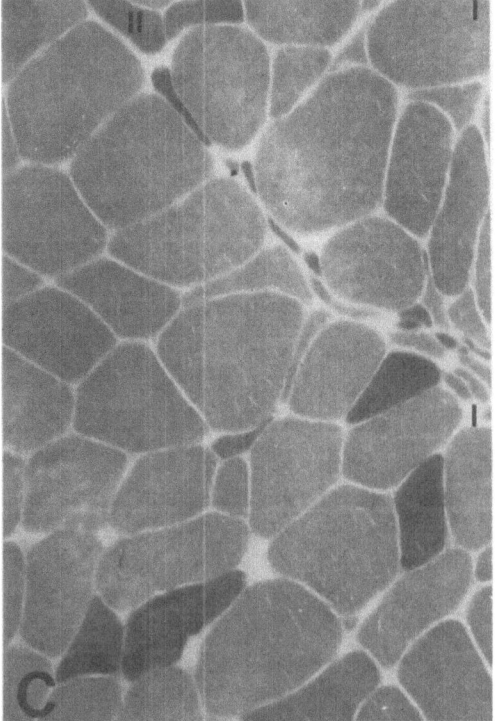

Fig. 8-36. Juvenile spinal muscular atrophy in an 8-year-old girl. In neurogenic atrophy, small, angulated fibers (arrows) often display strong activity in the NADH (A, ×200) and the MAG (B, ×200) preparations, but no reciprocity of histochemical enzyme activity, although atrophic fibers belong to type I and type II in the ATPase preparation (pH 10.4) (C, ×184).

preparations, which occasionally is the only sign of a neurogenic process. This alteration is particularly obvious when it is realized that reinnervated fibers may resume their original volume. "Target" fibers (Fig. 8-25), occurring chiefly in type I fibers, are presumably specific indicators of a neurogenic process, usually ascribed to denervation, but occasionally also ascribed to reinnervation.[64] In neurogenic atrophy, small angulated fibers frequently show strong activity of nonspecific esterase and of both NADH and MAG (Figs. 8-36A,B). The reactions of these latter two oxidative enzymes have been regarded as evidence of denervation,[68] although usually denervation affects both type I and type II fibers (Fig. 8-36C).

The presence of a neural-cell adhesion molecule at the surface of and within the myofiber may also identify denervated myofibers, (i.e., in late denervation after remote poliomyelitis).[43] Abnormalities or lack of axonal terminals at the motor endplate, however, have never been shown in such small angulated fibers as evidence of denervation. The strong reactions of both NADH and MAG enzymes in small angulated fibers is only circumstantial evidence, but not proof of denervation.

After long-standing denervation, myopathic features and loss of myofibers may dominate the morphologic picture, producing end-stage myopathy, which does not allow distinction between primarily neurogenic and primarily myopathic diseases. End-stage abnormalities occur in peroneal muscular atrophy, poliomyelitis, and juvenile spinal muscular atrophy. The changes of end-stage myopathy indicate that muscle fibers continue to undergo changes well beyond the initial phase after a brief single event of denervation.

Neurogenic processes visible in muscle biopsies usually comprise two groups: (1), spinal muscular atrophies and (2) neuropathies.

Spinal Muscular Atrophies

INFANTILE SPINAL MUSCULAR ATROPHY (ISMA)
This disorder occurs in two clinical forms: a rapidly progressive fatal form of perinatal onset, and an intermediate form that develops during the first or second year of life and has a more protracted course. The rapidly progressive malignant form of ISMA is called Werdnig-Hoffmann disease.

Muscle biopsy demonstrates group atrophy that may involve entire fascicles. Atrophic muscle fibers are usually round rather than polygonal and may be of type I and type II or predominantly type II (Figs. 8-37A,B). Among atrophic muscle fibers, large rounded type I fibers (Figs. 8-37A,B) are scattered or in groups. These large hypertrophic fibers are thought to be reinnervated. Fibrosis of the perimysium is more obvious than that of the endomysium. Necrosis and regeneration of muscle fibers is usually absent. Intramuscular nerve twigs, if present, may have few myelinated axons (Fig. 8-38).

In older children, small angulated fibers, disseminated or arranged in groups, may also occur. In the intermediate form of ISMA, these neurogenic features, resembling neurogenic atrophy in adults, may become more obvious; but during the first year of life, muscle biopsy findings do not allow precise distinction of prognosis between the two forms of ISMA.

In the early or preclinical stage of ISMA,[66] diagnostic separation of muscle fibers into atrophic or hypertrophic may not be as feasible as in later stages (Fig. 8-39). Sometimes, the pattern of fiber type disproportion develops, (i.e., predominance of type I

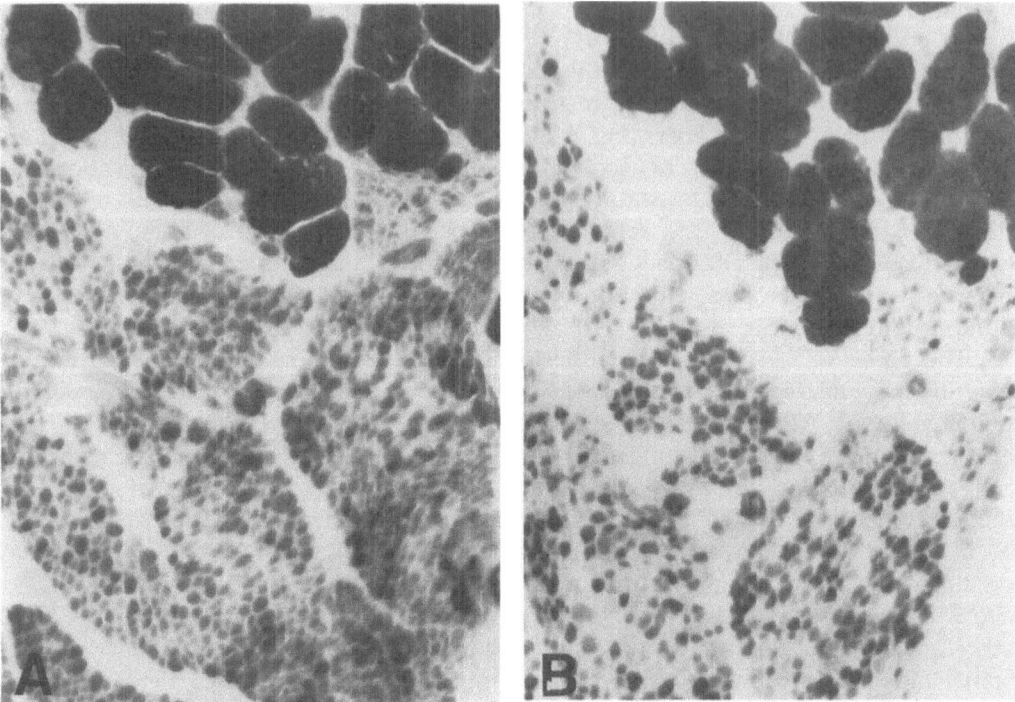

Fig, 8-37. The hypertrophic fibers belong to type I (dark); the atrophic fibers encompass type I and mainly type II, defying precise subtyping: 3½-year-old girl, infantile spinal muscular atrophy; quadriceps. [(A) ATPase preparation, pH 4.5; ×168. (B) ATPase preparation, pH 4.3; ×168].

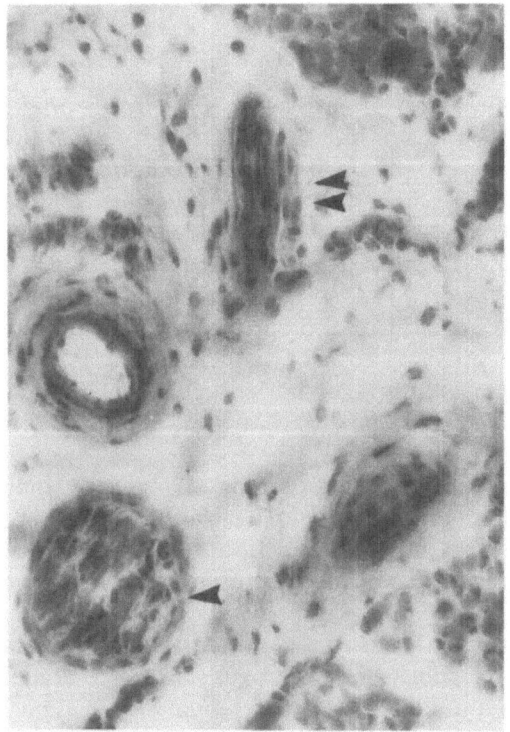

Fig. 8-38. Intramuscular nerve twigs either contain myelinated axons (arrow) or lack myelinated axons (double arrow): 3-week-old girl, infantile spinal muscular atrophy; quadriceps. (modified trichrome; ×200).

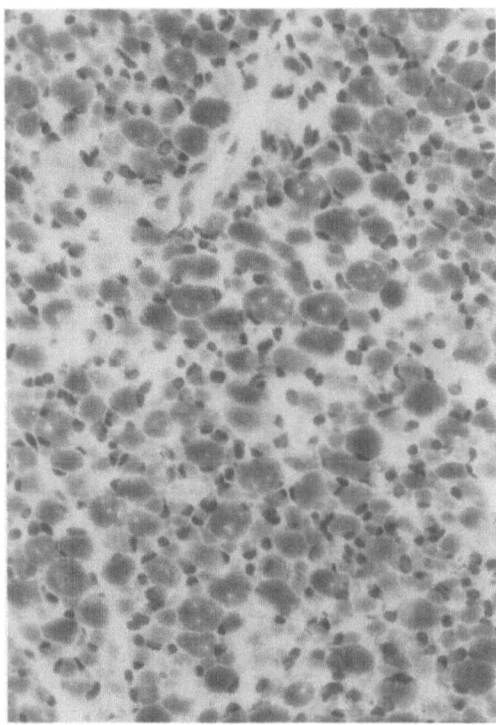

Fig. 8-39. In early infantile spinal muscular atrophy, fiber differences in size between hypertrophic and atrophic fibers are mild: 3½-week-old girl. Same biopsy as in Fig. 8-38. (Hematoxylin–eosin; ×225).

fibers and disproportion in fiber size between type I and type II fibers). This change may later revert to a neurogenic pattern. ISMA may also be difficult to diagnose in a muscle that includes only atrophic fibers. Measuring fiber size and comparing these values with age-matched controls, may be necessary to arrive at the correct diagnosis.

JUVENILE SPINAL MUSCULAR ATROPHY (WOHLFART–KUGELBERG–WELANDER DISEASE)

This chronic spinal muscular atrophy (JSMA) of late onset and protracted course usually has angulated or polygonal atrophic muscle fibers arranged in small or large groups (Fig. 8-40). In addition, myopathic features such as endomysial fibrosis, hypertrophy of muscle fibers, muscle fiber splitting, and occasional necrosis and regeneration of muscle fibers may be visible. Myopathic features may prevail to such an extent that morphologic distinction between JSMA and limb girdle dystrophy or Becker's muscular dystrophy is difficult. Hypertrophic fibers are frequently of type II.

ADULT SPINAL MUSCULAR ATROPHY (LOWER MOTOR NEURON DISEASE, SPINAL MUSCULAR ATROPHY, DUCHENNE-ARAN, AND AMYOTROPHIC LATERAL SCLEROSIS)

Spinal muscular atrophy of adult onset also is characterized by groups of atrophic polygonal muscle fibers of both types, often with hypertrophy of adjacent fibers. These large fibers, often type II, represent compensatory hypertrophy, but they may also be an early stage of denervation. Necrosis and regeneration of muscle fibers may be associated with rapid progression of the disease, particularly in amyotrophic lateral sclerosis.

OTHER SPINAL MUSCULAR ATROPHIES

Other neuromuscular disorders affecting the lower motor neuron have been identified. They include: progressive juvenile bulbar palsy of Fazio–Londe; myopathia distalis juvenilis of Biemond, previously regarded as a myopathy[119] (Fig. 8-41), and scapulopero-

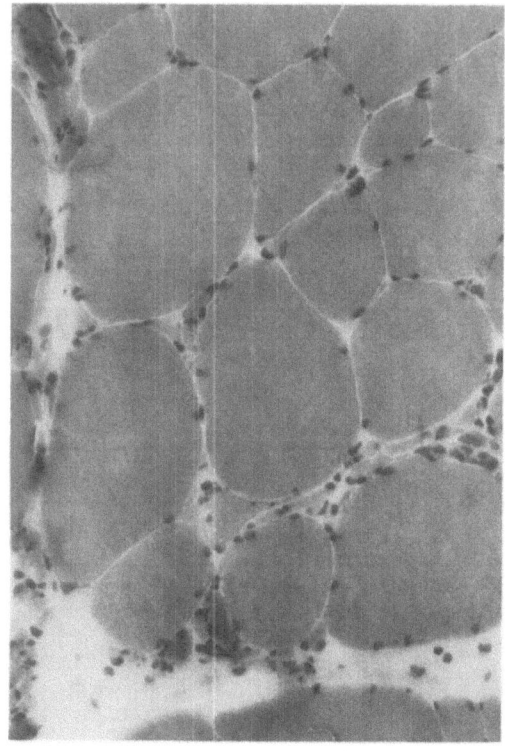

Fig. 8-40. Groups of atrophic fibers: 8-year-old girl, juvenile spinal muscular atrophy. Same biopsy as in Figs. 8-36A–C. (Haematoxylin–eosin; ×200).

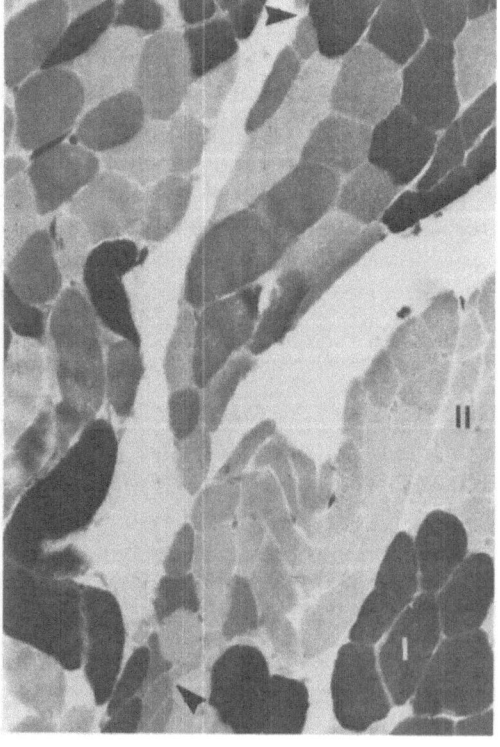

Fig. 8-41. This neurogenic disease is marked by atrophic fibers (arrows) and type grouping of type I and type II fibers: 38-year-old woman, myopathia distalis juvenilis hereditaria (Biemond); biceps. (ATPase preparation, pH 4.5; ×122.5).

neal atrophy or facioscapulohumeral atrophy. Charcot–Marie–Tooth disease or peroneal muscular atrophy has been divided into a demyelinating form (hereditary motor and sensory neuropathy I (HMSN I)[69] and a neuronal form (hereditary motor and sensory neuropathy II (HMSN II)[69] on the basis of clinical, electrophysiologic, and structural (peripheral nerve) criteria. The neuronal form of Charcot–Marie–Tooth disease (HMSN II) may be a type of spinal muscular atrophy. The muscle in peroneal muscular atrophy has shown neurogenic features and numerical increase of internal nuclei, termed chronic familial neuropathy,[68] but distinction between the demyelinating form and the neuronal form of peroneal muscular atrophy was not attempted in those studies.[68]

CONGENITAL MYOPATHIES

Congenital myopathies (CM) are a group (Table 8-8) of slowly progressive, often familial neuromuscular disorders, manifest mostly in childhood (Table 8-9), and are identified by specific muscle abnormalities. Separation from other groups of neuromuscu-

Table 8-8.
Congenital Myopathies

Structural Changes	
Central core disease	Shy and Magee, 1956[194]
Multi-core disease	Engel et al., 1971[79]
Mini-core disease	Currie et al., 1974[54]
Nemaline myopathy	Shy et al., 1963[193]
Myotubular myopathy	Spiro et al., 1966[196]
Centronuclear myopathy	Sher et al., 1967[192]
Fingerprint body myopathy	Engel et al., 1972[77]
Zebra body myopathy	Lake and Wilson, 1975[139]
Cytoplasmic body myopathy	Goebel et al., 1981[106]
Spheroid body myopathy	Goebel et al., 1978[104]
Sarcotubular myopathy	Jerusalem et al., 1973[125]
Tubular aggregate myopathy	Morgan-Hughes et al., 1970[161]
Cylindrical spiral myopathy	Bove et al., 1980[26]
Myofibrillar lysis myopathy	Cancilla et al., 1971[38]
Satellite cell myopathy	Beckmann et al., 1971[14]
Granulofilamentous myopathy	Fardeau et al., 1978[86]
Selective myosin degeneration myopathy	Yarom and Shapira, 1977[212]
Abnormal myomuscular junction myopathy	Bormioli, et al, 1980[25]
Trilaminar fiber myopathy	Ringel, et al, 1978[178]
Reducing body myopathy	Brooke and Neville, 1972[35]
Intermediate filament and sarcoplasmic body myopathy	Edström, et al. 1980[71]
"Cap disease"	Fidzianska, et al, 1981[88]
Tubulomembraneous inclusion myopathy	Fukuhara, et al, 1981[90]
Nucleodegenerative myopathy	Schröder, 1982[186]

Nonstructured Types	
Congenital fiber type disproportion	Brooke, 1973[32]
"Benign myopathy" with autosomal-dominant inheritance	Bethlem and Van Wijngaarden, 1976[19]
Microfiber myopathy	Hanson et al., 1977[112]
Type I myofiber hypotrophy without central nuclei	Prince et al., 1972[172]
"Benign congenital hypotonia"	Walton, 1956[208]
Type II muscle fiber hypoplasia	Matsuoka et al., 1974[150]
Minimal change myopathy	Dubowitz, 1980[67]

Table 8-9.
Floppy Infant Syndrome

Infantile spinal muscular atrophy
Congenital myopathies
Metabolic myopathies
Congenital muscular dystrophy
Benign congenital hypotonia
Infantile dystrophic myotonia
Cerebral hypotonia
Prader–Willi syndrome
Neonatal or congenital myasthenia
Hereditary hypertrophic neuropathy (HSMN III)
Connective tissue disorders

lar disorders has been made possible by the application of histochemical and electron-microscopic techniques.[65] The individual forms are defined by morphologic criteria, hence muscle biopsy is essential for the diagnosis. CM often has an autosomal-dominant or autosomal recessive mode of inheritance; therefore, nonaffected family members should be examined, sometimes even by muscle biopsy. The morphologic criteria of individual so-called "structured" CM are inclusions, such as rods or cytoplasmic bodies, on lesions of myofibrils as central, and multi- and mini-cores. CM often shows predominance of type I fibers, type uniformity of muscle fibers, and type I fiber atrophy.[36] The classification of CM according to disease-specific features has been challenged[36] because type I fiber predominance and type I fiber atrophy may be encountered in several forms of CM. Disease-specific features such as rods or central cores may occur with various frequencies within the same biopsied muscle, and in several biopsied muscles of the same patient[20] or in muscles biopsied in several affected family members.[15] In addition, disease-specific features overlap. Multi-cores and central nuclei of centronuclear myopathy[141] or central core disease and rod myopathy have appeared within the same family,[1] and certain CM-specific morphologic features, such as rods or cores, may also be present in non-CM neuromuscular diseases.

In addition to CM with disease-specific morphologic abnormalities, nonspecific myopathies with similar clinical symptoms are frequently encountered in children. Often, only type I fibers predominate with or without type I fiber atrophy. These conditions are called "nonstructured,"[143] indicating CM without specific structural features.

Central Core Disease (CCD)

CCD is a frequent and the first identified congenital myopathy.[194] Skeletal muscle fibers have single or a few cores centrally, occasionally eccentrically, or peripherally located "cores." These cores are best seen in NADH preparations (Fig. 8-42). They are areas of deficient substrate within the sarcoplasmic network of cross-sectioned muscle fibers. They extend over numerous sarcomeres, and may be seen also as smudgy regions in modified trichrome or nonspecific esterase preparations. In ATPase preparations, the structured cores are dark, but the "nonstructured" cores show faint staining defects. Cores occur chiefly in type I fibers. Ultrastructurally, a structured core[163] is composed of regular sarcomeres more contracted than the surrounding ones (Fig. 8-43). The fine

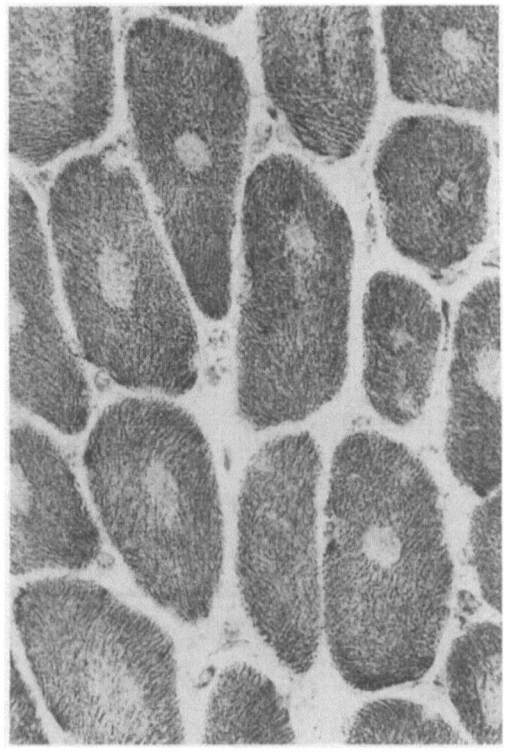

Fig. 8-42. The central cores are free of substrate in the NADH preparation and are of various sizes: 5-year-old girl, central core disease; quadriceps (×370).

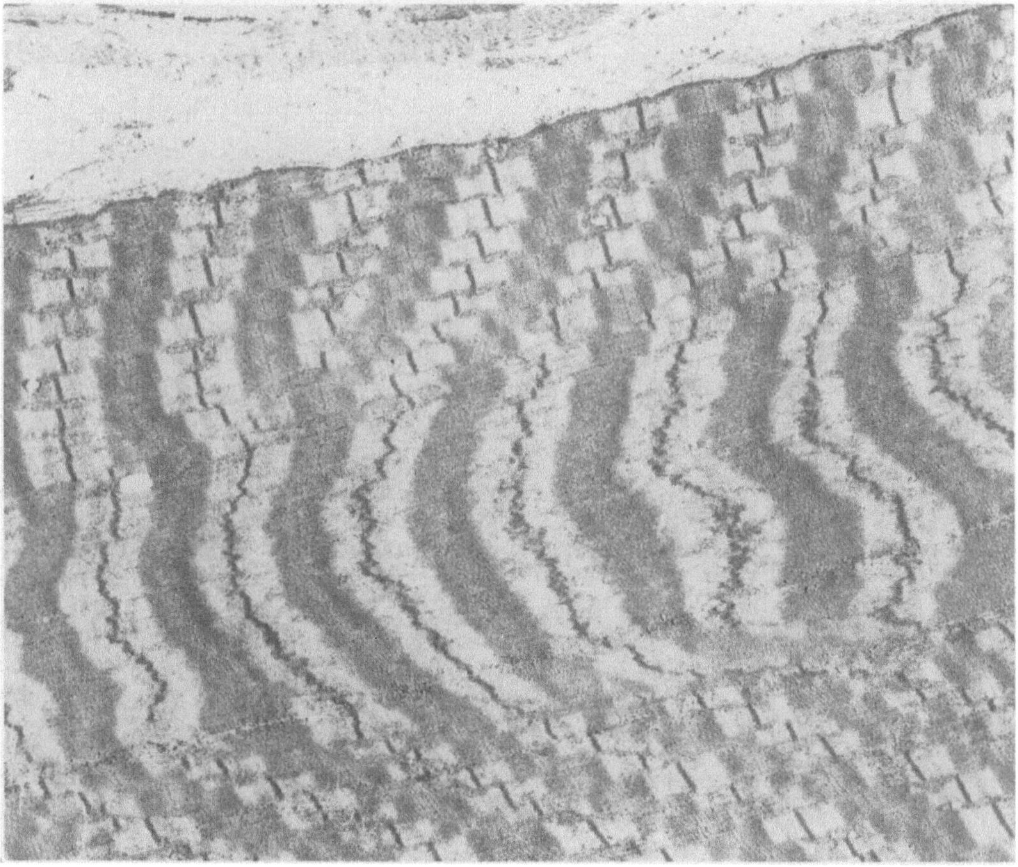

Fig. 8-43. In the "structured" core (×6,650), the sarcomeres of the core are in different register than the surrounding sarcomeres. Same biopsy as in Fig. 8-42.

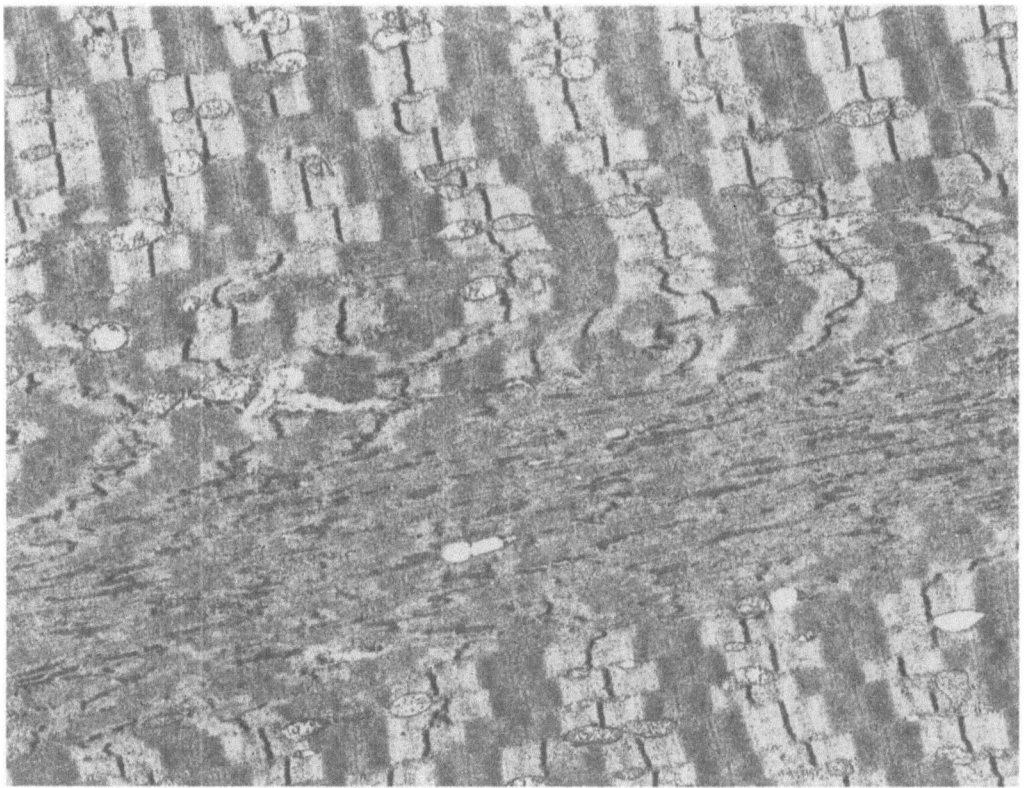

Fig. 8-44. An "unstructured" core shows marked blurring of the sarcomeres and paucity of mitochondria. Same biopsy as in Fig. 8-42 (×6,840).

structure of the sarcomeres is normal. In nonstructured cores (Fig. 8-44), there is considerable disintegration of Z-band material, smearing of Z-bands, and loss of myofilaments in the core area. In this respect, nonstructured cores resemble targetoid fibers. Contrary to earlier reports, both types of cores may occur in the same patient, muscle, and myofiber (Figs. 8-43, 8-44). Mitochondria are usually absent from central cores, attesting to the substrate-free area in the NADH preparation. Apart from these core lesions, there is usually type I fiber predominance or a uniform enzyme-histochemical reaction of muscle fibers. This type I fiber predominance may occur without cores. In such instances, cores may be present in muscle from other affected relatives. CCD may often also be associated with malignant hyperthermia.[89]

Cores have been produced experimentally by tenotomy and local tetanus intoxication,[49,191] and core-like lesions may occur in human muscle after rupture of the muscle tendon (Fig. 8-45), although evidence is not available that patients afflicted with CCD have clinical findings similar to tenotomy or local tetanus intoxication.

Multi-core or Mini-core Disease (MCD)

Multi-cores[79] or mini-cores[140] similar or identical to "focal loss of cross-striation,"[20] are small, smudgy lesions in the modified trichrome preparation (Fig. 8-46A), substrate-deficient in the NADH preparation, frequently in type I myofibers, but also in type

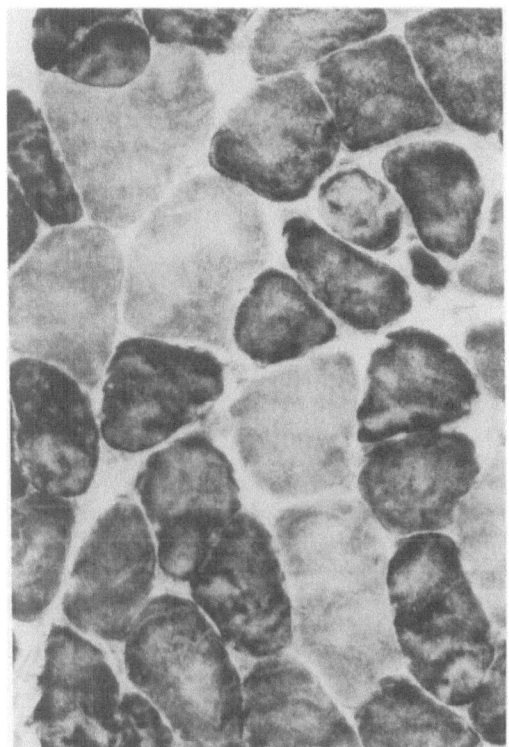

Fig. 8-45. Numerous substrate-free "core"-like lesions in a biceps muscle; rupture of tendon. (NADH preparation; ×148).

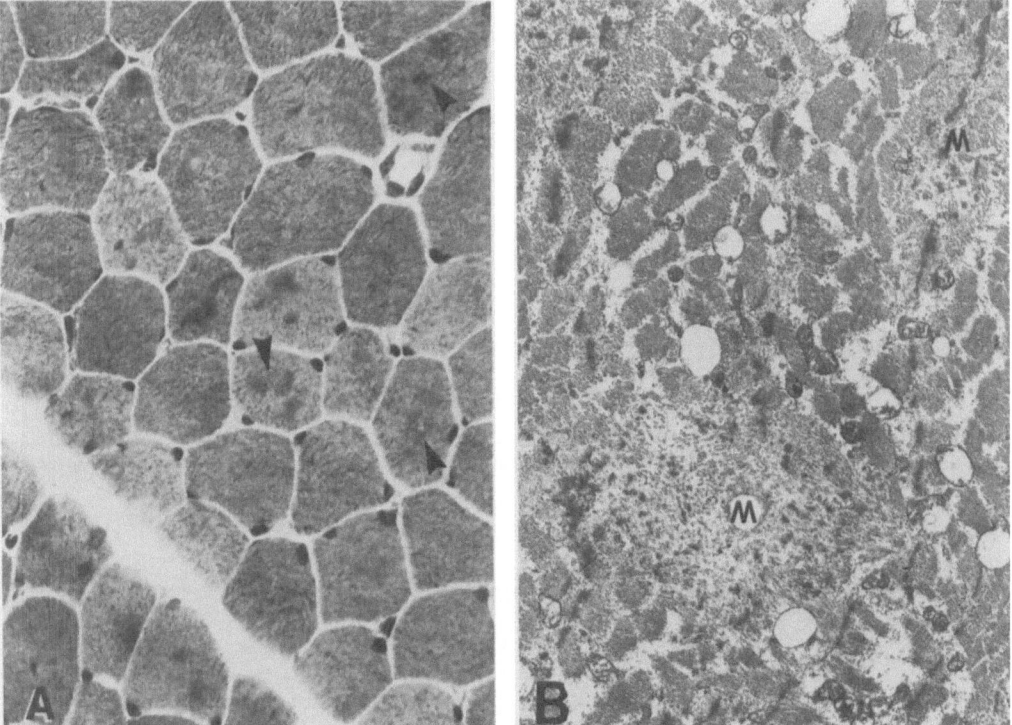

Fig. 8-46. Mini- (multi-) core disease in an 8-year-old girl; quadriceps. (A) Numerous small, "smudgy" foci (arrows) in cross-sectioned muscle fibers are the minicores. (Modified trichrome; ×370). (B) multiple minicores (M) are marked by disruption of sarcomeres (×6,993).

II, and occur in sporadic and familial neuromuscular disorders of childhood.[79,140] Multi- or mini-cores usually occur simultaneously within an affected myofiber. Electron microscopically, mini-cores are foci of sarcomeric lesions (Fig. 8-46B) similar to "streaming of the Z-disk." A lack of mitochondria is noted in these mini-core regions. Multi- or mini-cores also resemble moth-eaten defects and targetoid lesions.

Nemaline (Rod) Myopathy

This CM occurs frequently among primary muscle disorders.[193] Muscle fibers are studded with innumerable rods (Fig. 8-8) stained red in modified trichrome preparations. They may be present across the entire muscle fiber or confined to peripheral sectors. These small, wedge-shaped inclusions, randomly arrayed, are separated giant Z-disks (Fig. 8-47). Often, one may encounter enlarged Z-disks (Fig. 8-47) within intact sarcomeres that show arrow-like protrusions into adjacent I-bands. Larger Z-disks may have only remnants of thin myofilaments, but no connection to regularly arranged sarcomeres.

Type I fiber predominance and type I fiber atrophy are additional features of nemaline myopathy. Rods of identical fine structure have also been described in cases of polymyositis.[39]

Centronuclear or Myotubular Myopathy

Neuromuscular disorders described under these terms are probably the same disorder,[192,196] although clinically, and particularly, genetically different forms may occur

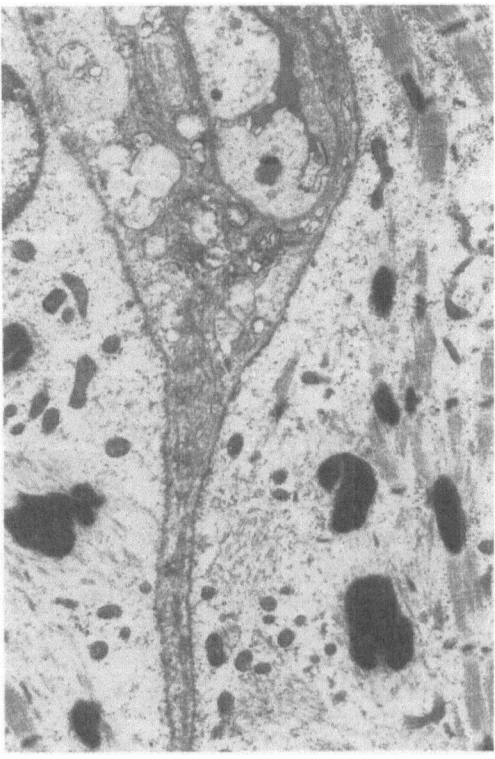

Fig. 8-47. Numerous large, dark inclusions in two adjacent muscle fibers with considerable degeneration of sarcomeres represent rods (nemaline bodies): 1½-year-old girl, nemaline myopathy; quadriceps. Same muscle as in Fig. 8-8 and (×6,734).

as autosomal-dominant, autosomal-recessive, and sex-linked-recessive and probably malignant forms.[10] Single, centrally located (Figs. 8-48, 8-49), often large, "juicy" (Fig. 8-50) nuclei are present in many muscle fibers. Peripheral nuclei in such myofibers may be numerically decreased or absent. A perinuclear halo free of myofilaments may (Fig. 8-51*A*) or may not (Fig. 8-51*B*) be present. Sometimes paranuclear sarcomeres may be thinner than those located distant to the nuclei.

Occasionally, multi- or mini-cores may be present in the muscle fibers of centronuclear myopathy[141] (Fig. 8-52). Type I fiber predominance and type I fiber atrophy may prevail (Fig. 8-49) and may be so conspicuous that two separate fiber populations may be noted even in non-enzyme-histochemical preparations. Fat cells are frequently found among muscle fibers.

Congenital Fiber Type Disproportion (CFTD)

CFTD is a neuromuscular disorder of childhood.[32] It is a nonstructured CM, because particular ultrastructural features, except an occasional "streaming of the Z-disk,"[142] are not seen. The characteristic pattern of the lesion is clearly elucidated (Fig. 8-53) in enzyme-histochemical preparations. These reveal type I fiber predominance and type I fiber atrophy (Fig. 8-53*A*), type I fiber predominance and type II fiber hypertrophy, or both. Differences between muscle fiber diameters of type I and type II fibers, which are of equal size in normal children, are greater than 13%. Type I fibers dominate by more than 50%. Subtyping of type II fibers may be difficult, and variations in type II

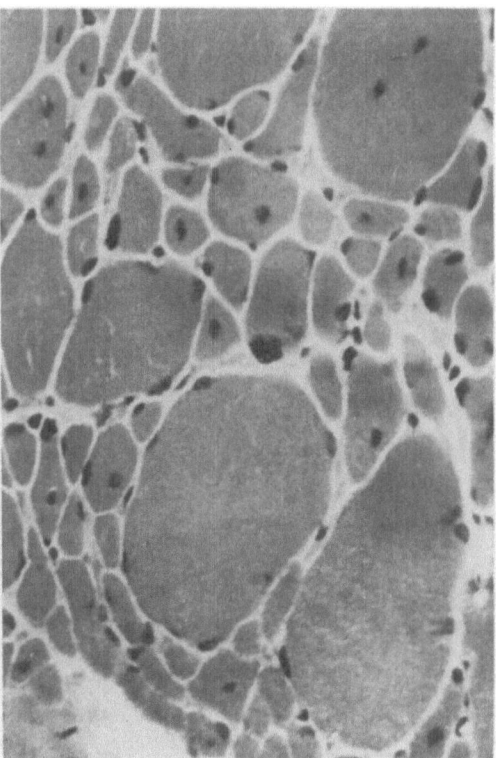

Fig. 8-48. There are numerous internal nuclei in small and large muscle fibers: 22-year-old man, centronuclear myopathy; deltoid. (Hematoxylin–eosin; ×378).

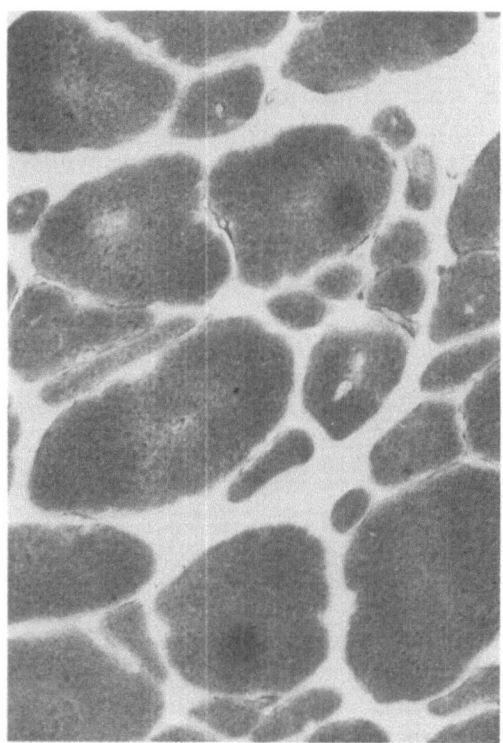

Fig. 8-49. Fibers with centrally located nuclei lack enzymatic activity; all muscle fibers depicted, both large and small ones are type I. Same patient as in Fig. 8-48 at the age of 28 years; deltoid. (ATPase preparation, pH 4.5; ×216).

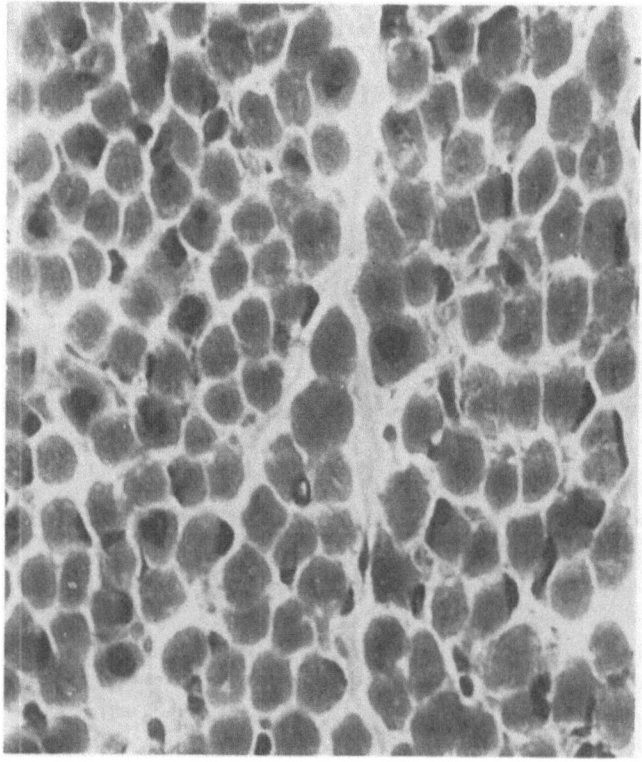

Fig. 8-50. Large "juicy" central nuclei in round muscle fibers: 4-month-old boy, centronuclear or myotubular myopathy of X-linked type. His brother died with respiratory insufficiency. Rectus abdominis. (Modified trichrome; ×620).

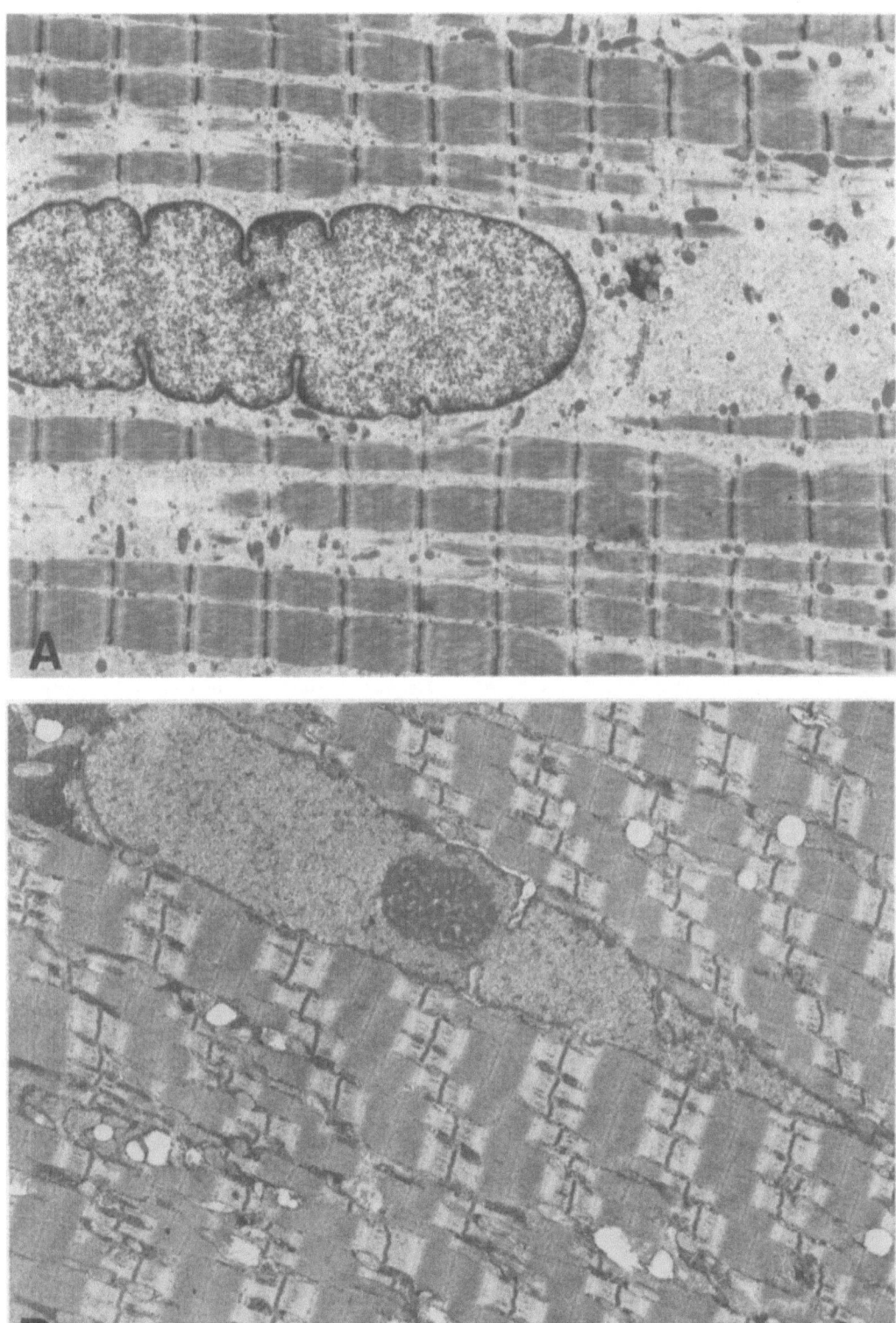

Fig. 8-51. Centronuclear myopathy in the same patient as in Fig. 8-48; deltoid. (A) The paranuclear region is devoid of sarcomeres (×5,700); (B) other centrally located nuclei are in intimate contact with surrounding sarcomeres (×6,840).

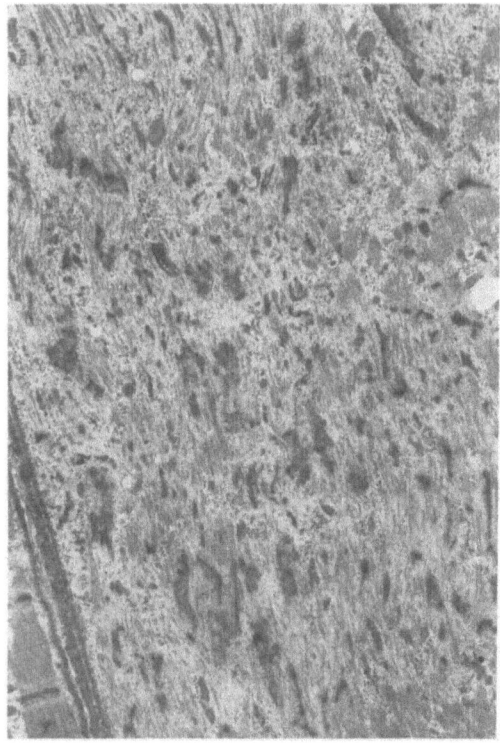

Fig. 8-52. A "core" lesion in centronuclear myopathy. Same muscle biopsy as in Fig. 8-48 (×5,959).

fiber subtypes may differ regionally (Figs. 8-53C,D). This morphologic pattern of fiber type disproportion may be similar to histochemical patterns of other CM associated with disease-specific features. There may thus be transitions between centronuclear myopathy and CFTD, e.g., muscle biopsies showing type I fiber atrophy without central nuclei[133] or with central nuclei.[190]

The morphologic pattern of muscle fiber type disproportion in CFTD is similar to that sometimes seen in preclinical infantile spinal muscular atrophy,[66] in Krabbe's leukodystrophy,[58,149] or early myotonic dystrophy. In preclinical infantile spinal muscular atrophy and myotonic dystrophy, this morphologic pattern of muscle fiber type disproportion is probably transient. Such observations, and that of fiber type disproportion in Krabbe's globoid cell leukodystrophy, cast some doubt upon the nosological specificity of CFTD.

The rigid spine syndrome, clinically defined by impaired flexion of the spine and elbows,[66] may also show a CFTD muscle pattern and IIB fiber deficiency (Figs. 8-54A,B) in the biceps muscle;[103,189] nonspecific myopathic features and endomysial fibrosis prevail in spinal muscles.

Miscellaneous CM

There are other CM (Table 8-8) that show disease-specific abnormalities. The clinical terms "floppy infant" syndrome (Table 8-9) and "amyotonia congenita of Oppenheim" may reflect a congenital myopathy. Benign congenital hypotonia may occasionally show

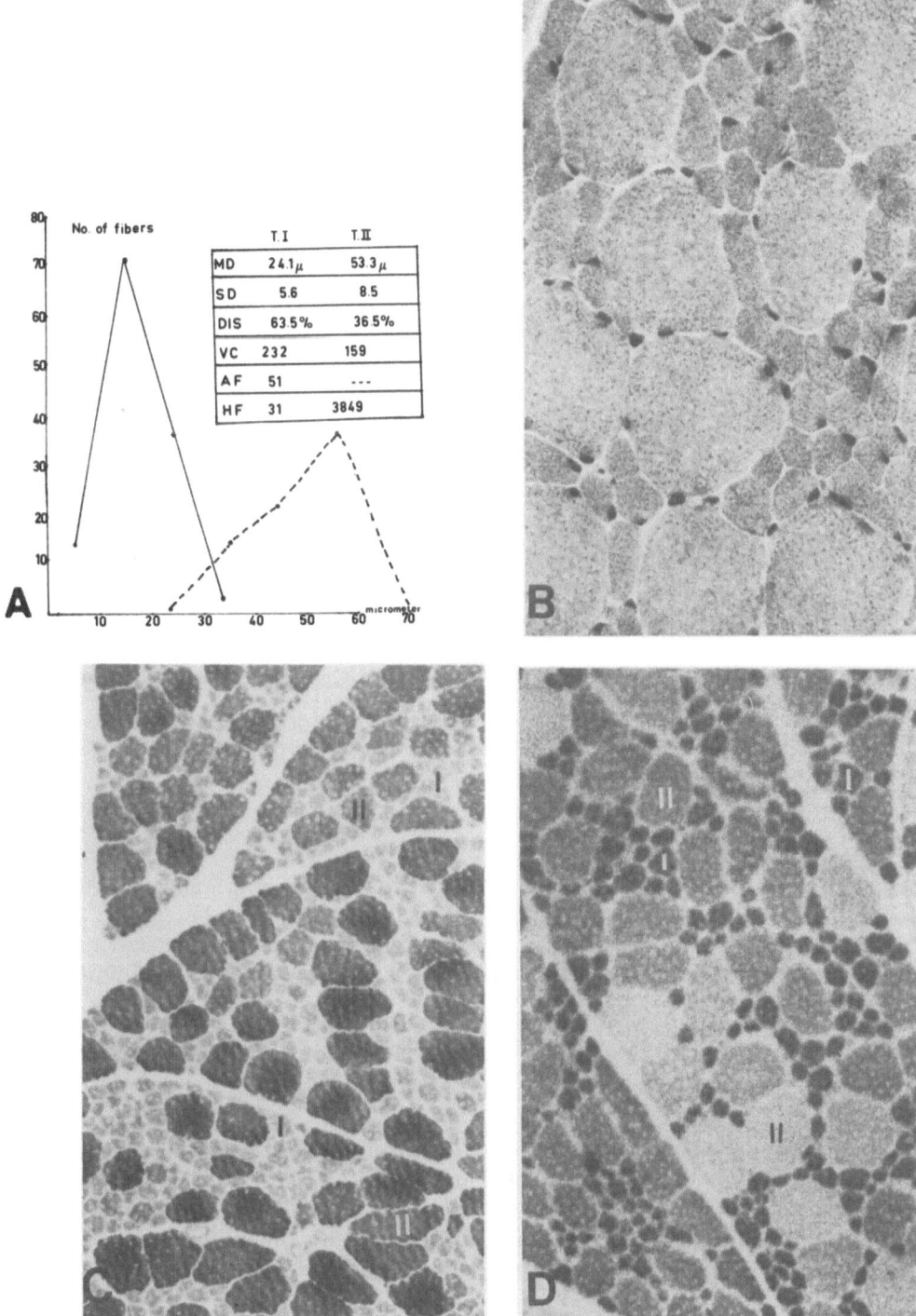

Fig. 8-53. Congenital fiber type disproportion in a 4-year-old boy; quadriceps. (A) A histogram shows type I fiber atrophy, type I fiber predominance, type II fiber hypertrophy. (B) Two populations of fibers, a few hypertrophic and numerous atrophic ones. (Modified trichrome; ×400). (C) Small fibers are of type I, the large fibers of type II. (ATPase preparation, pH 9.3; ×180.) (D) The type II fibers show variously intense enzyme histochemical activities, but the small type I fibers are uniformly dark. (ATPase preparation, pH 4.2; ×260).

255

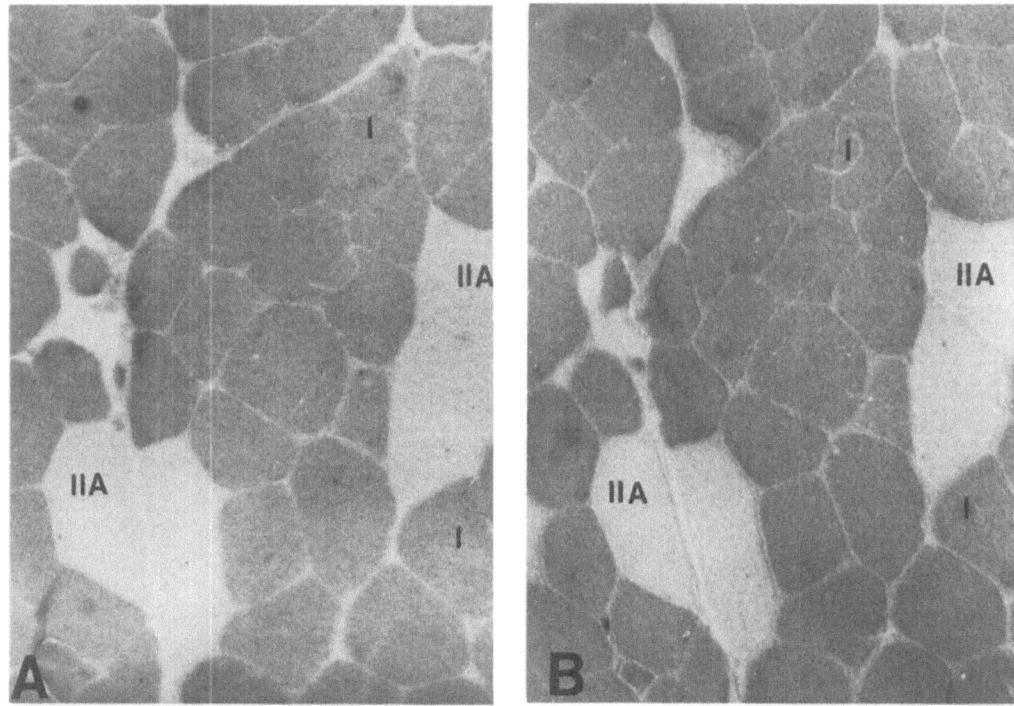

Fig. 8-54. Type I fiber predominance, type I fiber atrophy, and type II fiber deficiency are typical: 15-year-old girl, rigid spine syndrome; biceps. [(A) ATPase preparation, pH 4.5; ×250. (B) ATPase preparation, pH 4.3; ×216.] Serial sections.

type I fiber predominance[84] or muscle changes may be absent. Some of these patients, and those who have what is called nonstructured CM, may be similar to patients having minimal change myopathy.[66] This term refers to certain patients having a myopathy, clinically regarded as congenital, whose muscles have no or only minimal, nonspecific abnormalities.

Inflammatory Myopathies and Collagen Vascular Diseases

Inflammation in skeletal muscle may be a consequence of (1) non-infectious, idiopathic, probably autoimmune-mediated processes; (2) associated nonspecific features of noninflammatory neuromuscular disease; or (3) local or generalized infections. The most important group comprises noninfectious myositis, mainly polymyositis.

Polymyositis and Dermatomyositis

Classification of polymyositis and dermatomyositis is based on clinical criteria. Usually, the pathologist establishes or eliminates the morphologic diagnosis of myositis and leaves further subclassification to the clinician. One list[22] indicates five groups of polymyositis:

1. Primary idiopathic polymyositis.
2. Primary idiopathic dermatomyositis.
3. Dermatomyositis (or polymyositis) associated with neoplasms.
4. Childhood dermatomyositis (or polymyositis) associated with vasculitis.
5. Polymyositis (or dermatomyositis) associated with collagen-vascular disease.

Another group[210] considers three types of polymyositis:

1. Polymyositis as organ-specific autoimmune disease.
2. Polymyositis or dermatomyositis as part of autoimmune disease, not organ-specific,
3. Polymyositis or dermatomyositis occurring possibly as a conditioned autoimmune response in malignant disease.

By light microscopy, dermatomyositis is often marked by a conspicuous perifascicular atrophy (Fig. 8-55). Such perifascicular damage of muscle fibers may also occur in enzyme-histochemical preparations, especially NADH and ATPase, which reveal defects of the respective substrates sometimes amounting to ghost fibers.

Perifascicular atrophy is probably caused by local ischemia related to damage of intramuscular capillaries. In childhood dermatomyositis, necrosis and regeneration of intramuscular capillaries have been demonstrated by both light[9] and electron microscopy[8,41] (Fig. 8-56). Such capillaries often show undulating tubules within membrane-bound spaces (Fig. 8-57) of endothelial cells, lymphocytes, pericytes, and other cells,[41] similar to the undulating tubules observed in lupus erythematosus.

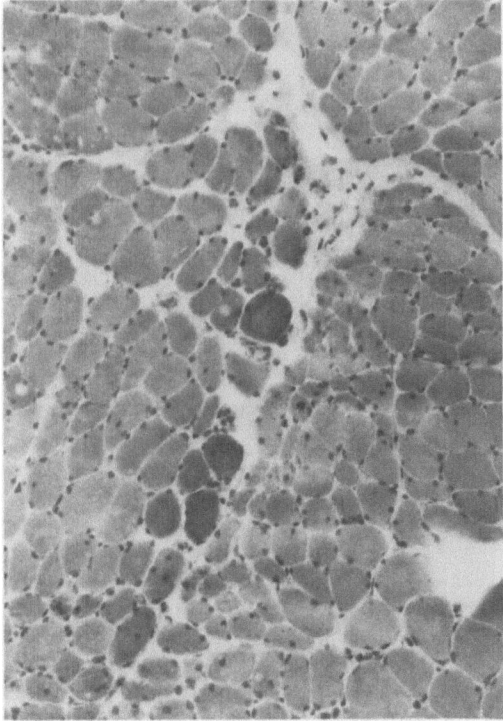

Fig. 8.55. Perifascicular atrophy and numerical increase of internal nuclei are characteristic: 57-year-old woman, dermatomyositis; deltoid. (Hematoxylin–eosin; ×115).

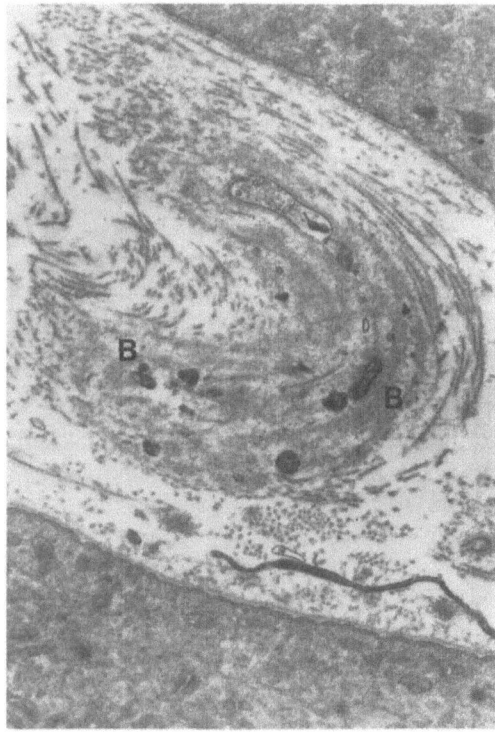

Fig. 8-56. Basement membrane (B) material visible between two muscle fibers, represents remnants of a necrotic capillary: 7-year-old boy, dermatomyositis; quadriceps (×13,100).

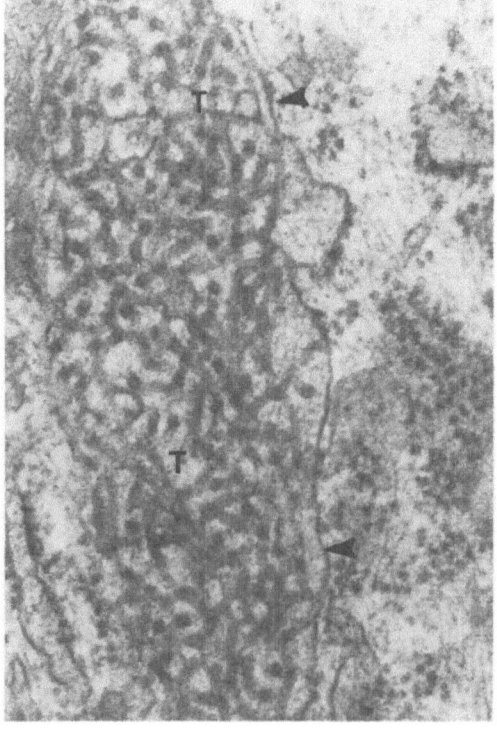

Fig. 8-57. Numerous undulating tubules (T) are surrounded by a membrane (arrows) within endothelial cells. Same muscle biopsy as in Fig. 8-56 (×6,850).

Aggregates of lymphocytes, mononuclear cells, and occasionally acid phosphatase-positive histiocytes, may be present among and within muscle fascicles. When they are absent, the perifascicular location of the lesions is characteristic of this type of myositis. At a later stage, chronic myopathic features may prevail; inflammation may be either conspicuous or slight. Atrophic, rounded muscle fibers are embedded in dense endomysial fibrosis (Fig. 8-58), but hypertrophic fibers are said to be absent.[68] Necrosis, phagocytosis, and regeneration of muscle fibers occur, occasionally to such an extent that rhabdomyolysis and myoglobinuria are associated with fulminant polymyositis. In other instances, the myositis may resemble a necrotizing myopathy with slight inflammation.

Polymyositis and dermatomyositis are now considered by pathogenetic criteria as different conditions or groups of conditions, the latter a vascular immune-mediated disorder, the former an autoimmune disease of muscle fibers.[177] Distribution of inflammatory cell types differs,[2,5] and direct attacks by lymphocytes against normal appearing muscle fibers have been documented as an early event in polymyositis.[3,4,78]

The causes of polymyositis and dermatomyositis are unknown, but viral infections have been suspected, largely because of electron-microscopic observations. Myxo and picorna virus-like particles have been found[46] in the nuclei and cytoplasm of muscle fibers. The myxo virus-like structures, however, are probably the intranuclear tubules or filaments seen in inclusion body myositis; the picorna-like particles may be aggregates of glycogen because they are not shown by an RNA stain,[46] but may be digested by amylase.[132] Unequivocal evidence of a viral cause for polymyositis or dermatomyositis has not appeared.

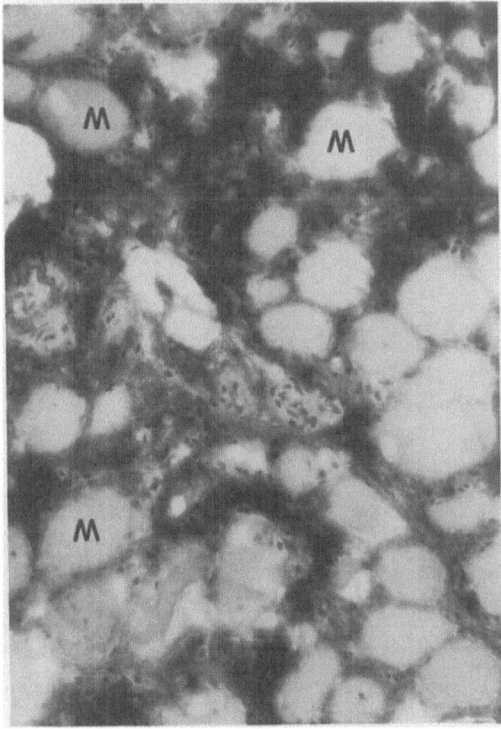

Fig. 8-58. Muscle fibers (M) surrounded by fibrotic endomysium: 43-year-old woman, chronic myositis; quadriceps. (Elastic van Gieson; ×180).

260   *Hans H. Goebel*

Cytoplasmic bodies or nemaline rods may occur in polymyositis as a nonspecific feature. If inflammation is absent, if myopathic features are mild and nemaline rods abound, and if the patient is an adult and a relative is not similarly diseased, the differentiation between chronic myositis and adult-onset sporadic nemaline myopathy may be difficult.

Another differential diagnostic problem may arise between chronic myositis with little inflammation and muscular dystrophy, either of the limb girdle type or the facio-scapulohumeral type, especially because inflammation may be present in the latter form of muscular dystrophy. In these instances, the muscle pathology has to be interpreted in light of the clinical and genetic history.

Abnormally structured mitochondria, particularly those containing crystal inclusions, have occurred in polymyositis.[45] Immune deposits in intramuscular capillary walls have not been seen in polymyositis,[116] but they may be present in other disorders associated with myositis, such as lupus erythematosus and dermatomyositis.[116] Neurogenic features may be encountered in myositis,[117] indicating involvement of the intramuscular nerve twigs by inflammation.

Inclusion body myositis is a separate type of inflammatory myopathy,[42] marked by intranuclear and intracytoplasmic filaments measuring 15–18 nm (Fig. 8–59). Another characteristic feature is rimmed vacuoles (Fig. 8-23). Immunohistologically it resembles

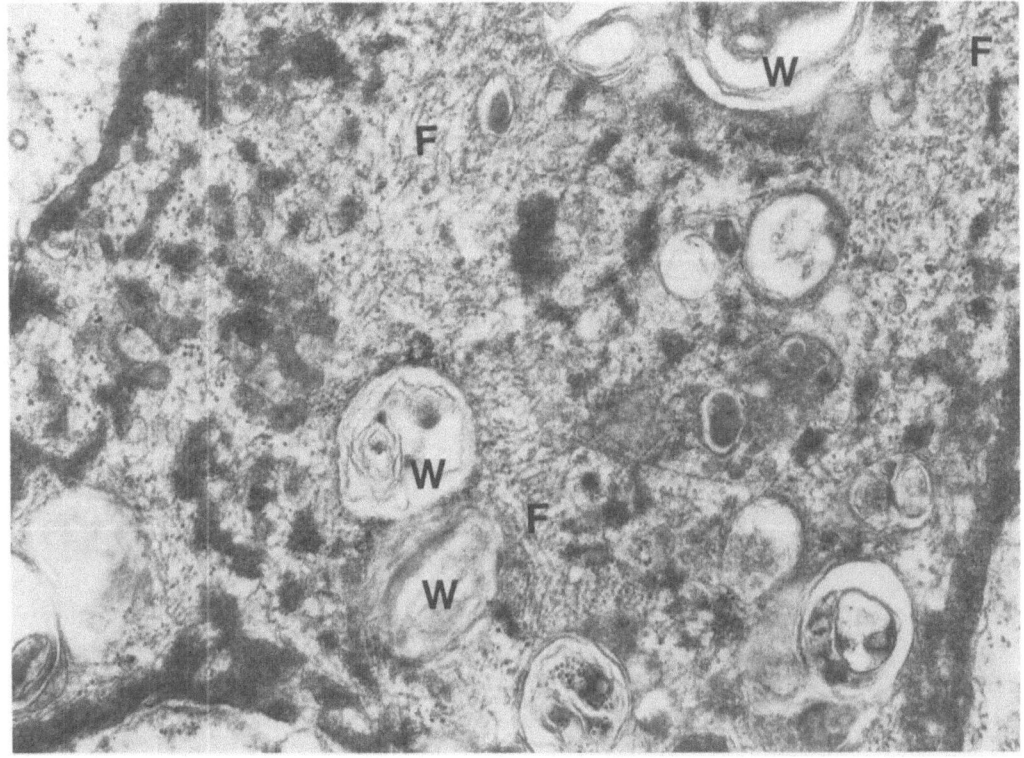

Fig. 8-59. A nucleus contains numerous filaments (F) and membranous whorls (W): 47-year-old woman, inclusion body myositis; biceps (×26,400).

polymyositis[5,78] but its myopathology differs quantitatively.[177] It has recently been related to a remote infection by the mumps virus.[47]

The differential diagnosis between inclusion body myositis, which may occur without inflammatory infiltrates, and oculopharyngeal muscular dystrophy may be difficult on morphologic grounds. Rimmed vacuoles and intranuclear filaments occur in both entities, though the intranuclear filaments in inclusion body myositis are usually larger than the 8–10 nm intranuclear filaments of oculopharyngeal muscular dystrophy. Small 7 nm intranuclear filaments also occur, however, in polymyositis.[185] The cause of inclusion body myositis is unknown, but adenovirus type 2 has recently been isolated from muscle biopsy specimens in inclusion body myositis.[155]

In the *acquired immunodeficiency syndrome (AIDS)*, the skeletal muscle may be affected by a myositis,[55] and the inflammatory infiltrate may contain giant cells[7] and even HIV-positive cells.[55] Rods or nemaline bodies may prominently figure in AIDS-affected muscle tissue.[55,109] Involvement of the peripheral nervous system in the AIDS process may result in secondary neurogenic atrophy[55] while type II muscle fiber atrophy[55] may be a non-specific feature.

Myositis Associated with Collagen Vascular Diseases and Related Disorders

Polymyalgia rheumatica is frequently associated with giant cell arteritis of the temporal artery; type II fiber atrophy, particularly of the IIB type, may be pronounced (Fig. 8-60).[34] In rheumatoid arthritis, in addition to nonspecific myopathic features and inflammation, type II fiber atrophy in earlier stages is followed by type I fiber atrophy in

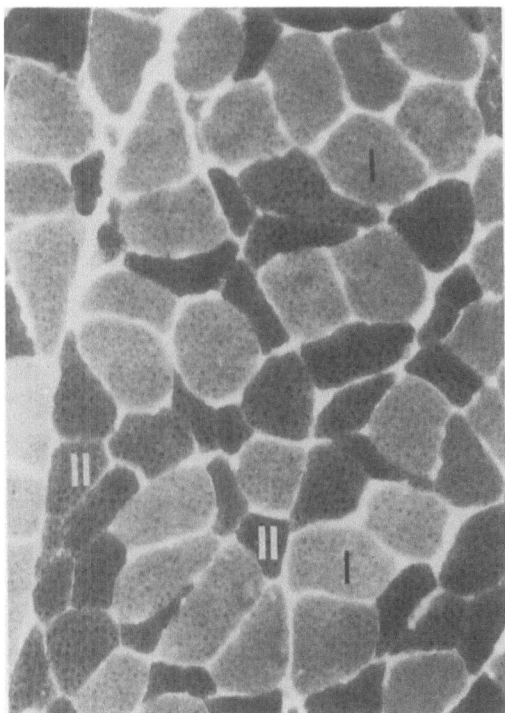

Fig. 8-60. Type II fibers are smaller than type I fibers, indicating pronounced selective type II atrophy: 79-year-old woman, polymyalgia rheumatica; biceps. (ATPase preparation, pH 10.4; × 168).

later stages of the disease.[34] In systemic sclerosis and lupus erythematosus, light-microscopic muscle changes are nonspecific; undulating tubules have been seen by electron microscopy in the latter condition.

Granulomatous Myositis

Granulomas within skeletal muscle may form a distinct feature related to many inflammatory myopathies, including polymyositis, tertiary syphilis, myasthenia gravis, rheumatoid arthritis, miliary tuberculosis, toxoplasmosis, and carcinoma.[144] Sarcoidosis is one of the diseases featuring granulomatous myositis (Fig. 8-61). The granulomas contain giant cells and others having strong acid phosphatase activity, as well as monocytes and epitheloid cells. Hypertrophy of muscle cells, even those located distant to the granulomas, may be prominent. The granulomas of polymyositis and sarcoidosis cannot be distinguished from one another on the basis of structural features.[118]

In myositis ossificans, bone is formed apart from dense connective tissue within muscle fascicles. Localized forms have been reported[153]; a generalized form, the Münchmeyer syndrome, is also called universal calcinosis.

Viral Myositis

Skeletal muscle may be involved in systemic viral infections, most often transiently. Muscle biopsy is not warranted. Myositis, myoglobinemia, and myoglobinuria may

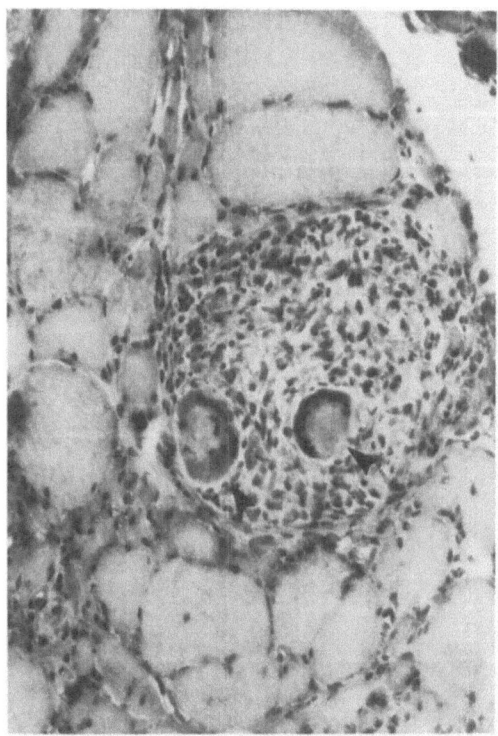

Fig. 8-61. A granuloma contains two giant cells (arrows): 57-year-old man, granulomatous myositis in sarcoidosis; biceps. (Elastic van Gieson: ×180).

occur[124]; Coxsackie virus adenovirus has been isolated in chronic myopathy[198] and in inclusion body myositis,[155] respectively.

Bacterial Myositis

This type of myositis may occur with surgical procedures followed by infection, usually a focal phenomenon. As a general disease, pyomyositis is rare in nontropical countries; it is frequent in tropical areas.[108]

Parasitic Infections

Skeletal muscles may be infested by protozoa and worms,[97] of which trichinosis is relevant to temperate climates. Myositis as well as the presence of larvae within necrotic muscle fibers, which may later result in calcification, can be observed.[110]

Quadriceps Myopathy

This type of myopathy, also called the "quadriceps syndrome," may be related to myositis.[159] It may have other causes, such as diabetes, and is then called diabetic amyotrophy.

IX. Metabolic Myopathies

Metabolic myopathies may be inherited or acquired. Enzyme deficiencies of lipid and glycogen metabolism and periodic paralyses are examples of the former group; endocrine disorders and sequelae of drug therapy or intoxication (for instance, alcohol) are examples of the latter conditions. Among the inherited disorders, the morphologic alterations of entities such as carnitine deficiency, type II glycogenoses, and certain lysosomal diseases are characteristic and suggestive of the underlying disease. Phosphorylase deficiency may be diagnosed by demonstrating absence of enzyme activity. Phosphorylase deficiency is also one of the few neuromuscular diseases, in which enzyme histochemical and biochemical findings are parallel. In congenital lethal hypophosphatasia, alkaline phosphatase is absent, both biochemically and histochemically in intramuscular vessel walls.[107] This condition does not produce neuromuscular symptoms.

Electron microscopy may aid in the diagnosis of some metabolic diseases, (e.g., type II glycogenosis, mucolipidosis IV, periodic paralysis, and mitochondrial myopathies). Acquired metabolic diseases do not induce specific muscle alterations, and a correct diagnosis is usually arrived at in conjunction with clinical and other nonmorphologic findings. The diagnosis of inherited metabolic diseases should be confirmed by biochemical investigation of the diseased muscle or other tissues. Lysosomal storage or repetitive necrosis and regeneration of myofibers suggest some metabolic myopathies.

Glycogenoses

There are 11 forms of biochemically defined glycogenoses.[123] Among these different forms, only a few affect skeletal muscle: types II, III, IV, V, and VII.

Glycogen accumulates either in the cytoplasm or within the lysosomal compartments, and in many instances, glycogen granules are more evident by electron microscopy than by light microscopy. Loss of glycogen during preparation of muscle specimens may result in a vacuolar appearance. The myopathies of glycogenoses may therefore be a form of vacuolar myopathy.[75]

Type II Glycogenoses

This disease may become manifest as infantile (Pompe's disease), juvenile, or adult forms and is transmitted autosomal-recessively.[80] All three variants are marked by severe deficiency of acid maltase (alpha-glucosidase), best determined biochemically in muscle, but also demonstrable in circulating leukocytes and urine.

The deficiency of acid maltase results in intralysosomal accumulation of glycogen because of a block in glycogen catabolism. Glycogen-filled vacuoles in type II glycogenosis thus have strong acid phosphatase activity (Fig. 8-62A), the marker enzyme of lysosomes. The deposition of glycogen in type II glycogenosis is widespread, hence glycogen accumulates within (Figs. 8-24 and 8-62B) and outside muscle fibers (e.g., in mural cells of intramuscular vessels) (Fig. 8-62C). The vacuolar appearance of muscle fibers is conspicuous in infantile type II glycogenosis (Fig. 8-62D). In addition, modified trichrome preparations may show purple material of unidentified origin. In addition to intralysosomal glycogen, sarcoplasmic glycogen increases, and the glycogen accumulating in mural cells of intramuscular vessels can be seen chiefly within lysosomes (Fig. 8-62B). The glycogen is strongly stained by the PAS method and is digestible with diastase.

Vacuolization and destruction of muscle fibers is milder in the juvenile and adult forms of type II glycogenosis. Frequently, only small membrane-bound sacs of lysosomal glycogen may be encountered among regularly arranged myofibrils (Fig. 8-62B). In addition, rimmed vacuoles are present. Glycogen deposits in lysosomes are nonspecific and may be found in lysosomal glycogen storage with normal acid maltase activity.[56,175] Acid maltase deficiency must be demonstrated biochemically to establish the diagnosis.

Type III glycogenosis is a rare variant occurring in children and adults.[61] It is biochemically defined by a glycogen debrancher deficiency (amylo-1,6-glucosidase) and morphologically by excessive sarcoplasmic glycogen.

Type IV glycogenosis (amylopectinosis) affects skeletal muscle, liver, and nervous system. It is the result of a deficiency of the branching enzyme alpha-1,4-glucan:alpha-1,4-glucan-6-glucosyl transferase, leading to deposition of granulofibrillar material and cytoplasmic glycogen.[152]

In polyglucosan body or polysaccharide storage myopathy,[200] a similar complex of fibrillar granular material accumulates within muscle fibers, but an enzyme deficiency is not known. The fibrillar material accumulating in type IV glycogenosis, in polyglucosan body myopathy, and in Lafora bodies is antigenetically similar.[100,213]

Type V glycogenosis (McArdle's disease) is the expression of myophosphorylase deficiency. This condition results in accumulation of cytoplasmic glycogen, digested by diastase. The myophosphorylase deficiency can be demonstrated by the absence of histoenzymatic activity in muscle fibers (Figs. 8-63A,B), although phosphorylase activity

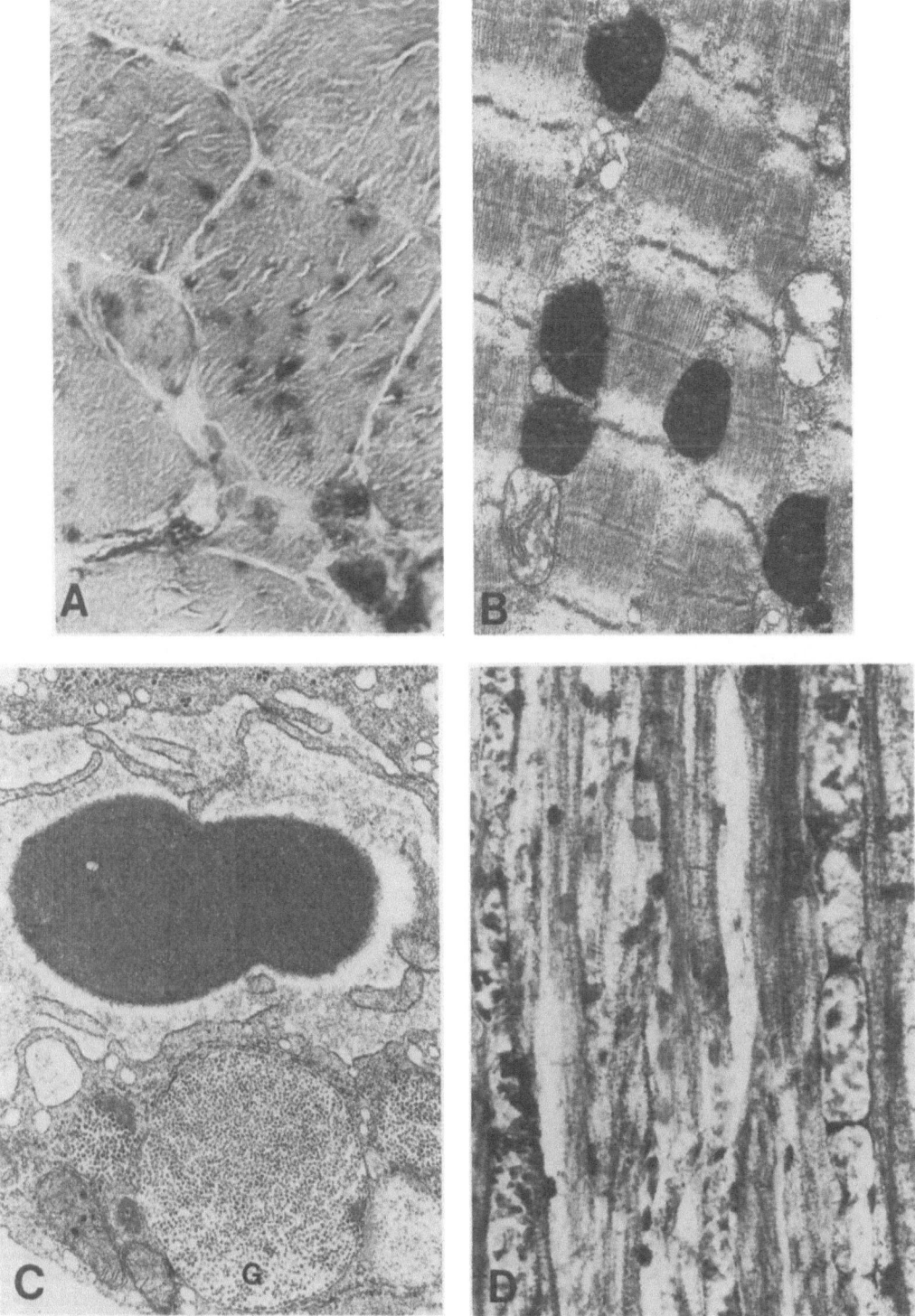

Fig. 8-62. Type II glycogenosis. (A) Increased acid phosphatase activity (dark dots) indicates enlargement of the lysosomal compartment: 30-year-old man, adult form; quadriceps (×530). (B) Numerous dark lysosomal bodies are filled with glycogen, indicative of lysosomal glycogen storage disease. Same biopsy as in Fig. 8-62A (×15,720). (C) Lysosomal glycogen (G) is found within an endothelial cell: 7-month-old girl, infantile type; gastrocnemius (×24,000). (D) There is severe vacuolation of muscle fibers in the infantile form. Same biopsy as in Fig. 8-62C. (Modified trichrome; ×420).

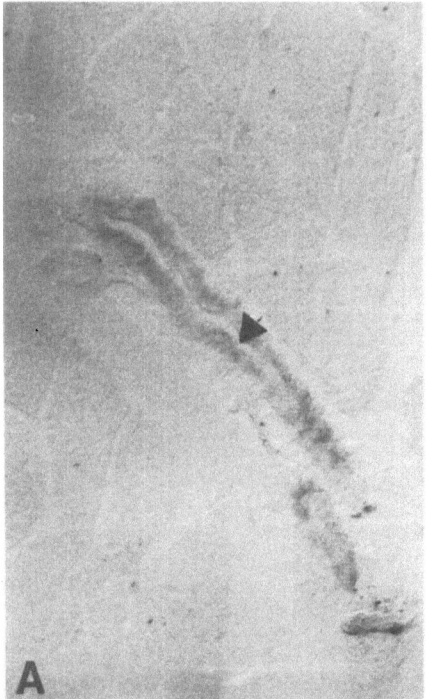

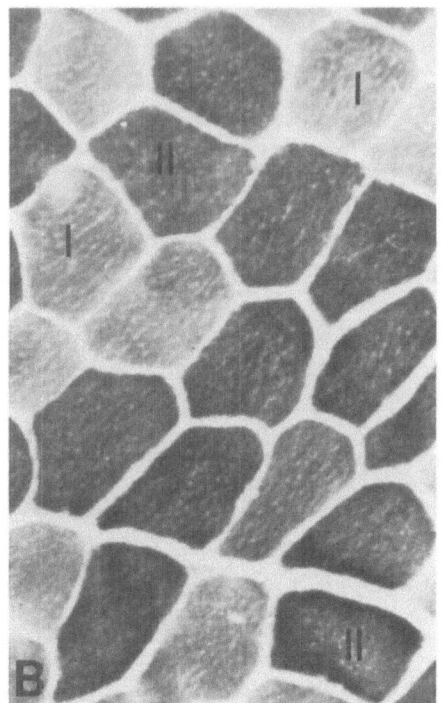

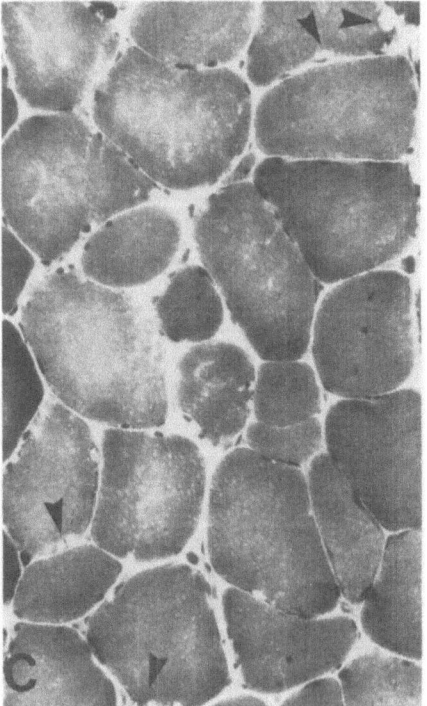

Fig. 8-63. Type V glycogenosis. (A) There is no myophosphorylase activity in muscle fibers, but faint
activity in intramuscular vessel (arrow) walls:
23-year-old man, no biochemical phosphorylase
activity in muscle; quadriceps (×212). (B) Activity
of myophosphorylase allows fiber typing in a
control section: 35-year old man; normal biceps
muscle (×212). (C) Several small, round or angular fibers, increase of internal nuclei, and hypertrophy of muscle fibers as well as few subsarcolemmal vacuoles (arrows) indicate vacuolar
myopathy. 56-year old man, biochemically
proven myophosphorylase deficiency; biceps
(Modified trichrome; ×164).

in mural cells of intramuscular vessels is faint but definite (Fig. 8-63*A*). The demonstration of phosphorylase in mural cells serves as an internal control.

The amylophosphorylase method[68] is preferred to the use of alpha-glucan-phosphorylase[18]; the former method depends on the phosphorylase activity, but the latter is based on PAS-positive material related to the presence of glycogen.

Phosphorylase deficiency may result in repetitive bouts of rhabdomyolysis and myoglobinuria after brief exertion. Disseminated muscle fiber necrosis, phagocytosis, and regeneration may be encountered in the biopsy. With increasing duration of the disease, a chronic nonspecific myopathy may ensue (Fig. 8-63C). Vacuoles occasionally may be seen beneath the sarcolemma (Fig. 8-63C), but they are of nonlysosomal origin.

Type VII glycogenosis is related to phosphofructokinase (PFK) deficiency, which may be expressed clinically in a manner similar to type V glycogenosis. Sarcoplasmic glycogen, sometimes of a fibrillar nature, nonspecific myopathy, or evidence of muscle fiber necrosis may be encountered. A double substrate–histochemical technique demonstrates the presence or absence of PFK.[23]

Lipid myopathies. Increased numbers of lipid particles in skeletal muscle fibers may be a nonspecific finding. The reason for the increased lipid content usually is not known. Type I fibers generally contain more lipid droplets than type II fibers.

In carnitine deficiency, lipid droplets within skeletal muscle fibers may exceed the normal range (Fig. 8-64), both in the myopathic and the systemic forms.[51] Abnormally structured mitochondria, (e.g., with crystal inclusions), may be also encountered.

In carnitine-palmityl-transferase deficiency, lipids within muscle fibers may be within normal range or slightly increased. This disorder is clinically marked by bouts of myoglo-

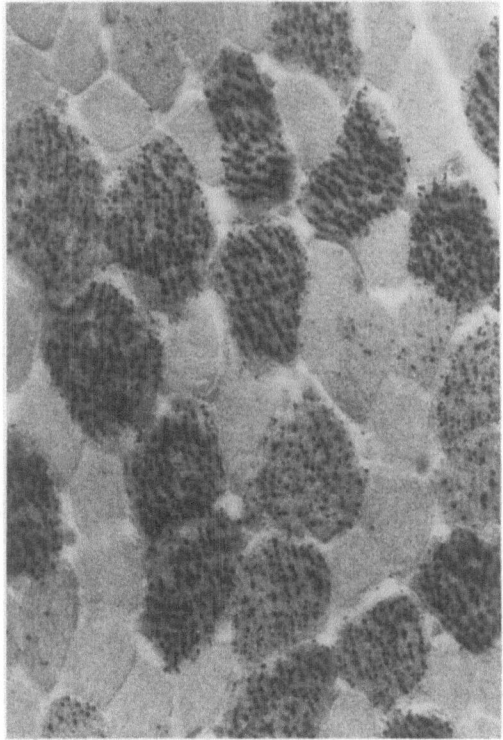

Fig. 8-64. Considerable increase of fat droplets (dark dots) in type I fibers: 6-year-old boy, biochemically confirmed carnitine deficiency; quadriceps (Oil red O; ×359).

binuria because of necrosis of muscle fibers. Disseminated necrosis, phagocytosis, and muscle fiber regeneration are more characteristic of this disorder than is the increase of lipid. Alternatively, the muscle may have nonspecific changes. Carnitine deficiency and carnitine-palmityl-transferase deficiency must be ascertained through appropriate biochemical methods.

Lysosomal diseases are progressive disorders characterized by intralysosomal accumulation of compounds that cannot be catabolized because of a disease-specific lysosomal enzyme deficiency. Certain lysosomal disorders show morphologic manifestations in skeletal muscle: infantile, late infantile, and juvenile neuronal ceroid lipofuscinoses (Figs. 8-65A,B); infantile, juvenile, and adult type II glycogenoses (Fig. 8-62); and mucolipidosis IV (Fig. 8-66). Lysosomal diseases are marked by accumulation of lysosomes and increased activity of acid phosphatase (Figs. 8-62A, 8-65A, and 8-66). Increased activity of acid phosphatase in otherwise normal-appearing muscle fibers may indicate lysosomal diseases affecting skeletal muscle (Figs. 8-62A, 8-65A, 8-66). Electron microscopy is necessary to identify the nature of the accumulated compounds (Figs. 8-62B and 8-65B).

Rhabdomyolysis causing increased serum myoglobin and myoglobinuria is a nonspecific feature (Table 8-10) of metabolic disorders such as phosphorylase deficiency and carnitine-palmityl-transferase deficiency; it also develops in hyperpyrexia, acute myositis, and acute alcohol intoxication. Depending on the duration of the disease, necrosis,

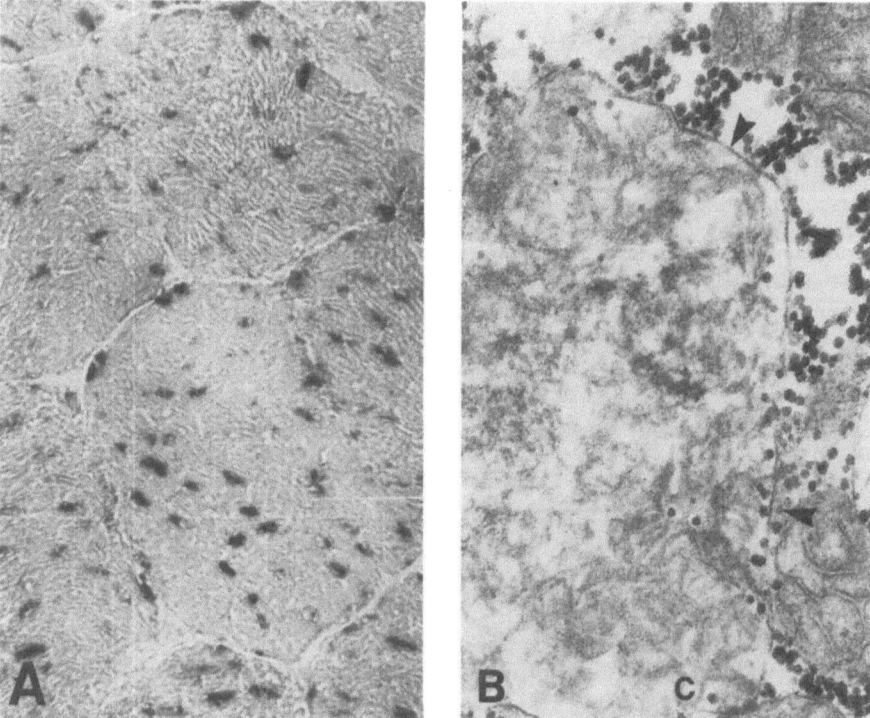

Fig. 8-65. Juvenile neuronal ceroid-lipofuscinosis in a 7-year-old boy; deltoid. (A) Numerous dark dots represent sites of lysosomal activity for acid phosphatase (×530). (B) Electron microscopically, the dark dots represent membrane-bound (arrows) curvilinear (C) profiles (×54,000).

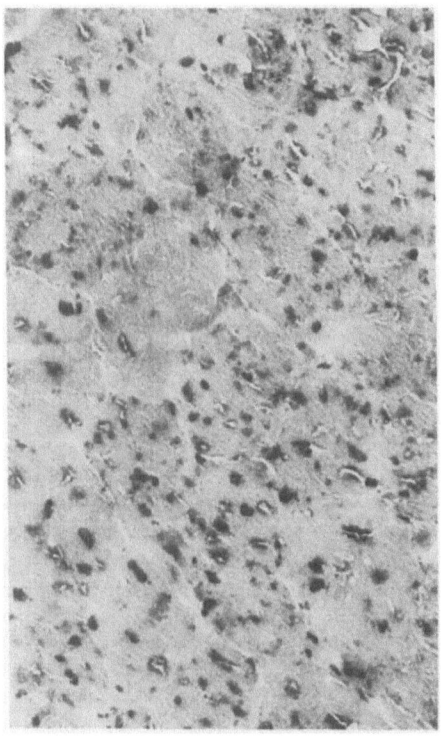

Fig. 8-66. Numerous dark dots represent sites of increased activity for lysosomal acid phosphatase: 14-year-old girl, mucolipidosis IV; quadriceps (×530).

phagocytosis (Fig. 8-67), and regeneration of disseminated muscle fibers may be seen in addition to nonspecific chronic myopathic features. The morphologic diagnosis would read "necrotizing myopathy," a nonspecific descriptive term. The cause or underlying biochemical defect of rhabdomyolysis is not apparent in muscle biopsies except for certain enzyme deficiencies or myositis. CK values also tend to be greatly elevated. In spite of greatly elevated CK levels in serum, muscle biopsies may show few abnormalities.

Table 8-10.
Causes of Myoglobinuria

Paroxysmal myoglobinuria (Meyer–Betz)
  I (familial, young males, induced by exercise)
  II (sporadic, children, induced by infections)
Glycogenosis (e.g., phosphorylase and phospho-
  fructokinase deficiencies)
Carnitine-palmityl-transferase deficiency
Mitochondrial myopathies
Trauma (e.g., crush)
Ischemia (e.g., tibialis-anterior syndrome, vascular
  occlusion)
Intoxication (e.g., alcohol, barbiturates, heroin, car-
  bon monoxide, amphotericin B, licorice, hornet
  venom, Haff disease)
Malignant hyperthermia
Acute polymyositis

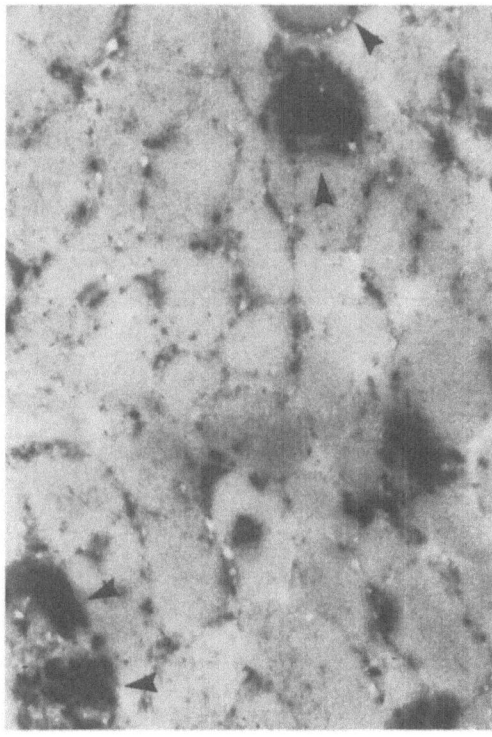

Fig. 8-67. Abundant acid phosphatase activity within macrophages marks phagocytosis of disseminated necrotic myofibers (arrows): 66-year-old woman, rhabdomyolysis and myoglobinuria, hyperosmolar diabetic coma, CK 26,000 U/l; biceps ($\times$208).

This finding is not confined to instances where rhabdomyolysis is localized, as in an ischemic work test or compression of a limb. Muscle changes may also be scant or absent in cases of generalized rhabdomyolysis. Can CK be released from non-necrotic myofibers, perhaps as a result of increased permeability of the plasma membrane, or are biopsied muscle specimens not representative samples of the entire skeletal musculature?

Characteristic or pathognomonic morphologic features of malignant hyperthermia (hyperpyrexia; heat stroke) are lacking. Muscle biopsy may not confirm this diagnosis if the disorder occurred in an incomplete form or if it was aborted early in generalized anesthesia. Muscle appearance in malignant hyperthermia may be either normal or consistent with nonspecific, chronic myopathy with or without signs of muscle fiber breakdown. The latter features are usually temporally related to the bout of malignant hyperthermia. Chronic myopathic changes[174] in this condition attest to the fact that the muscle is chronically diseased even in the absence of malignant hyperthermia. "Cores," indistinguishable from those of central core disease, have been demonstrated in many patients and their relatives.

Periodic paralyses. These acquired or inherited (in general, autosomal-dominant) metabolic disorders are usually accompanied by impaired potassium metabolism. They are classified as hypokalemic, hyperkalemic, or normokalemic periodic paralyses (PP) comprising different clinical complexes. The sarcoplasmic reticulum and the T-tubules are primarily involved in the disease. Swelling of the triads or terminal sacs of the sarcoplasmic reticulum (SR) first occur during the paralytic attacks, often resulting in vacuolated myofibers (Figs. 8-68*A,B*). With increasing duration of the disorder, SR proliferates, often with mineralization.[75] Hypokalemic PP has the most conspicuous changes. Tubular

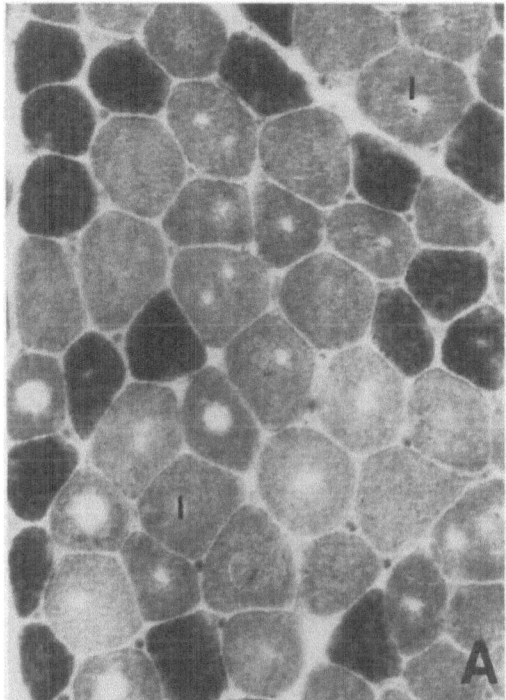

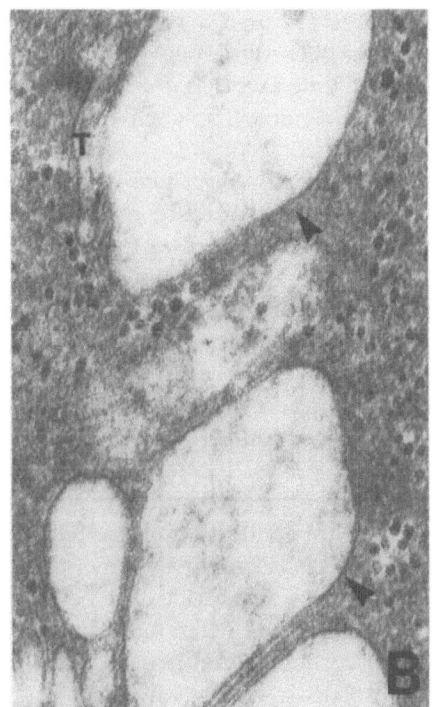

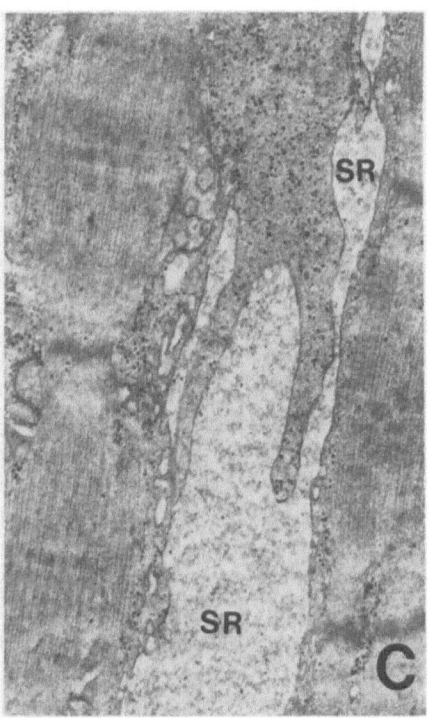

Fig. 8-68. Hypokalemic periodic paralysis in an 18-year-old woman; gastrocnemius. (A) Numerous vacuoles are present in type I fibers. (MAG preparation; ×228). (B) Numerous large, membrane-bound (arrows) vacuoles, one adjacent to a possible T-tubule (T) (×70,500). (C) Dilatation of the sarcoplasmic reticulum (SR) parallel to the long axis of the sarcomeres (×20,000).

aggregates are also a typical feature (Fig. 8-18). Less well-defined SR abnormalities have also been described.[75] Occasionally, dilatation of the terminal sac or SR cisternae along the long axis (Fig. 8-68C) of the sarcomeres may be the only morphologic evidence of PP. Light-microscopic appearances may be normal, particularly in secondary transient hypokalemia.

Mitochondrial myopathies are an ill-defined group of neuromuscular disorders,[60,62,130,148] marked by electron-microscopic evidence of abnormal structure of mitochondria (Figs. 8-17A,B). The mitochondria lack cristae and have circular arrangements of some cristae and crystal inclusions as well as electron-dense spheroids. Abnormal mitochondria are often increased in size and number. If clusters of mitochondria become large, they produce "ragged red fibers" (Figs. 8-15, 8-16). In certain mitochondrial myopathies, biochemical defects have been detected, often associated with lactic acidosis; this warrants the classification of mitochondrial myopathies as metabolic myopathies. In other mitochondrial myopathies, especially the oculocraniosomatic or Kearns–Sayre syndrome, precise biochemical lesions have often not been identified. The clinical range of mitochondrial myopathies is so great that precise classification of an individual mitochondrial myopathy requires all available clinical, serologic, and biochemical data. The term "mitochondrial myopathy" thus is morphologic and should be retained only until mitochondrial myopathies are better understood.

Myoadenylate deaminase deficiency is a recent but nosologically not yet completely defined condition that is associated with numerous other neuromuscular diseases but may also occur without them.[98] Then, it may be related to exercise-induced myalgia. The enzyme defect can be detected by enzymehistochemical and biochemical techniques.

Vitamin E deficiency in humans is usually without effect on skeletal muscle. Experimentally, vitamin E deficiency may cause necrosis of muscle fibers. Lack of vitamin E, an antioxidant, may occasionally result in increased amounts of lipopigments (Figs. 8-69A & B) in otherwise normal-appearing, nonatrophic muscle fibers.[37] Vitamin E deficiency may occur as a secondary phenomenon in children afflicted with biliary cirrhosis,[111] cystic fibrosis, or possibly malabsorption syndromes. It has also been associated with a-beta-lipoproteinemia, the Bassen–Kornzweig syndrome.[136]

A growing number of patients has been reported, afflicted with a spinocerebellar syndrome, who displayed vitamin E deficiency of unknown origin, though of a treatable form.[214]

Endocrine disorders. The following endocrine diseases may have clinical and morphologic neuromuscular lesions: hyper- and hypothyroidism, hyper- and hypo-parathyroidism, acromegaly, Cushing's disease, and hyperaldosteronism. Hyperthyroidism or thyrotoxicosis is the endocrine disease most frequently affecting skeletal muscle. Abnormally structured mitochondria occasionally occur in diseased myofibers.[74] On the whole, pathognomonic or even specific muscle lesions are lacking in endocrine disorders. Type I and type II[135] myofiber atrophies occur, particularly in Cushing's syndrome, or after steroid drug therapy. Primary hypothyroidism is now thought to be the cause of "hypertrophia muscularis vera," also called the Kocher–Debré–Sémélaigne syndrome.[195]

Excessive alcohol ingestion may produce nonspecific, acute, and chronic myopathic features.[147] As there is no specific morphologic picture, the correct diagnosis can be made only in association with clinical and other information.

Certain drugs may produce neuromuscular diseases: penicillamine = myositis or myasthenia; steroids = type II myofiber atrophy; chloroquine = vacuolar lysosomal myopathy; ipecac syrup, epsilon-amino-caproic acid, rifampicin = nonspecific myopathies.

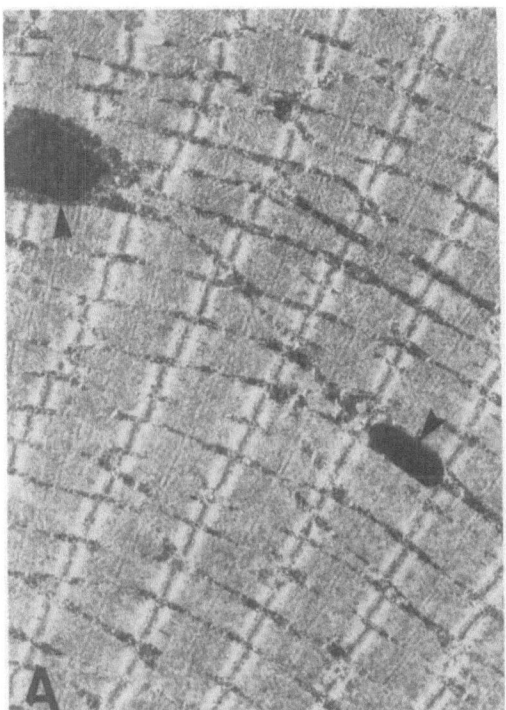
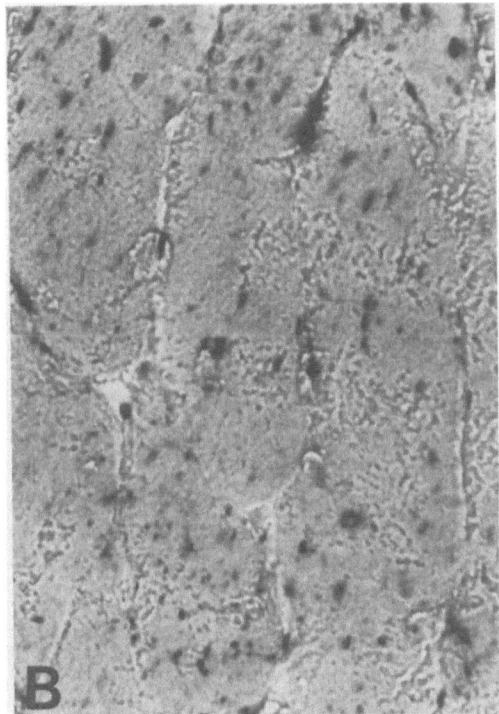

Fig. 8-69. Vitamin E deficiency: vitamin E serum lowered to 10% of normal, in an 8-year-old boy; gastrocnemius. (A) Dark membrane-bound lysosomal inclusions (arrows) are autofluorescent lipopigments (×7,600). (B) The autofluorescent lipopigments display increased activity of acid phosphatase (dark dots) (×600).

Myasthenia Gravis and Myasthenic Syndromes

Myasthenia gravis and the myasthenic syndromes are diseases of the neuromuscular junction or motor endplate. They are usually diagnosed by clinical, electromyographic, and pharmacologic investigations. Histopathologic examination plays a minor role in diagnosing these disorders, and precise diagnosis of any of these diseases cannot be reliably made with the light microscope. Pathologic changes may be present, however, in muscle biopsies in myasthenia gravis, such as type II atrophy (Fig. 8-70A); denervation atrophy, usually consisting of small groups of atrophic fibers, occasionally also of large groups; single necrotic fibers and "lymphorrhages."[85,134,183] Occasionally, myasthenia may be associated with polymyositis[59] or it may be induced by penicillamine. This drug is used in the treatment of rheumatoid arthritis, a disease that itself may be associated with muscle lesions.

Adequate morphologic study of disease-specific features in myasthenia gravis and myasthenic syndromes necessitates electron-microscopic evaluation of motor endplates. Myasthenia gravis is thought to represent an immune-mediated degeneration of post-synaptic acetylcholine *receptors* and postsynaptic *junctional folds*. Electron microscopy may show considerable atrophy of the postsynaptic part of the motor endplate (Fig. 8-70B): (i.e., shorter junctional folds, remnants of degenerating fold material, loops of basal lamina indicating presence of former junctional folds, and enlarged primary clefts

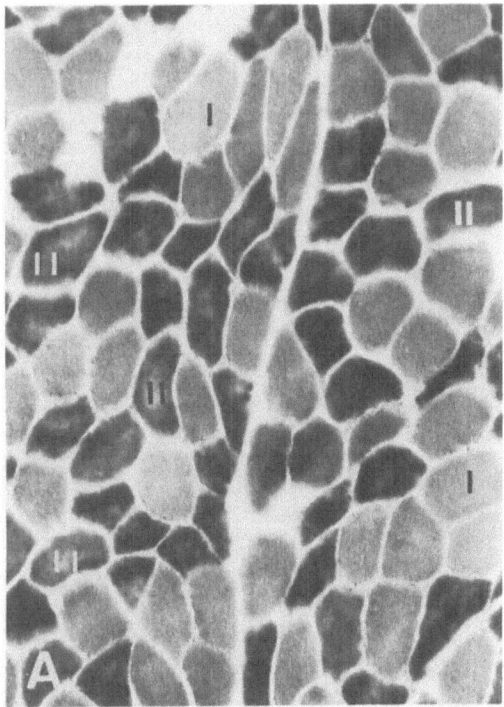

Fig. 8-70. Myasthenia gravis in a 25-year-old woman; biceps. (A) Conspicuous type II myofiber atrophy. (MAG preparation; ×156). (B) Subneural apparatus of motor endplate in untreated myasthenia gravis in a 23-year-old man; intercostal muscle (×12,000). (C) Hypertrophic subneural folds of motor endplate in myasthenic syndrome associated with bronchial carcinoma in a 68-year-old man; intercostal muscle (×17,800). (Figs. 9-70b and 9-70c courtesy of S.M. Chou, M.D., Cleveland, OH).

between the presynaptic and postsynaptic parts of the motor end plate).[76] These qualitative changes have been quantified.[83]

Such studies have been augmented by subsequent morphologic and immunopathologic investigations concerning the acetylcholine receptors and the presence of complement and immunoglobulins at the motor endplate region, in both human myasthenia gravis and experimentally induced autoimmune myasthenia gravis.[82] With the improvement of morphologic techniques, application of such electron-microscopic and immunopathologic methods to the diagnosis of myasthenia gravis and myasthenic syndromes is feasible.

Combined clinical, electromyographic, and electron-microscopic studies have also enabled separation of congenital myasthenic syndromes of various types[81] as well as the distinction between myasthenic or Eaton–Lambert syndrome[91] another autoimmune disease (92), and myasthenia gravis (Fig. 8-70C).

Myotonias

Clinical myotonia is the impairment of relaxation of muscles after contraction. Percussion myotonia and the electromyographic features of myotonia are so characteristic that some hereditary neuromuscular disorders have been classified according to the presence of myotonia. A morphologic equivalent of the myotonia has not been detected by light or electron microscopy.

The neuromuscular disorders grouped as myotonias include autosomal-dominant dystrophic myotonia (myotonic dystrophy or atrophy); congenital myotonia of autoso-

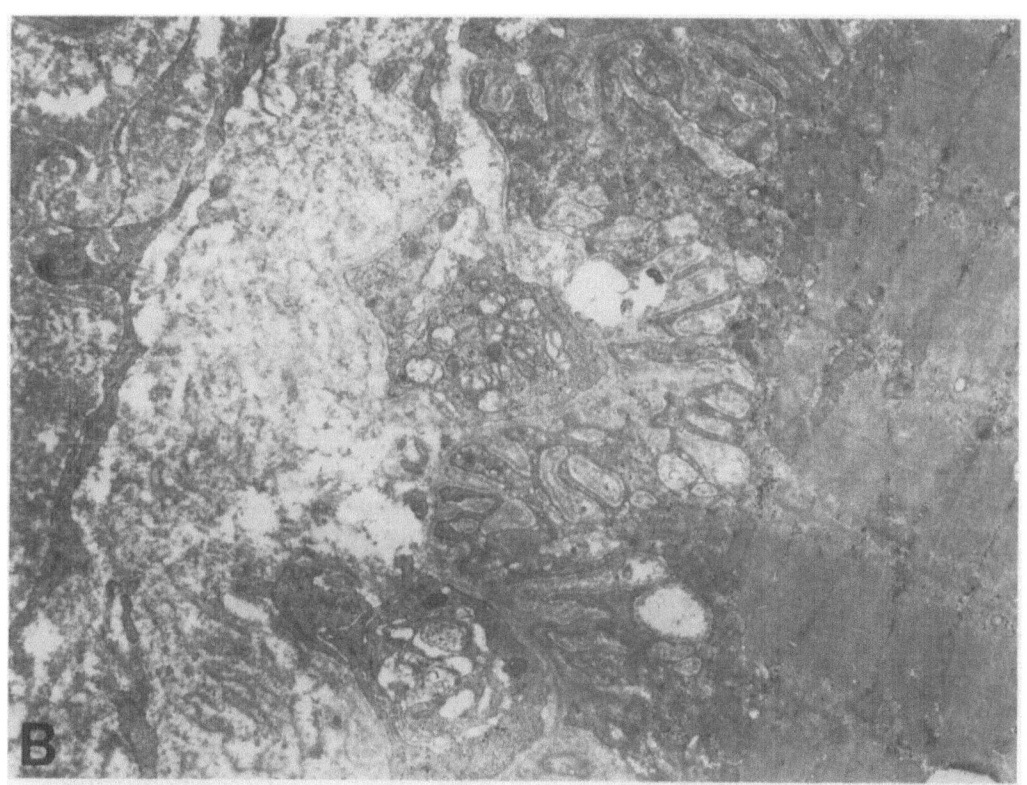

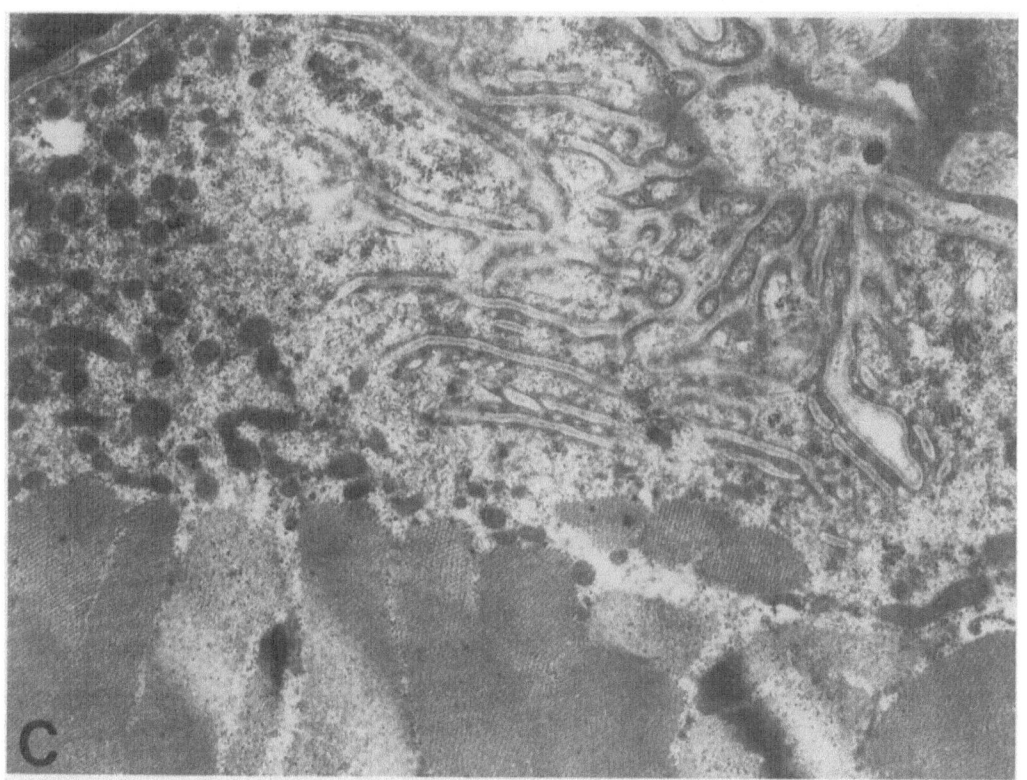

mal-dominant type, one of which is Thomsen's disease, but other subgroups have recently been defined on clinical grounds;[13] congenital myotonia of autosomal-recessive type; and paramyotonia or Eulenburg's disease.

Dystrophic or atrophic myotonia (myotonic dystrophy). In the early stages of this disease, muscles may show selective type I fiber atrophy and type I fiber predominance (Fig. 8-71) as well as hypertrophy of type II fibers (Fig. 8-72). This change is particularly noticeable in the biceps but it can also be seen in the deltoid and other limb muscles. This morphologic pattern of fiber type disproportion may resemble that seen in congenital fiber type disproportion (Fig. 8-53). The mean fiber diameters of type I and type II fibers differ considerably. Dystrophic myotonia is largely a disease of adults, but congenital fiber type disproportion is a disorder of children. This morphologic pattern of myofiber type disproportion may later disappear. In infantile and juvenile dystrophic myotonia, type I fiber atrophy (or possibly hypotrophy) may also be present (Fig. 8-73).[131] Internally located nuclei may greatly increase but ringbinden and sarcoplasmic masses (Figs. 8-74A,B) only develop later in the disease. Finally, at the end of the disease (Fig. 8-74C), muscles may show "end-stage myopathy," marked by extensive loss of myofibers, replacement by fat cells, and fibrosis.

Pyknotic nuclear clumps and occasional angulated fibers suggest a neurogenic origin of dystrophic myotonia. Morphologic evidence of denervation of dystrophic myotonia either has remained unconfirmed[171] or has been regarded as independent.[168] Because of excessive splitting, intrafusal myofibers may be numerous.[114,197] Electron microscopy may reveal abundant lesions,[187] but they are diagnostically nonspecific.

Congenital myotonia. Morphologically, there are discrete, nonspecific abnormal find-

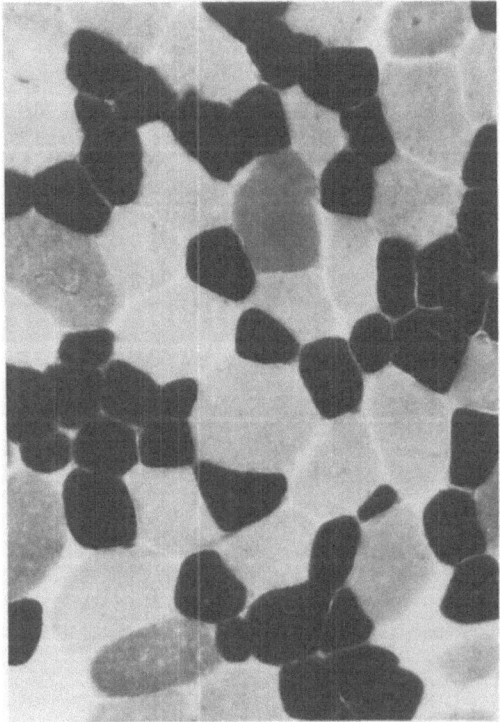

Fig. 8-71. Selective type I fiber (dark) atrophy and type I fiber predominance early in the disease: 20-year-old woman, myotonic dystrophy; biceps. (ATPase preparation, pH 4.5; ×180).

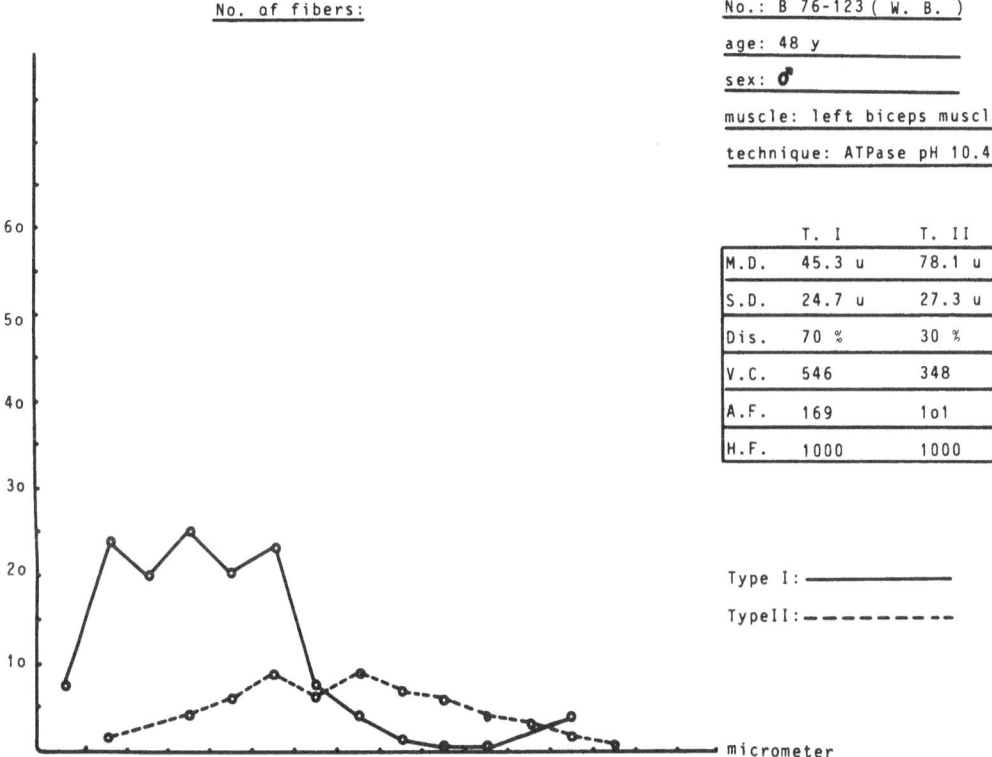

No. of fibers:

No.: B 76-123 (W. B.)

age: 48 y

sex: ♂

muscle: left biceps muscle

technique: ATPase pH 10.4

	T. I	T. II
M.D.	45.3 u	78.1 u
S.D.	24.7 u	27.3 u
Dis.	70 %	30 %
V.C.	546	348
A.F.	169	1o1
H.F.	1000	1000

Type I : —————————

TypeII : — — — — — — —

micrometer

Fig. 8-72. The histogram reveals the morphologic pattern of fiber type disproportion (type I fiber atrophy and predominance, type II fiber hypertrophy) early in the disease: 40-year-old man, myotonic dystrophy; biceps.

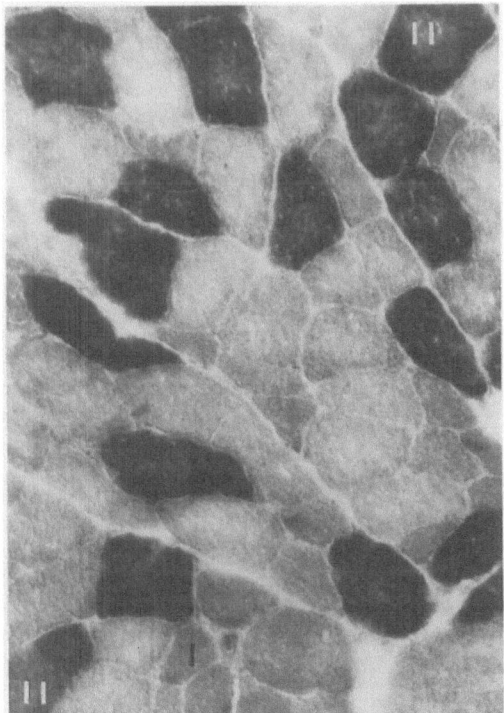

Fig. 8-73. Type I fiber predominance and atrophy occurs also in the juvenile form: 16-year-old boy, juvenile myotonic dystrophy; deltoid. (MAG preparation; ×192).

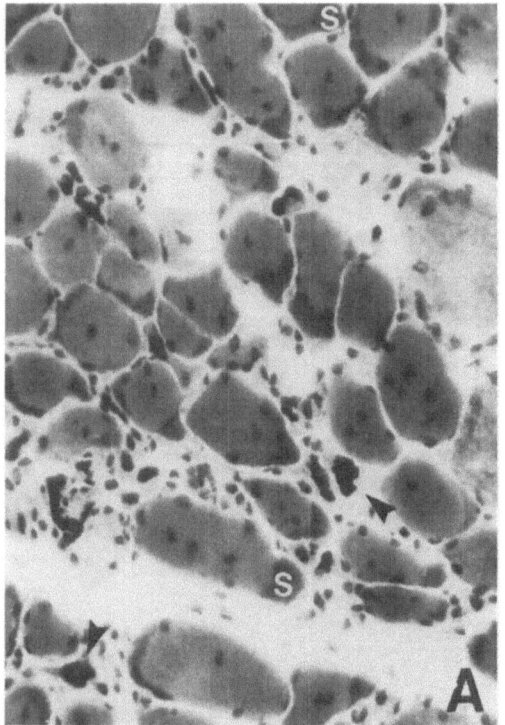

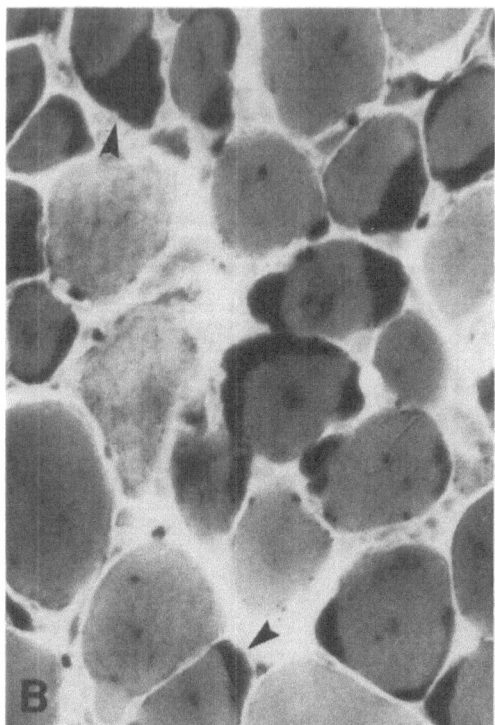

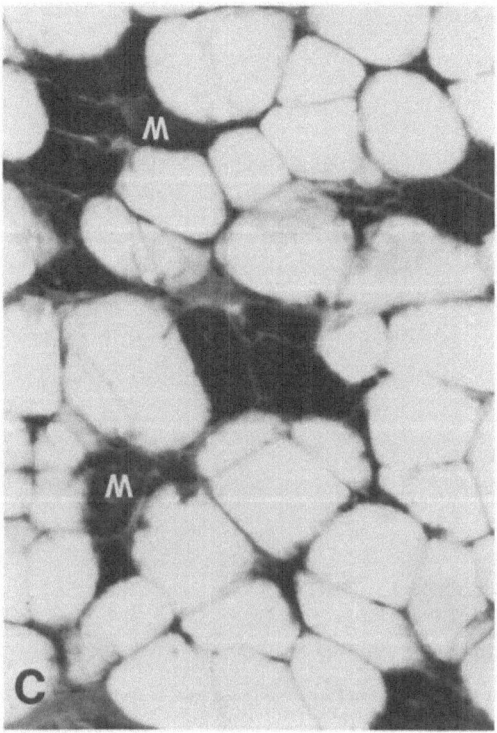

Fig. 8-74. Myotonic dystrophy in a 57-year-old woman, postmortem tissue. (A) Numerous internally located nuclei, peripheral sarcoplasmic masses (S), and several pyknotic nuclear clumps (arrows) are typical of the late stage of the disease; tibialis anterior (×220). (B) The sarcoplasmic masses are highly positive in the nonspecific esterase preparation (arrows); tibialis anterior (×260). (C) In the "endstage" only a few myofibers (M) with internal nuclei are left within large aggregates of fat cells gastrocnemius. (Modified trichrome; ×216).

ings in muscles of patients afflicted with congenital myotonias. Separate hereditary clinical forms do not entail different morphologic features. These changes are usually confined to enzyme-histochemical abnormalities, a numerical increase of internally located nuclei, and ultrastructural features. Type I (Fig. 8-75A) or type II atrophy (Figs. 8-75B, 8-76) may be encountered. Hypertrophy of muscle fibers may also be found (Fig. 8-77), especially in the autosomal-dominant type or Thomsen's disease, reflecting the heavy build of the patient. It has been previously emphasized[53] that type IIB fiber deficiency is characteristic of congenital myotonia, irrespective of the genetic subtype. This statement may be correct when studying the biceps muscle, as the authors[53] did, but type IIB fibers are present in other muscles, such as the quadriceps muscle of myotonic patients[115] (Fig. 8-77).

Paramyotonia of Eulenburg. This autosomal-dominant neuromuscular disorder may show few lesions: usually single fiber atrophy, sometimes more of type I, sometimes more of type II (Fig. 8-78), and a few degenerating fibers. Type IIB fibers, thought to be deficient in the biceps,[53] are present in the quadriceps muscle.[115]

Ocular Myopathies

Human extraocular muscle (EOM) differ from limb skeletal muscles in that the former show particular layering of myofibers and separate so-called coarse fibers,[179]

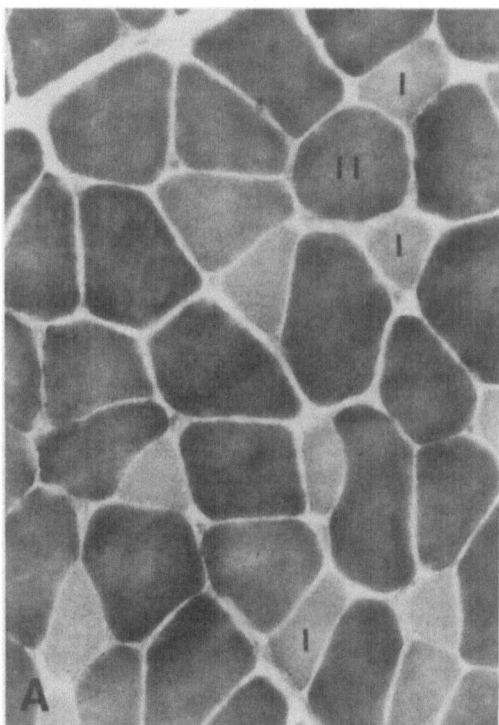 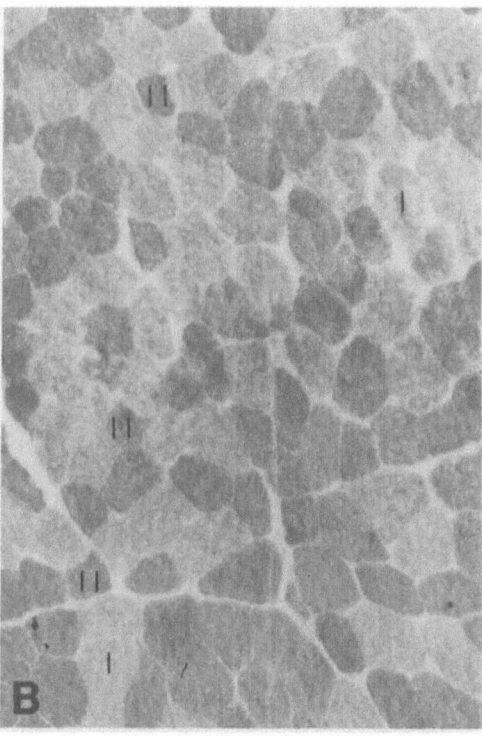

Fig. 8-75. Autosomal-recessive congenital myotonia; quadriceps. (A) Type I fibers are smaller than type II fibers: 7-year-old boy. (MAG preparation; ×216). (B) Type II fibers are smaller than type I fibers. Younger brother of previous patient was 7 years old at the time of biopsy. (ATPase preparation, pH 10.4; ×192).

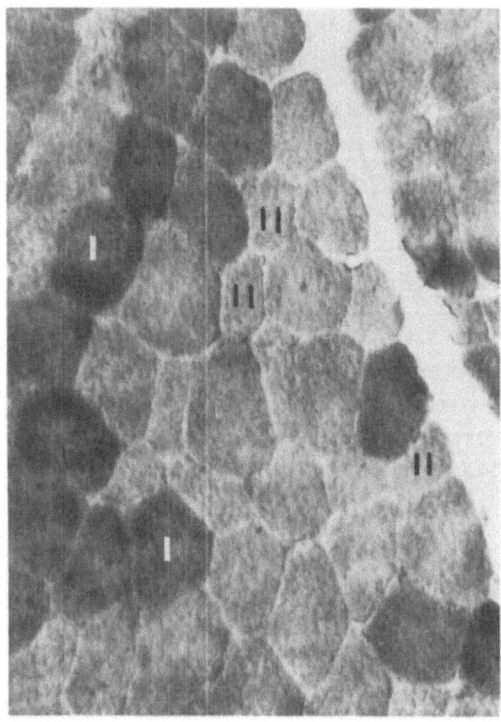

Fig. 8-76. Type II fibers are smaller than type I fibers: 13-year-old boy, autosomal-dominant congenital myotonia (Thomsen's disease); quadriceps. (NADH preparation; ×204).

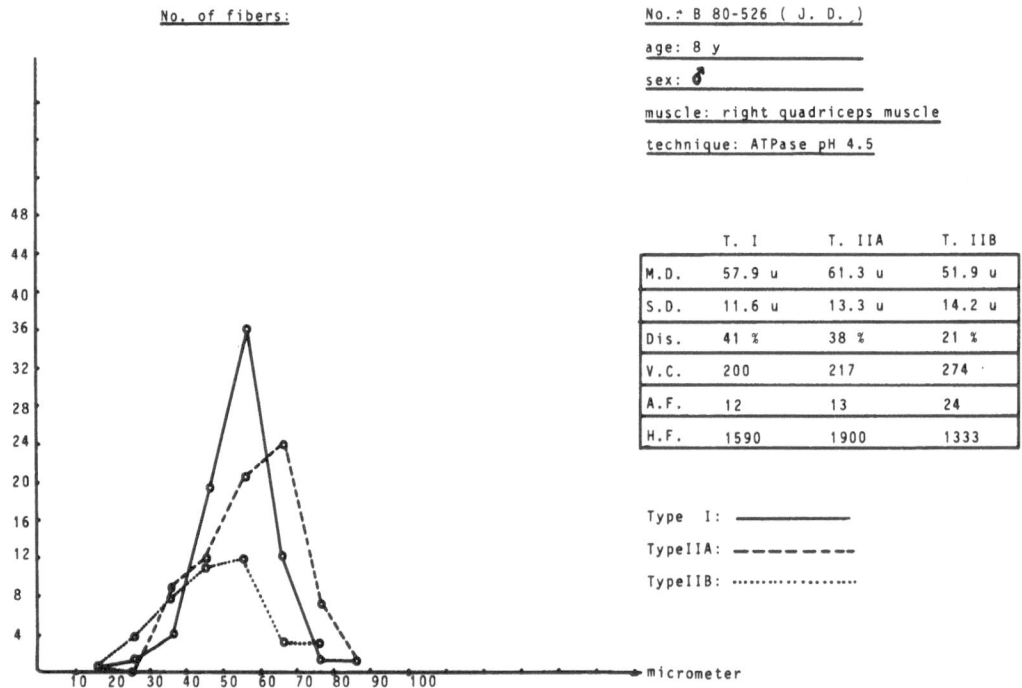

No. of fibers:

No.: B 80-526 (J. D.)

age: 8 y

sex: ♂

muscle: right quadriceps muscle

technique: ATPase pH 4.5

	T. I	T. IIA	T. IIB
M.D.	57.9 u	61.3 u	51.9 u
S.D.	11.6 u	13.3 u	14.2 u
Dis.	41 %	38 %	21 %
V.C.	200	217	274
A.F.	12	13	24
H.F.	1590	1900	1333

Type I: ──────────

TypeIIA: ─ ─ ─ ─ ─ ─

TypeIIB: ·····················

Fig. 8-77. The histogram shows conspicuous hypertrophy of type I, type IIA, and type IIB myofibers, no type IIB deficiency: 8-year-old boy, congenital myotonia; quadriceps.

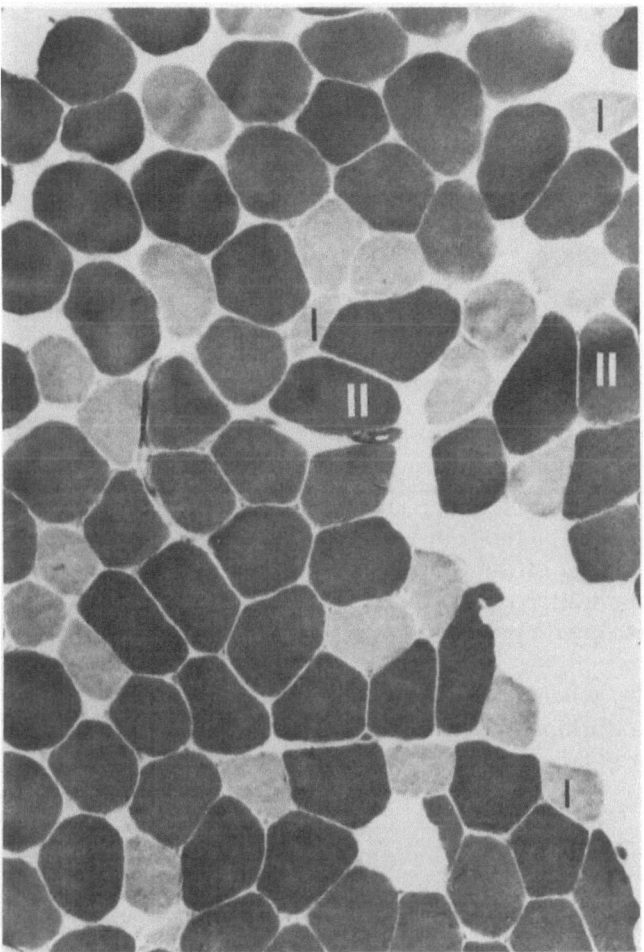

Fig. 8-78. Type I fiber atrophy: 20-year-old man, paramyotonia of Eulenburg; quadriceps. (ATPase preparation, pH 10.4; ×127.5)

in addition to fiber types, called fine and granular, that probably correspond to type I and type II fibers of limb muscles, respectively.[179] In the human inferior oblique muscle, fiber types could actually be compared to type I, IIA, IIB, and IIC myofibers of limb muscles.[121] Apart from smaller diameters of 17.5–20 μm, EOM fibers also present ultra-structural differences in that inclusions, such as filamentous bodies, zebra bodies and nemaline bodies, may occur in normal EOM.[145]

Clinically, ocular muscle symptoms, ptosis, and external ophthalmoplegia occur in many neuromuscular disorders (Table 8-11). In some, such as polymyositis, dystrophic myotonia, myasthenia gravis, or thyroid myopathies, the findings may differ among individual patients. In other diseases, ocular muscle weakness is an early or prominent sign, as in centronuclear myopathy, oculopharyngeal muscular dystrophy, or the oculo-craniosomatic syndrome. Whether an isolated ocular myopathy actually exists is doubtful. Nevertheless, the term "ocular muscular dystrophy" is still occasionally used.

Ocular muscle symptoms are often associated with clinical involvement of limb

Table 8-11.
Causes of Ocular Muscle Weakness

Ocular muscular dystrophy/myopathy
Oculocraniosomatic syndrome Kearns–Sayre
Other mitochondrial myopathies
Oculopharyngeal dystrophy
Oculopharyngodistal myopathy (Satoyoshi)
Centronuclear myopathy
Congenital fiber type disproportion
Ocular myositis
Myasthenia gravis
Thyroid myopathy
Central core disease

muscles, hence muscle biopsies are usually taken from limb muscles. Recently,[180] muscle biopsies from patients afflicted with chronic progressive external ophthalmoplegia have shown features similar to those in limb muscles obtained from the same patient at the same time. Knowledge of the changes in diseased extraocular muscles, however, still remains scant. Application of enzyme-histochemical techniques, and to a limited extent, of electron microscopy, to postmortem EOM specimens may further enlarge knowledge of diseased EOM.

Unfortunately, when muscle specimens, largely of the levator palpebrae muscle, become available during corrective surgery, the tissue is fibrotic and usually contains only remnants of EOM, resembling "end-stage myopathy."

Miscellaneous

Lesions of muscle may occur in many other disorders, but such conditions do not usually require muscle biopsy, as in trauma and traumatic denervation, ischemia, viral infections, meningomyelocele, other malformations, or several syndromes. Their myopathological spectrum is only incompletely known.

Acknowledgments

The author is grateful to the many contributors, who have aided in the preparation of this manuscript: to the "Stiftung Volkswagenwerk" for financial support (Az. I/36 303), to Ms. M. Schlie for light-microscopic preparations; to Mrs. F. Schulz and Ms. R. Kosswig for electron-microscopic and photographic work; to T. Baier and W. Holzapfel for histographic analyses; to Mrs. G. Ropte and Ms. E. Sabin for secretarial and editorial assistance; and foremost to the clinical colleagues for continual cooperation.

References

1. Afifi AK, Smith JW, Zellweger H: Congenital nonprogressive myopathy. Central core disease and nemaline myopathy in one family. Neurology 15:371–381, 1965
2. Arahata K, Engel AG: Monoclonal antibody analysis of mononuclear cells in myopathies. I: Quantitation

of subsets according to diagnosis and sites of accumulation and demonstration and counts of muscle fibers invaded by T cells. *Ann Neurol* 16:193–208, 1984

3. Arahata K, Engel AG: Monoclonal antibody analysis of mononuclear cells in myopathies. III: Immunoelectron microscopy aspects of cell-mediated muscle fiber injury. *Ann Neurol* 19:112–125, 1986

4. Arahata K, Engel AG: Monoclonal antibody analysis of mononuclear cells in myopathies. IV: Cell-mediated cytotoxicity and muscle fiber necrosis. *Ann Neurol* 23:168–173, 1988

5. Arahata K, Engel AG: Monoclonal antibody analysis of mononuclear cells in myopathies. V: Identification and quantitation of T8$^+$ cytotoxic and T8$^+$ suppressor cells. *Ann Neurol* 23:493–499, 1988

6. Bailey RO, Marzulo DC, Hans MB: Infantile facioscapulohumeral muscular dystrophy: New observations. *Acta Neurol Scand* 74:51–58, 1986

7. Bailey RO, Turok DI, Jaufmann BP, et al: Myositis and acquired immunodeficiency syndrome. *Hum Pathol* 18:749–751, 1987

8. Banker BQ: Dermatomyositis of childhood. Ultrastructural alterations of muscle and intramuscular blood vessels. *J Neuropathol Exp Neurol* 34:46–75, 1975

9. Banker BQ, Victor M: Dermatomyositis (systemic angiopathy) of childhood. *Medicine* 45:261–289, 1966

10. Barth PG, Van Wijngaarden GK, Bethlem J: X-linked myotubular myopathy with fatal neonatal asphyxia. *Neurology* 25:531–536, 1975

11. Bautista, J, Rafel E, Castilla JM, Alberca R: Hereditary distal myopathy with onset in early infancy. Observation of a family. *J Neurol Sci* 37:149–158, 1978

12. Becker PE: Two new families of benign sex-linked recessive muscular dystrophy. *Rev Can Biol* 21:551–566, 1962

13. Becker PE: Myotonia congenita and syndromes associated with myotonia. Clinical–genetic studies of the nondystrophic myotonias. In Becker PE, Lenz W, Vogel F, et al (eds): *Topics in Human Genetics, Vol. 3*, Stuttgart, Thieme, 1977

14. Beckmann R, Freund-Mölbert E, Ketelsen UP: Eine Myopathie unklarer Genese mit Degeneration von "Satellitzellen". *Pathol Eur* 6:161–171, 1971

15. Bender AN, Willner JP: Nemaline (rod) myopathy: The need for histochemical evaluation of affected families. *Ann Neurol* 4:37–42, 1978

16. Ben Hamida M, Fardeau M, Attia N: Severe childhood muscular dystrophy affecting both sexes and frequent in Tunisia. *Muscle & Nerve* 6:469–480, 1983

17. Bernat JL, Ochoa JL: Muscle hypertrophy after partial denervation: A human case. *J Neurol Neurosurg Psychiatry* 41:719–725, 1978

18. Bethlem J: *Muscle Pathology. Introduction and Atlas.* North-Holland Publishing, Amsterdam, London; American Elsevier Publishing, New York, 1970

19. Bethlem J, Van Wijngaarden GK: Benign myopathy, with autosomal dominant inheritance—A report on three pedigrees. *Brain* 99:91–100, 1976

20. Bethlem J, Arts WF, Dingemans KP: Common origin of rods, cores, miniature cores, and focal loss of cross-striations. *Arch Neurol* 35:555–566, 1978

21. Bodensteiner JB, Engel AG: Intracellular calcium accumulation in Duchenne dystrophy and other myopathies: A study of 567,000 muscle fibers in 114 biopsies. *Neurology* 28:439–446, 1978

22. Bohan A, Peter JB: Polymyositis and dermatomyositis. *N Engl J Med* 292:344–347, 403–407, 1975

23. Bonilla E, Schotland DL: Histochemical diagnosis of muscle phosphofructokinase deficiency. *Arch Neurol* 22:8–12, 1970

24. Borg K, Borg J, Lindblom U: Sensory involvement in distal myopathy (Welander). *J Neurol Sci* 80:323–332, 1987

25. Bormioli SP, Lucke S, Angelini C: Abnormal myomuscular junctions and AChE in a congenital neuromuscular disease. *Muscle Nerve* 3:240–247, 1980

26. Bove KE, Iannaccone ST, Hilton PK, Samaha F: Cylindrical spirals in a familial neuromuscular disorder. *Ann Neurol* 7:550–556, 1980

27. Bradley WG: The limb-girdle syndromes, in Vinken PJ, Bruyn GW (eds): *Handbook of Clinical Neurology. Vol. 40, Part I*, Amsterdam North-Holland Publishing Company, 1979, 433–469

28. Bradley WG, Fulthorpe JJ: Studies of sarcolemmal integrity in myopathic muscle. *Neurology* 28:670–677, 1978

29. Bradley WG, Hudgson P, Larson PF, et al: Structural changes in the early stages of Duchenne muscular dystrophy. *J Neurol Neurosurg Psychiatry* 35:451–455, 1972

30. Bradley WG, Jones MZ, Fawcett PRW: Becker-type muscular dystrophy. *Muscle & Nerve* 1:111–132, 1978

31. Brooke MH: The pathologic interpretation of muscle histochemistry, in Pearson CM, Mostofi FK, (eds): *The Striated Muscle*, Baltimore, Williams & Wilkins, 1973, 86–122

284   *Hans H. Goebel*

32. Brooke MH: Congenital fiber type dysproportion, in Kakulas BA (ed): *Clinical Studies in Myology, Part 2*, Excerpta Medica, Amsterdam; New York, American Elsevier, 1973, 147–159
33. Brooke MH, Engel WK: The histographic analysis of human muscle biopsies with regard to fiber types. 4. Children's biopsies. *Neurology* 19:591–605, 1969
34. Brooke MH, Kaplan H: Muscle pathology in rheumatoid arthritis, polymyalgia rheumatica, and polymyositis. A histochemical study. *Arch Pathol Lab Med* 94:101–118, 1972
35. Brooke MH, Neville HE: Reducing body myopathy. *Neurology* 22:829–840, 1972
36. Brooke MH, Carroll JE, Ringel SP: Congenital hypotonia revisited. *Muscle & Nerve* 2:84–100, 1979
37. Burck U, Goebel HH, Kuklendahl, HD, et al: Neuromyopathy and vitamin E deficiency in man. *Neuropediatrics* 12:267–278, 1981
38. Cancilla PA, Kalyanaraman K, Verity MA, et al: Familial myopathy with probable lysis of myofibrils in type I fibers. *Neurology* 21:579–585, 1971
39. Cape CA, Johnson WW, Pitner SE: Nemaline structures in polymyositis. *Neurology* 20:494–502, 1970
40. Carpenter S, Karpati G: Duchenne muscular dystrophy. Plasma membrane loss initiates muscle cell necrosis unless it is repaired. *Brain* 102:147–161, 1979
41. Carpenter S, Karpati G, Rothman S, et al: The childhood type of dermatomyositis. *Neurology* 26:952–962, 1976
42. Carpenter S, Karpati G, Heller I, et al: Inclusion body myositis: A distinct variety of idiopathic inflammatory myopathy. *Neurology* 28:8–17, 1978
43. Cashman NR, Maselli R, Wollmann RL, et al: Late denervation in patients with antecedent paralytic poliomyelitis. *N Engl J Med* 317:7–12, 1987
44. Chijiiwa T, Nishimura M, Inomata H, et al: Ocular manifestations of congenital muscular dystrophy (Fukuyama type). *Ann Ophthalmol* 15:921–928, 1983
45. Chou SM: "Megaconial" mitochondria observed in a case of chronic polymyositis. *Acta Neuropathol (Berlin)* 12:68–89, 1969
46. Chou SM: Prospects of viral etiology in polymyositis, in Kakulas BA (ed): *Clinical Studies in Myology, Part 2*, Excerpta Medica, Amsterdam, 1973, 17–28
47. Chou SM: Inclusion body myositis: A chronic persistent mumps myositis? *Hum Pathol* 17:765–777, 1986
48. Chou SM, Nonaka I: Satellite cells and muscle regeneration in diseased human skeletal muscles. *J Neurol Sci* 34:131–145, 1977
49. Chou SM, Chou TM, Mori M: The "core" myofibers induced by local tetanus and tenotomy in rats. *J Neuropathol Exp Neurol* 40:300, 1981
50. Coërs C, Woolf AL: *The Innervation of Muscle.* Blackwell Scientific Publications, Oxford, 1959
51. Cornelio F, Di Donato S, Peluchetti D, et al. Heterogenity of carnitine deficiency. Clinicopathological aspects of eight cases. *Perspect Inherited Metabol Dis* 3:129–150, 1979
52. Craig ID, Allen IV, McCormick D: A biochemical, histological and electron microscopical study of possible carriers in Duchenne muscular dystrophy. *Irish J Med Sci* 147:125–133, 1978
53. Crews J, Kaiser KK, Brooke MH: Muscle pathology of myotonia congenita. *J Neurol Sci* 28:449–457, 1976
54. Currie S, Noronha M, Harriman D: "Minicore" disease. In *Third International Congress on Muscle Diseases*, Excerpta Medica, Amsterdam, 1974, 12 (Abstract)
55. Dalakas MC, Pezeshkpour GH: Neuromuscular diseases associated with human immunodeficiency virus infection. *Ann Neurol* 23: S38–S48, 1988
56. Danon MJ, Oh SJ, DiMauro S, et al: Lysosomal glycogen storage disease with normal acid maltase. *Neurology* 31:51–57, 1981
57. DeGirolami U, Smith TW: Pathology of skeletal muscle diseases. *Am J Pathol* 107:235(1)–276(42), 1982 (Monograph)
58. Dehkharghani F, Sarnat HB, Brewster MA, et al: Congenital muscle fiber-type disproportion in Krabbe's leukodystrophy. *Arch Neurol* 38:585–587, 1981
59. DeReuck J, Thiery E, DeCoster W, et al: Myasthenic syndrome in polymyositis. *Eur Neurol* 14:275–284, 1976
60. DiMauro S, Bonilla E, Zeviani M, et al: Mitochondrial myopathies. *Ann Neurol* 17:521–538, 1985
61. DiMauro S, Hartwig GB, Hays A, et al: Debrancher deficiency: Neuromuscular disorder in 5 adults. *Ann Neurol* 5:422–436, 1979
62. DiMauro S, Miranda AF, Sakoda S, et al: Metabolic myopathies. *Am J Med Genet* 25:635–651, 1986
63. Dubowitz V: Progressive muscular dystrophy of the Duchenne type in females and its mode of inheritance. *Brain* 83:432–439, 1960
64. Dubowitz V: *Developing and Diseased Muscle.* (S.I.M.P. Research Monograph No. 2.) New York, Spastics International Medical Publications, 1968

65. Dubowitz V: The "new" myopathies. *Neuropediatries* 1: 137–148, 1969
66. Dubowitz V: *Muscle Disorders in Childhood*. Philadelphia WB Saunders, 1978
67. Dubowitz V: The floppy infant. In *Clinics in Developmental Medicine No. 76* (2nd Ed.). Philadelphia Spastics, International Medical Publications, 1980
68. Dubowitz V, Brooke, MH: *Muscle Biopsy: A Modern Approach*. Philadelphia, WB Saunders 1973
69. Dyck PJ: Inherited neuronal degeneration and atrophy affecting peripheral motor, sensory, and autonomic neurons. In *Peripheral Neuropathy, Vol. II*, (2nd ed.) Dyck PJ, Thomas PK, Lambert EH; et al (eds): Philadelphia, WB Saunders, 1984, 1600–1655
70. Edström, L: Histochemical and histopathological changes in skeletal muscle in late-onset hereditary distal myopathy (Welander). *J Neurol Sci* 26:147–157, 1975
71. Edström L, Thornell LE, Eriksson A: A new type of hereditary distal myopathy with characteristic sarcoplasmic bodies and intermediate (skeletin) filaments. *J Neurol Sci* 47:171–190, 1980
72. Emery AEH, Burt D: Intracellular calcium and pathogenesis and antenatal diagnosis of Duchenne muscular dystrophy. *Br Med J* 1:355–357, 1980
73. Emery AEH, Dreifuss FE: Unusual type of benign X-linked muscular dystrophy. *J Neurol Neurosurg Psychiatry* 29:338–342, 1966
74. Engel AG: Neuromuscular manifestations of Graves' disease. *Mayo Clin Proc* 47:919–925, 1972
75. Engel AG: Vacuolar myopathies: Multiple etiologies and sequential structural studies, in Pearson CM, Mostofi FK, (eds), *The Striated Muscle*, Baltimore, Williams & Wilkins, 1973, 301–341
76. Engel, AG: Myasthenia gravis, in Vinken PJ, Bruyn GW (eds): *Handbook of Clinical Neurology, Vol. 41, Part II*, Amsterdam North-Holland Publishing Company, 1979, 95–145
77. Engel AG, Angelini C, Gomez MR: Fingerprint body myopathy. A newly recognized congenital muscle disease. *Mayo Clin Proc* 47:377–388, 1972
78. Engel AG, Arahata K: Monoclonal antibody analysis of mononuclear cells in myopathies. II: Phenotypes of autoinvasive cells in polymyositis and inclusion body myositis. *Ann Neurol* 16:209–215, 1984
79. Engel AG, Gomez MR, Groover RV: Multicore disease. A recently recognized congenital myopathy associated with multifocal degeneration of muscle fibers. *Mayo Clin Proc* 46:666–681, 1971
80. Engel AG, Gomez RM, Seybold ME, et al: The spectrum and diagnosis of acid maltase deficiency. *Neurology* 23:95–106, 1973
81. Engel AG, Lambert EH, Mulder DM, et al: Recently recognized congenital myasthenic syndromes. *Ann NY Acad Sci* 377:614–639, 1981
82. Engel AG, Sahaski K, Lambert EH, et al: The ultrastructural localization of the acetylcholine receptor, immunoglobulin G and the third and ninth complement components at the motor end-plate and their implications for the pathogenesis of myasthenia gravis, in Aguayo AJ, Karpati G (eds): *Current Topics in Nerve and Muscle Research*, Eds. (International Congress Series No. 455.) Amsterdam Excerpta Medica, 1979, 111–122
83. Engel AG, Santa T: Motor end plate fine structure, in Desmedt JE (ed): *New Developments in EMG and Clinical Neurophysiology, Vol. 1*, Karger, Basel, 1973, 196–228
84. Engel WK, Borenstein A: Benign congenital hypotonia: Histochemical basis of proposed pathogenesis. *J Histochem Cytochem* 20:849, 1972
85. Engel WK, McFarlin DE: Discussion of "muscle lesions in myasthenia gravis." *Ann NY Acad Sci* 135:68–78, 1966
86. Fardeau M, Bodet-Guillain J, Tomé FMS, et al: Une nouvelle affection musculaire familiale, définie par l'accumulation intra-sarcoplasmique d'un matériel granulo-filamenteux dense en microscopie électronique. *Rev Neurol (Paris)* 134:411–425, 1978
87. Farrants GW, Hovmöller S, Stadhouders AM: Two types of mitochondrial crystals in diseased human skeletal muscle fibers. *Muscle & Nerve* 11:45–55, 1988
88. Fidzianska A, Badurska B, Ryniewicz B, et al: "Cap disease": New congenital myopathy. *Neurology* 31:1113–1120, 1981
89. Frank JP, Harati Y, Butler IJ, et al: Central core disease and malignant hyperthermia syndrome. *Ann Neurol* 7:11–17, 1980
90. Fukuhara N, Kumamoto T, Hirahara H, et al: A new myopathy with tubulomembranous inclusions. *J Neurol Sci* 50:95–107, 1981
91. Fukuhara N, Takamori M, Gutmann L, et al: Eaton–Lambert syndrome. Ultrastructural study of the motor end-plates. *Arch Neurol* 27:67–78, 1972
92. Fukuoka T, Engel AG, Lang B, et al: Lambert-Eaton myasthenic syndrome: I. Early morphological effects of IgG on the presynaptic membrane active zones. Ann Neurol 22:193–199, 1987
93. Fukuyama Y, Osawa M, Suzuki H: Congenital progressive muscular dystrophy of the Fukuyama type—Clinical, genetic and pathologic considerations. *Brain Dev* 3:1–29, 1981

94. Furukawa T, Toyokura Y: Congenital, hypotonic-sclerotic muscular dystrophy. *J Med Genet* 14:426–429, 1977

95. Gambarelli D, Hassoun J, Pelissier JF, et al: Concentric laminated bodies in muscle pathology. *Pathol Eur* 9:289–296, 1974

96. Gardner-Medwin D, Johnston HM: Severe muscular dystrophy in girls. *J Neurol Sci* 64:79–87, 1984

97. Garnham PCC: *The Structure and Function of Muscle, Vol. IV* (2nd ed.). New York, Academic Press, 1973, 249–288

98. Goebel HH, Bardosi A: Myoadenylate deaminase deficiency. *Klin Wochenschr* 65:1023–1033, 1987

99. Goebel HH, Fidzianska A, Lenard HG, et al: A morphological study of non-Japanese congenital muscular dystrophy associated with cerebral lesions. *Brain Dev* 5:292–301, 1983

100. Goebel HH, Gullotta F, Yokota T: Polyglucosan myopathy—a Lafora body-like neuromuscular disorder. *J Neuropathol Exp Neurol* 47:311, 1988

101. Goebel HH, Muller J: The unusual features of traumatic neurogenic muscular atrophy in the infant: An anatomic study. *Neuropediatrics* 8:274–285, 1977

102. Goebel HH, Muller J, DeMyer W: Myopathy associated with Marfan's syndrome. *Neurology* 23:1257–1268, 1973

103. Goebel HH, Lenard HG, Görke W, et al: Fibre type disproportion in the rigid spine syndrome. *Neuropediatrics* 8:467–477, 1977

104. Goebel HH, Muller J, Gillen HW, et al: Autosomal dominant "spheroid body myopathy." *Muscle & Nerve* 1:14–26, 1978

105. Goebel HH, Prange H, Gullotta F, et al: Becker's X-linked muscular dystrophy. Histological, enzyme-histochemical, and ultrastructural studies of two cases, originally reported by Becker. *Acta Neuropathol (Berlin)* 46:69–77, 1979

106. Goebel HH, Schloon H, Lenard HG: Congenital myopathy with cytoplasmic bodies. *Neuropediatrics* 12:166–180, 1981

107. Goebel HH, Schlie M, Burck U: Fetal congenital lethal hypophosphatasia: Histochemical absence of alkaline phosphatase activity in endothelial cells of intramuscular capillaries. *Acta Neuropathol (Berlin)* 57:236–238, 1982

108. Goldberg JS, London WL, Nagel DM: Tropical pyomyositis: A case report and review. *Pediatrics* 63:298–300, 1979

109. Gonzales MF, Olney RK, So YT, et al: Subacute structural myopathy associated with human immunodeficiency virus infection. *Arch Neurol* 45:585–587, 1988

110. Gross B, Ochoa J: Trichinosis: Clinical report and histochemistry of muscle. *Muscle & Nerve* 2:394–398, 1979

111. Guggenheim MA, Ringel SP, Silverman A, et al: Progressive neuromuscular disease in children with chronic cholestasis and vitamin E deficiency: Diagnosis and treatment with alpha tocopherol. *J Pediatr* 100:51–58, 1982

112. Hanson PA, Mastrianni AF, Post L: Neonatal ophthalmoplegia with microfibers: A reversible myopathy? *Neurology* 27:974–980, 1977

113. Harriman D: Histology of the motor end-plate (motor-point muscle biopsy). In *Physical Medicine Library, Vol. 1* (2nd ed.), S. Licht, (ed) E. Licht, New Haven, 1961, 134–152

114. Heene R: Histological and histochemical findings in muscle spindles in dystrophia myotonica. *J Neurol Sci* 18:369–372, 1973

115. Heene R, Gabriel R: Histochemische und histometrische Untersuchungen bei Myotonia und Paramyotonia congenita. In *Fortschritte der Myologie, Bd. 5,* Ed. Deutsche Gesellschaft "Bekämpfung der Muskelkrankheiten," Freiburg, 1978, 266–268

116. Heffner RR, Jr., Barron SA, Jenis EH, et al: Skeletal muscle in polymyositis. *Arch Pathol Lab Med* 103:310–313, 1979

117. Heffner RR, Jr., Barron SA: Denervating changes in focal myositis, a benign inflammatory pseudotumor. *Arch Pathol Lab Med* 104:261–264, 1980

118. Hewlett RH, Brownell B: Granulomatous myopathy: Its relationship to sarcoidosis and polymyositis. *J Neurol Neurosurg Psychiatry* 38:1090–1099, 1975

119. Heyck H, Schaefer K: "Myopathia distalis juvenilis hereditaria" (Biemond), a neurogenic disease. In *Third International Congress on Muscle Diseases.* Excerpta Medica, Amsterdam, 1974, 86 (Abstract)

120. Hoffman EP, Fischbeck KH, Brown RH, et al: Characterization of dystrophin in muscle-biopsy specimens from patients with Duchenne's or Becker's muscular dystrophy. *N Engl J Med* 318:1363–1368, 1988

121. Hoogenraad TU, Jennekens FGI, Tan KEWP: Histochemical fibre types in human extraocular muscles, an investigation of inferior oblique muscle. *Acta Neuropathol (Berlin)* 45:73–78, 1979

122. Hopkins LC, Jackson JA, Elsas LJ: Emery–Dreifuss humeroperoneal muscular dystrophy: An X-linked myopathy with unusual contractures and bradycardia. *Ann Neurol* 10:230–237, 1981
123. Hug G: Glycogen storage diseases. *Birth Defects* 12:145–175, 1976
124. Jehn UW, Fink MK: Myositis, myoglobinemia, and myoglobinuria associated with enterovirus echo 9 infection. *Arch Neurol* 37:457–458, 1980
125. Jerusalem F, Engel AG, Gomez MR: Sarcotubular myopathy. A newly recognized, benign, congenital, familial muscle disease. *Neurology* 23:897–906, 1973
126. Jerusalem F, Engel AG, Gomez MR: Duchenne dystrophy. I. Morphometric study of the muscle microvasculature. *Brain* 97:115–122, 1974
127. Johnson MA, Polgar J, Weightman D, et al: Data on the distribution of fiber types in thirty-six human muscles. An autopsy study. *J Neurol Sci* 18:111–129, 1973
128. Julien J, Vital C, Vallat JM, et al: Oculopharyngeal muscular dystrophy. A case with abnormal mitochondria and "fingerprint" inclusions. *J Neurol Sci* 21:165–169, 1974
129. Kamieniecka Z, Schmalbruch H: Myopathies with abnormal mitochondria: A clinicopathologic classification. *Muscle & Nerve* 1:413–415, 1978
130. Kamieniecka Z, Schmalbruch H: Neuromuscular disorders with abnormal muscle mitochondria. *Int Rev Cytol* 65:321–357, 1980
131. Karpati G, Carpenter S, Watters GV, et al: Infantile myotonic dystrophy. Histochemical and electron microscopic features in skeletal muscle. *Neurology* 23:1066–1077, 1973
132. Katsuragi S, Miyayama H, Takeuchi T: Picornavirus-like inclusions in polymyositis—aggregation of glycogen particles of the same size. *Neurology* 31:1476–1480, 1981
133. Kinoshita M, Satoyoshi E, Kumagai M: Familial type I fiber atrophy. *J Neurol Sci* 25:11–17, 1975
134. Kinoshita M, Nakazato H, Wakata N, et al: Myasthenic neuromyopathy. An unusual neuromuscular disorder. *Eur Neurol* 21:52–58, 1982
135. Korenyi-Both A, Korenyi-Both I, Kayes, BC: Thyrotoxic myopathy. Pathomorphological observations of human material and experimentally induced thyrotoxicosis in rats. *Acta Neuropathol* (Berlin) 53:237–248, 1981
136. Kott E, Delpre G, Kadish U, et al: Abeta-lipoproteinemia (Bassen–Kornzweig syndrome). Muscle involvement. *Acta Neuropathol* (Berlin) 37:255–258, 1977
137. Krijgsman JB, Barth PG, Stam FC, et al: Cogenital muscular dystrophy and cerebral dysgenesis in a Dutch family. *Neuropediatrics* 11:108–120, 1980
138. Kumamoto T, Fukuhara N, Nagashima M, et al: Distal myopathy. Histochemical and ultrastructural studies. *Arch Neurol* 39:367–371, 1982
139. Lake BD, Wilson J: Zebra body myopathy. Clinical, histochemical and ultrastructural studies. *J Neurol Sci* 24:437–446, 1975
140. Lake BD, Cavanagh N, Wilson J: Myopathy with minicores in siblings. *Neuropathol Appl Neurobiol* 3:159–167, 1977
141. Lee YS, Yip WCL: A fatal congenital myopathy with severe type I fibre atrophy, central nuclei and multicores. *J Neurol Sci* 50:277–290, 1981
142. Lenard HG, Goebel HH: Congenital fibre type disproportion. *Neuropediatrics* 6:220–231, 1975
143. Lenard HG, Goebel HH: Congenital muscular dystrophies and unstructured congenital myopathies. *Brain Dev* 2:119–125, 1980
144. Lynch PG, Bansal DV: Granulomatous polymyositis. *J Neurol Sci* 18:109, 1973
145. Mair WGP, and Tomé FMS: *Atlas of the Ultrastructure of Diseased Human Muscle.* Edinburgh-London, Churchill Livingstone, 1972
146. Markesbery WR, Griggs RC, Herr B: Distal myopathy: Electron microscopic and histochemical studies. *Neurology* 27:727–735, 1977
147. Martin FC, Slavin G, Levi AJ: Alcoholic muscle disease. *Br Med Bull* 38:53–56, 1982
148. Martin JJ: Generalized mitochondrial disturbances and myopathies. In Busch HGM, Jennekens FGI, HR Scholte HR (eds): *Mitochondria and Muscular Diseases*, Mefar b.v., Beetsterzwaag, 1981, 219–223
149. Martin JJ, Clara R, Ceuterick C, et al: Is congenital fibre type disproportion a true myopathy? *Acta Neurol Belg* 76:335–344, 1976
150. Matsuoka Y, Gubbay SS, Kakulas BA: A new myopathy with type II muscle fibre hypoplasia. *Proc Aust Assoc Neurol* 11:155–159, 1974
151. Maunder-Sewry CA, Dubowitz V: Needle muscle biopsy for carrier detection in Duchenne muscular dystrophy. Part 1. Light microscopy—Histology, histochemistry and quantitation. *J Neurol Sci* 49:305–324, 1981
152. McMaster KR, Powers JM, Hennigar GR, Jr., et al: Nervous system involvement in type IV glycogenosis. *Arch Pathol Lab Med* 103:105–111, 1979

153. Meffert O, Weber HG: Beitrag zur Myositis ossificans localisata. *Dtsch Med Wochenschr* 98:653–656, 1973
154. Meola G, Scarpini E, Silani V, et al: Manifesting carrier of X-linked Duchenne muscular dystrophy. *J Neurol Sci* 49:455–463, 1981
155. Mikol J, Felten-Papaiconomou A, Ferchal F, et al: Inclusion-body myositis: Clinicopathological studies and isolation of an adenovirus type 2 from muscle biopsy specimen. *Ann Neurol* 11:576–581, 1982
156. Milhorat AT, Goldstone L: Muscular dystrophy of Duchenne type in females. In *Progress in Neurogenetics, Vol. 1*, Barbeau A, Brunette JR, (eds): Excerpta Medica, Amsterdam, 1969, 148–152
157. Milhorat AT, Shafiq SA, Goldstone L: Changes in muscle structure in dystrophic patients, carriers and normal siblings seen by electron microscopy; correlation with levels of serum creatinephosphokinase (CPK). *Ann NY Acad Sci* 138:246–292, 1966
158. Miyoshi K, Iwasa M, Kawai H, et al: Autosomal recessive distal muscular dystrophy—A new variety of distal muscular dystrophy predominantly seen in Japan. *Nippon Rinsho (Tokyo)* 35:3922–3928, 1977
159. Mohr PD, Knowlson TG: Quadriceps myositis: An appraisal of the diagnostic criteria of quadriceps myopathy. *Postgrad Med J* 53:757–760, 1977
160. Mokri B, Engel AG: Duchenne dystrophy: Electron microscopic findings pointing to a basic or early abnormality in the plasma membrane of the muscle fiber. *Neurology* 25:1111–1120, 1975
161. Morgan-Hughes JA, Mair WGP, Lascelles PT: A disorder of skeletal muscle associated with tubular aggregates. *Brain* 93:873–880, 1970
162. Morris CJ, Raybould JA: Histochemically demonstrable fibre abnormalities in normal skeletal muscle and in muscle from carriers of Duchenne muscular dystrophy. *J Neurol Neurosurg Psychiatry* 34:348–352, 1971
163. Neville HE, Brooke MH: Centreal core fibers: Structured and unstructured. In *Basic Research in Myology, Part 1*, Kakulas BA (ed) Excerpta Medica, Amsterdam, 1973, 497–511
164. Nonaka I, Chou SM: Congenital muscular dystrophy. In *Handbook of Clinical Neurology, Vol. 41, Part II*, Vinken PJ, Bruyn GW, (eds): Amsterdam North-Holland Publishing Company, 1979, 27–50
165. Nonaka I, Sunohara N, Ishiura S, et al: Familial distal myopathy with rimmed vacuole and lamellar (myeloid) body formation. *J Neurol Sci* 51:141–155, 1981
166. Nonaka I, Takagi A, Sugita H: The significance of type 2C muscle fibers in Duchenne muscular dystrophy. *Muscle & Nerve* 4:326–333, 1981
167. Nonaka I, Sugita H, Takada K, et al: Muscle histochemistry in congenital muscular dystrophy with central nervous system involvement. *Muscle & Nerve* 5:102–106, 1982
168. Panayiotopoulos CP, Scarpalezos S: Dystrophia myotonica. A model of combined neural and myopathic muscle atrophy. *J Neurol Sci* 31:261–268, 1977
169. Pearson CM: Histopathological features of muscle in the preclinical stages of muscular dystrophy. *Brain* 85:109–120, 1962
170. Polgar J, Johnson MA, Weightman D, et al: Data on the fiber size in thirty-six human muscles. An autopsy study. *J Neurol Sci* 19:307–318, 1973
171. Pollock M, Dyck PJ: Peripheral nerve morphometry in myotonic dystrophy. *Arch Neurol* 33:33–39, 1976
172. Prince AD, Engel WK, Warmolts JR: Type I myofiber smallness without central nuclei or myotonia. *Neurology* 22:401, 1972
173. Raitta C, Lamminen M, Santavuori P, et al: Ophthalmological findings in a new syndrome with muscle, eye and brain involvement. *Acta Ophthalmol* 56:465–472, 1978
174. Reske-Nielsen E: Malignant hyperthermia in Denmark: Survey of a family study and investigations into muscular morphology in ten additional cases. In *Malignant Hyperthermia*, Aldrete JA, Britt BA, (eds): New York, Grune & Stratton, 1978, 287–327
175. Riggs JE, Schochet SS, Gutmann L, et al: Lysosomal glycogen storage disease without acid maltase deficiency. Neurology 33:873–877, 1983
176. Ringel SP, Carroll JE, Schold SC: The spectrum of mild X-linked recessive muscular dystrophy. *Arch Neurol* 34:408–416, 1977
177. Ringel SP, Kenny CE, Neville HE, et al: Spectrum of inclusion body myositis. *Arch Neurol* 44:1154–1157, 1987
178. Ringel SP, Neville HE, Duster MC, et al: A new congenital neuromuscular disease with trilaminar muscle fibers. *Neurology* 28:282–289, 1978
179. Ringel SP, Wilson WB, Barden MT, et al: Histochemistry of human extraocular muscle. *Arch Ophthalmol* 96:1067–1072, 1978
180. Ringel SP, Wilson WB, Barden MT: Extraocular muscle biopsy in chronic progressive external ophthalmoplegia. *Ann Neurol* 6:326–339, 1979

181. Rowland LP, Fetell M, Olarte M, et al: Emery–Dreifuss muscular dystrophy. *Ann Neurol* 5:111–117, 1979
182. Roy S, Dubowitz V: Carrier detection in Duchenne muscular dystrophy. A comparative study of electron microscopy, light microscopy and serum enzymes. *J Neurol Sci* 11:65–79, 1970
183. Russell DS: Histological changes in the striped muscles in myasthenia gravis. *J Pathol* 65:279–289, 1953
184. Schmalbruch H: Muscle fibre splitting and regeneration in diseased human muscle. *Neuropathol Appl Neurobiol* 2:3–19, 1976
185. Schochet SS Jr, McCormick WF: Polymyositis with intranuclear inclusions. *Arch Neurol* 28:280–283, 1973
186. Schröder JM: *Pathologie der Muskulatur.* Berlin, Springer, 1982
187. Schröder JM, Adams RD: The ultrastructural morphology of the muscle fiber in myotonic dystrophy. *Acta Neuropathol (Berlin)* 10:218–241, 1968
188. Schröder JM, Becker PE: Anomalien des T-Systems und des sarkoplasmatischen Reticulums bei der Myotonie, Paramyotonie und Adynamie. *Virchows Arch (Pathol Anat)* 357:319–344, 1972
189. Seay AR, Zityer FA, Petajan JH: Rigid spine syndrome. A type I fiber myopathy. *Arch Neurol* 34:119–122, 1977
190. Serratrice G, Pellissier JF, Faugere MC, et al: Centronuclear myopathy: Possible central nervous system origin. *Muscle & Nerve* 1:62–69, 1978
191. Shafiq SA, Gorycki MA, Asidu SA, et al: Tenotomy. Effect on the fine structure of the soleus of the rat. *Arch Neurol* 20:625–632, 1969
192. Sher JH, Rimalovski AB, Athanassiades TJ, et al: Familial centronuclear myopathy: A clinical and pathological study. *Neurology* 17:727–742, 1967
193. Shy GM, Engel WK, Somers JE, et al: Nemaline myopathy. A new congenital myopathy. *Brain* 86:793–810, 1963
194. Shy GM, Magee KR: A new congenital non-progressive myopathy. *Brain* 79:610–621, 1956
195. Spiro AJ, Hirano A, Beilin RL, et al: Cretinism with muscular hypertrophy (Kocher–Debré–Sémélaigne syndrome). Histochemical and ultrastructural study of skeletal muscle. *Arch Neurol* 23:340–349, 1970
196. Spiro AJ, Shy GM, Gonatas NK: Myotubular myopathy. Persistence of fetal muscle in an adolescent boy. *Arch Neurol* 14:1–14, 1966
197. Swash M, Fox KP: Abnormal intrafusal muscle fibres in myotonic dystrophy: A study using serial sections. *J Neurol Neurosurg Psychiatry* 38:91–99, 1975
198. Tang TT, Sedmak GV, Siegesmund KA, et al: Chronic myopathy associated with Coxsackie virus type A9. A combined electron microscopical and viral isolation study. *N Engl J Med* 292:608–611, 1975
199. Tassin S, Walter GF, Brucher JM, et al: Histochemical and ultrastructural analysis of the mitochondrial changes in a familial mitochondrial myopathy. *Neuropathol Appl Neurobiol* 6:337–347, 1980
200. Thompson AJ, Swash M, Cox EL, et al: Polysaccharide storage myopathy. *Muscle & Nerve* 11:349–355, 1988
201. Tomé FMS, Fardeau M: Nuclear inclusions in oculopharyngeal dystrophy. *Acta Neuropathol (Berlin)* 49:85–87, 1980
202. Toop J, Emery AEH: Muscle histology in fetuses at risk for Duchenne muscular dystrophy. *Clin Genet* 5:230–233, 1974
203. Towfighi J, Sassani JW, Suzuki K, et al: Cerebro-ocular dysplasia-muscular dystrophy (COD-MD) syndrome. *Acta Neuropathol (Berlin)* 65:110–123, 1984
204. Turkel SB, Howell R, Iseri AL, et al: Ultrastructure of muscle in fetal Duchenne's dystrophy. *Arch Pathol Lab Med* 105:414–418, 1981
205. Van der Does de Willebois AEM, Bethlem J, Meyer AEFH, et al: Distal myopathy with onset in early infancy. *Neurology* 18:383–390, 1968
206. Voit T, Krogmann O, Lenard HG, et al: Emery-Dreifuss muscular dystrophy: Disease-spectrum and differential diagnosis. *Neuropediatrics* 19:62–71, 1988
207. Walthard KM, Tchialoff M: Motor points, in *Physical Medicine Library, Vol. 1* (2nd ed.), Licht S (ed), Licht, New Haven, Licht Publishers, 1961, 153–170
208. Walton JN: Amyotonia congenita. A follow-up study. *Lancet* 1:1023–1027, 1956
209. Walton JN: Thomas PK: World Federation of Neurology Research Committee Research Group on Neuromuscular Diseases *J Neurol Sci* 86:333–360, 1988
210. Walton JN, Hudgson P: Inflammatory myopathies and related diseases. In *Vol. 2,* Goldensohn ES, Appel SH, (eds): *Scientific Approaches to Clinical Neurology,* Philadelphia, Lea & Febiger, 1977, 1866–1783
211. Winn KJ, Heller RH: Pathologic diagnosis of Duchenne muscular dystrophy in an aborted fetus. *Clin Genet* 13:335–338, 1978
212. Yarom R, Shapira Y: Myosin degeneration in a congenital myopathy. *Arch Neurol* 34:114–115, 1977

213. Yokota T, Ishihara T, Kawano H, et al: Immunological homogeneity of Lafora body, corpora amylacea, basophilic degeneration in heart, and intracytoplasmic inclusions of liver and heart in type IV glycogenosis. *Acta Pathol Japon* 37:941–946, 1987
214. Yokota T, Wada Y, Furukawa T, et al: Adult-onset spinocerebellar syndrome with idiopathic vitamin E deficiency. *Ann Neurol* 22:84–87, 1987
215. Zellweger H, Afifi A, McCormick WF, et al: Benign congenital muscular dystrophy: A special form of congenital hypotonia. *Clin Pediatr* 6:655–663, 1967
216. Zellweger H, Afifi A, McCormick WF, et al: Severe congenital muscular dystrophy. *Am J Dis Child* 114:591–602, 1967

INDEX